Contemporary Stereotactic Radiosurgery

Technique and Evaluation

Edited by

Bruce E. Pollock, MD
Associate Professor
Department of Neurologic Surgery
Mayo Medical School and the Mayo Clinic and Foundation
Rochester, Minnesota

FUTURA

Futura Publishing Company, Inc.
Armonk, New York

Library of Congress Cataloging-in-Publications Data

Contemporary stereotactic radiosurgery : technique and evaluation / edited by Bruce E. Pollock.
p. ; cm.
Includes bibliographical references and index.
ISBN 0-87993-708-4
1. Radiosurgery. 2. Stereoencephalotomy. I. Pollock, Bruce E.
[DNLM: 1. Radiosurgery—methods. WL 368 T255 2002]
RD594.15 .T43 2002
617′.05—dc21

2002019267

Published by
Futura Publishing Company
135 Bedford Road
Armonk, NY 10504
www.futuraco.com

LC#: 2002019267
ISBN#: 0-87993-708-4

Printed in the United States of America on acid-free paper.

To my parents, Ruth and Eugene Pollock

Contributors

Aviva Abosch, MD, PhD Division of Neurological Surgery, University of Toronto, Toronto, Ontario, Canada

John R. Adler, Jr., MD Professor, Department of Neurosurgery, Stanford University, Medical Center, Palo Alto, CA, USA

Ossama Al-Mefty, MD Professor and Chairman, Department of Neurosurgery, University of Arkansas for Medical Sciences, Little Rock, AR, USA

Sepideh Amin-Hanjani, MD Neurological Service, Massachusetts General Hospital, Harvard Medical School, Boston, MA, USA

David W. Andrews, MD, FACS Associate Professor, Department of Neurosurgery, Jefferson Medical College, Philadelphia, PA, USA

Michael L. J. Apuzzo, MD Edwin M. Todd/Trent H. Wells, Jr., Professor, Neurological Surgery and Radiation Oncology, Biology, and Physics, Keck School of Medicine, University of Southern California, Los Angeles, CA, USA

Fred G. Barker II, MD Neurological Service, Massachusetts General Hospital, Harvard Medical School, Boston, MA, USA

Gene H. Barnett, MD Professor and Vice-Chairman, Department of Neurosurgery, The Cleveland Clinic, Cleveland, OH, USA

Daniel L. Barrow, MD MBNA/Bowman Professor and Chairman, Department of Neurosurgery, Emory University School of Medicine, Atlanta, GA, USA

Derald E. Brackmann, MD House Ear Clinic, Los Angeles, CA, USA

Paul D. Brown, MD Assistant Professor, Division of Radiation Oncology, Mayo Medical School and the Mayo Clinic and Foundation, Rochester, MN, USA

Kim J. Burchiel, MD John Raaf Professor and Chairman, Department of Neurological Surgery, Oregon Health Sciences University, Portland, OR, USA

Steven D. Chang, MD Assistant Professor, Department of Neurosurgery, Stanford University Medical Center, Palo Alto, CA, USA

Joseph C. T. Chen, MD, PhD Clinical Instructor, Department of Neurological Surgery, Keck School of Medicine, University of Southern California, Los Angeles, CA, USA

Christine Delsanti, MD Stereotactic and Functional Neurosurgery Department, Timone Hospital, Marseille, France

John C. Flickinger, MD Professor, Departments of Radiation Oncology and Neurological Surgery, University of Pittsburgh Medical Center, Pittsburgh, PA, USA

Robert L. Foote, MD Professor, Division of Radiation Oncology, Mayo Medical School and the Mayo Clinic and Foundation, Rochester, MN, USA

David M. C. Forster, MA, MB, Bchir, FRCS Consultant Neurosurgeon, Cromwell Hospital, London, UK

Jonathan A. Friedman, MD Resident, Department of Neurologic Surgery, Mayo Medical School and the Mayo Clinic and Foundation, Rochester, MN, USA

Rick A. Friedman, MD, PhD House Ear Clinic, Los Angeles, CA, USA

Deborah A. Gorman, RN Associate, Department of Neurologic Surgery, Mayo Medical School and the Mayo Clinic and Foundation, Rochester, MN, USA

Philip H. Gutin, MD Chief, Neurosurgery Service, Fred Lebow Chair in Neuro-Oncology, Memorial Sloan-Kettering Cancer Center, New York, NY, USA

Michael G. Herman, PhD Assistant Professor, Division of Radiation Oncology, Head, Section of Radiation Physics, Mayo Medical School and the Mayo Clinic and Foundation, Rochester, MN, USA

Bengt Karlsson, MD, PhD Department of Neurosurgery, Karolinska Hospital, Stockholm, Sweden

Douglas Kondziolka, MD, MSc, FRCS(C), FACS Professor, Departments of Neurological Surgery and Radiation Oncology, University of Pittsburgh Medical Center, Pittsburgh, PA, USA

Alex M. Landolt, MD Neurosurgery Section, Klinik im Park, Zürich, Switzerland

Richard P. Levy, MD Department of Radiation Oncology, Stanford University Medical Center, Palo Alto, CA, USA

Michael J. Link, MD Assistant Professor, Department of Neurologic Surgery, Mayo Medical School and the Mayo Clinic and Foundation, Rochester, MN, USA

Mark E. Linskey, MD Associate Professor, Department of Neurological Surgery, University of Arkansas for Medical Sciences, Little Rock, AR, USA

Jay S. Loeffler, MD Neurological Service and Department of Radiation Oncology, Massachusetts General Hospital, Harvard Medical School, Boston, MA, USA

Nicoletta Lomax, MS Neurosurgery Section, Klinik im Park, Zürich, Switzerland

Andres M. Lozano, MD, PhD, FRCS (C) Professor of Surgery, Division of Neurological Surgery, University of Toronto, Tasker Chair in Functional Neurosurgery, Toronto, Ontario, Canada

L. Dade Lunsford, MD, FACS Lars Leksell Professor and Chairman, Department of Neurological Surgery, Professor of Radiation Oncology and Radiology, University of Pittsburgh Medical Center, Pittsburgh, PA, USA

David P. Martin, MD Department of Neurosurgery, Stanford University Medical Center, Palo Alto, CA, USA

Edwin C. McCullough, PhD Professor, Division of Radiation Oncology, Mayo Medical School and the Mayo Clinic and Foundation, Rochester, MN, USA

Fredric B. Meyer, MD Professor, Department of Neurologic Surgery, Mayo Medical School and the Mayo Clinic and Foundation, Rochester, MN, USA

Douglas A. Nichols, MD Associate Professor, Departments of Diagnostic Radiology and Neurologic Surgery, Mayo Medical School and the Mayo Clinic and Foundation, Rochester, MN, USA

Ajay Niranjan, MCh Departments of Neurological Surgery and Radiation Oncology, University of Pittsburgh Medical Center, Pittsburgh, PA, USA

William Pellet, MD OtoNeurosurgery Department, Sainte Marguerite Hospital, Marseille, France

Bruce E. Pollock, MD Associate Professor, Department of Neurologic Surgery, Mayo Medical School and the Mayo Clinic and Foundation, Rochester, MN, USA

Jean Régis, MD Stereotactic and Functional Neurosurgery Department, Timone Hospital Marseille, France

Pierre Hughes Roche, MD OtoNeurosurgery Department, Sainte Marguerite Hospital Marseille, France

C. Leland Rogers, MD Division of Radiation Oncology, Barrow Neurological Institute Phoenix, AZ, USA

Stefan G. Scheib, PhD Neurosurgery Section, Klinik im Park, Zürich, Switzerland

Paula J. Schomberg, MD Associate Professor and Chairman, Division of Radiation Oncology, Mayo Medical School and the Mayo Clinic and Foundation, Rochester, MN, USA

Edward G. Shaw, MD Professor and Chairman, Department of Radiation Oncology, Wake Forest University, Winston-Salem, NC, USA

Dhruv Singhal, BS Departments of Neurological Surgery and Radiation Oncology, University of Pittsburgh Medical Center, Pittsburgh, PA, USA

Kris A. Smith, MD Division of Neurological Surgery, Barrow Neurological Institute, Phoenix, AZ, USA

Outouma Soumare, MD OtoNeurosurgery Department, Sainte Marguerite Hospital, Marseille, France

Scott L. Stafford, MD Assistant Professor, Division of Radiation Oncology, Mayo Medical School and the Mayo Clinic and Foundation, Rochester, MN, USA

Gary K. Steinberg, MD, PhD Bernard and Ronni Lacroute-William Randolph Hearst, Professor of Neurosurgery and the Neurosciences, Chairman, Department of Neurosurgery, Stanford University Medical Center, Palo Alto, CA, USA

Robert D. Strang, MD Instructor, Department of Neurosurgery, University of Arkansas College of Medicine, Little Rock, AR, USA

John H. Suh, MD Associate Professor, Department of Radiation Oncology, The Cleveland Clinic, Cleveland, OH, USA

Jean Marc Thomassin, MD ENT Surgery, Timone Hospital, Marseille, France

Mary Lee Vance, MD Professor of Medicine and Neurosurgery, University of Virginia Health Sciences Center, Charlottesville, VA, USA

Masaaki Yamamoto, MD Katsuta Hospital Mito GammaHouse, Hitachi-naka, Ibargi, Japan

Preface

History has shown that advances in medicine tend to occur as quantum leaps rather than small incremental steps. This has been particularly true within neurological surgery. Over the past 40 years, we have witnessed three primary events that have transformed this field and our ability to care for patients with diseases affecting the nervous system. First, the introduction of the microscope into the operating room permitted surgeons to safely remove lesions with less morbidity than previously thought possible. Furthermore, with the advent of microscopy, the interest in and study of intracranial anatomy increased tremendously and was translated into new surgical approaches to previously inoperable regions. Second, the development of cross-sectional imaging, initially with computed tomography, and later, magnetic resonance imaging, allowed more accurate and less invasive preoperative diagnosis of patients. Progress in neuroimaging techniques continues to advance at a rapid pace, changing our practices on a seemingly day-to-day basis. Third, frame-based stereotactic techniques permitted localization of intracranial lesions with sub-millimetric accuracy, fostering the growth of functional neurosurgery. Today, frameless stereotactic procedures have become commonplace, increasing our ability to resect tumors and vascular malformations through smaller, precisely placed craniotomies with less chance of injuring the adjacent normal brain. At this point, I would submit that the introduction of stereotactic radiosurgery to neurosurgical practice is of the same magnitude as these earlier sentinel events.

Originally conceived by Dr. Lars Leksell in the 1950s as a method to treat intracranial lesions without having to open the skull, the concept coupled stereotactic localization and the energy of ionizing radiation to accurately destroy intracranial lesions. The past 50 years have brought remarkable advances within the field of radiosurgery and it is now a multidisciplinary specialty that involves not only neurosurgeons, but also radiation oncologists, medical physicists, and neuroradiologists. Testimony to the acceptance of radiosurgery within medicine is the exponential growth in the indications for and the number of centers performing stereotactic radiosurgery. In the mid-1980s, radiosurgery was performed at approximately 10 centers worldwide with the majority of patients having arteriovenous malformations. Currently, there are more than 200 centers within the USA alone. Radiosurgery is now commonly used to treat patients with benign and malignant brain tumors. Moreover, interest in using radiosurgery to manage patients with functional disorders such as trigeminal neuralgia and epilepsy continues to increase.

However, resistance within neurosurgery and other specialties to radiosurgery as an unproven and generally overutilized procedure has accompanied its increasing clinical application. In many cases, the arguments against radiosurgery are valid and based on a thoughtful evaluation of its long-term risks. Conversely, the anger expressed by many critics when discussing this technique testifies to the emotional component often encountered. Thus, to balance the scales per se, this book has provided recognized experts, most of whom do not perform radiosurgery, the opportunity to voice their opinions in commentary that follows each chapter. It is the sincere hope of the editor that readers will be able to decide for themselves, after reading this text, the role that radiosurgery should play in the management of patients with neurological disorders.

A number of people need to be acknowledged, because without their assistance, this book would not have been possible. First, Steven Korn of Futura Publishing, Inc., who patiently listened to my ideas and offered sound advice repeatedly throughout production of this book. Second, Marcy Kroll, also of Futura Publishing Company, for editing and layout ideas that allowed the submitted words and figures to actually take form. Third, Marylin J. Witts for her incredible patience in coordinating the ingoing and outgoing chapters, comments, and never-ending phone calls. Last, and most importantly, to my wife Kristen whose simple acts of kindness and affection inspire me each day to be a better person.

Bruce E. Pollock, MD
Rochester, Minnesota

Contents

Contributors v
Preface xi

1. Stereotactic Radiosurgery: Evolution, Lessons Learned, and Integration into Neurosurgical Practice 1
Bruce E. Pollock
Comment: *L. Dade Lunsford* 14

2. Physical Aspects of Cranial Stereotactic Radiosurgery 17
Michael G. Herman, Edwin C. McCullough
Comment: *Joseph C. T. Chen, Michael L. J. Apuzzo* 34

3. Radiobiological and Dosimetric Considerations in Stereotactic Radiosurgery 37
John C. Flickinger
Comment: *David W. Andrews* 46

4. Dose Selection and Prediction of Stereotactic Radiosurgery Outcomes 53
Bengt Karlsson
Comment: *David M.C. Forster* 70

5. Stereotactic Radiosurgery for Arteriovenous Malformations 75
Masaaki Yamamoto
Comment: *Fredric B. Meyer* 106

6. Stereotactic Radiosurgery for Dural Arteriovenous Fistulae 109
Michael J. Link, Bruce E. Pollock, Douglas A. Nichols, Jonathan A. Friedman, Deborah A. Gorman, Robert L. Foote, Scott L. Stafford
Comment: *Daniel L. Barrow* 137

7. Stereotactic Radiosurgery for Cavernous Malformation 139
Steven D. Chang, Richard P. Levy, David P. Martin, Gary K. Steinberg, John R. Adler, Jr.
Comment: *Fred G. Barker II, Sepideh Amin-Hanjani, Jay S. Loeffler* 153

8. Stereotactic Radiosurgery for Meningioma 157
Scott L. Stafford, Bruce E. Pollock, Robert L. Foote, Michael J. Link, Paula J. Schomberg
Comment: *Robert D. Strang, Ossama Al-Mefty* 172

9. Stereotactic Radiosurgery for Vestibular Schwannoma 181
Jean Régis, Pierre Hughes Roche, Christine Delsanti, Outouma Soumare, Jean Marc Thomassin, William Pellet
Comment: *Rick A. Friedman, Derald E. Brackmann* 206

10. Stereotactic Radiosurgery for Pituitary Adenoma 213
Alex M. Landolt, Nicoletta Lomax, Stefan G. Scheib
Comment: *Mary Lee Vance* 241

11. Stereotactic Radiosurgery for Brain Metastases 245
Bruce E. Pollock, Paul D. Brown
Comment: *Edward G. Shaw* 262

12. Stereotactic Radiosurgery for Glial Tumors 265
Gene H. Barnett, John H. Suh
Comment: *Philip H. Gutin* 280

13. Stereotactic Radiosurgery of Chordomas, Glomus Tumors, and Malignant Skull Base Tumors 283
Robert L. Foote, Bruce E. Pollock
Comment: *Mark E. Linskey* 304

14. Stereotactic Radiosurgery for Refractory Trigeminal Neuralgia 309
Kris A. Smith, C. Leland Rogers
Comment: *Kim J. Burchiel* 325

15. Stereotactic Radiosurgery for Epilepsy and Movement Disorders 327
Douglas Kondziolka, Dhruv Singhal, Ajay Niranjan, L. Dade Lunsford
Comment: *Aviva Abosch, Andres M. Lozano* 343

Index 347

Chapter 1

Stereotactic Radiosurgery:

Evolution, Lessons Learned, and Integration into Neurosurgical Practice

Bruce E. Pollock

Introduction

Stereotactic radiosurgery is the precise delivery of a single fraction of high-dose ionizing radiation to an imaging-defined target. Conceived by Lars Leksell in 1951,[1] the first radiosurgical procedure was performed using an orthovoltage x-ray tube coupled with a stereotactic device to treat a patient with trigeminal neuralgia. This pioneer believed that stereotactic radiosurgery would decrease the morbidity associated with conventional intracranial surgery. The past five decades have resulted in significant advances in this technology that have improved its safety and clinical applicability. A detailed history outlining the development of radiosurgery is beyond the scope and purpose of the present chapter; numerous resources are available that cover in detail the rich and fascinating events that shaped the field of radiosurgery.[2,3] However, the primary development that enabled the growth of radiosurgery was the introduction of computed tomography (CT) and magnetic resonance imaging (MRI). With the advent of axial, and later, multiplanar neuroimaging capability, radiosurgery was no longer limited to targets that could be defined by either plain skull radiographs or cerebral angiography. Radiosurgery has evolved into a multidisciplinary field that combines the expertise of neurosurgeons, radiation oncologists, medical physicists, and neuroradiologists. Today, radiosurgery is utilized in the management of

From Pollock BE (ed). *Contemporary Stereotactic Radiosurgery: Technique and Evaluation.* Armonk, NY, Futura Publishing Company, Inc. ©2002.

patients with a wide variety of vascular malformations, benign and malignant brain tumors, and functional disorders. Although clinical utilization now far exceeds our understanding of the radiobiology of radiosurgery,[4–7] research is under way to clarify the molecular effects of radiosurgery which should translate into improved patient outcomes in the near future.

This chapter will provide a general overview of how radiosurgery has evolved, current clinical indications, and potential uses of this technology. Later chapters in this book will offer further detail on each topic. In addition, the impact that radiosurgery has had on the way neurosurgeons think and practice will be discussed.

Evolution of Radiosurgery Practice

The early practice of radiosurgery was marked by exceptional patience and a conservative approach to its clinical usage. Typically, a small group of patients were treated for a particular indication and then observed over a period of years. Only when the treatment results for those patients became available for evaluation were similar patients considered for radiosurgery. This methodology took into account the delayed nature of complications that can occur after radiosurgery. Also, this wait-and-see approach was appropriate for the time because routine imaging after radiosurgery was often difficult to obtain and thus patient outcomes were primarily based on clinical follow-up. However, once the safety of radiosurgery became established and more information was available to neurosurgeons and radiation oncologists, the growth of the field was rapid. Throughout the 1970s and 1980s, expansion of radiosurgery was linear; in the last decade the growth of this technology has been exponential.

To account for this growth, new indications for radiosurgery have developed based, in part, on both clinical research and patient demand. This latter point is worthy of more discussion. In the past, patients arrived at their physician's office and, after evaluation, were informed of their diagnosis. The proper management, at least from the perspective of that doctor, was then outlined to the patient with little information provided to the patient regarding alternative forms of therapy. With the advent of patient advocacy groups and the Internet, medical information is now widely available to patients in regard to diseases, their treatment options, and expected outcomes. Because of these factors, patients now come for consultation with a great deal of data (much of it derived from non-peer reviewed sources) and the expectation that they will be intimately involved in the decision-making process regarding their care. This paradigm shift has had both good and bad effects on patient care. Generally well-informed patients will seek out centers or individual physicians based on published results, thus concentrating patients with particular diagnoses at "centers of excellence." Such segregation of heathcare delivery is no doubt beneficial to both the patient and third-party payers. Still, because the Internet has no review process, vast quantities of misinformation get passed on to patients as peer-reviewed data. The result is that much of the information provided to patients is biased and frequently false, but becomes accepted by patients as valid and reliable. The extreme of this distasteful trend is the actual solicitation of patients for a particular treatment based on a center's website. Unfortunately, this form of medical practice is rampant among many radiosurgical centers. As no enforceable method exists to monitor or police the activities of such academic impostors, it remains the responsibility of each physician to provide accurate information at the time of consultation.

Indications for Radiosurgery

Proper patient selection is critical for good patient outcomes after radiosurgery. Patients with larger lesions (>35 mm in average diameter) are typically not considered good candidates for radiosurgery for several reasons. One, at larger volumes the radiation fall-off into the surrounding normal tissues is not as steep and the risk of delayed radiation-related complications increases exponentially. Two, patients with larger lesions often have symptoms related to mass effect. For such patients, surgical resection is the preferred management strategy. Thus, the role of the neurosurgeon on the radiosurgical team is evident; patients referred for radiosurgery can be evaluated for the best treatment option available, rather than only radiosurgery. Conversely, some patients who are poor candidates for radiosurgery may benefit from fractionated radiation therapy. For these patients, the radiation oncologist on the radiosurgery team is able to provide appropriate further care. Table 1 lists the diagnoses of the first 1977 patients undergoing radiosurgery at the Mayo Clinic, Rochester, MN. Of these patients, 28% had vascular malformations, 32% had benign intracranial tumors, and 32% had malignant intracranial tumors. One hundred sixty-nine (97%) underwent radiosurgery for trigeminal neuralgia. It should be understood that these percentages are not static, as the indications for radiosurgery have changed significantly over the past decade.

Radiosurgery has been accepted as an integral tool for the management of patients with a wide variety of intracranial disorders. Nonetheless, a great deal of controversy remains regarding the role radiosurgery should play in managing certain patient groups. Table 2 assigns select diagnoses to three separate categories based on their incorporation into current neurosurgical practice. Established indications have withstood the test of time, and patient outcomes are comparable to, if not better than, other treatment options. Examples include select arteriovenous malfor-

Table 1
Gamma Knife Radiosurgery Patients at the Mayo Clinic from January 1990 to June 2001

Indication	*No. of Patients (%) (n=1977)*
Arteriovenous malformation	370 (19)
Dural arteriovenous fistula	126 (6)
Cavernous malformation	18 (1)
Vestibular schwannoma	195 (10)
Meningioma	271 (14)
Pituitary adenoma	115 (6)
Other schwannoma	27 (1)
Brain metastases	308 (15)
Glial tumor*	146 (7)
Hemangioblastoma	17 (1)
Other tumor†	215 (11)
Trigeminal neuralgia	169 (9)

*Includes patients with astrocytoma, anaplastic astrocytoma, glioblastoma multiforme, oligodendroglioma, ependymoma, medulloblastoma, neurocytoma, pilocytic astrocyoma.

†Includes patients with chordoma, chondrosarcoma, glomus tumor, craniopharyngioma, hemangiopericytoma, and nasopharyngeal carcinoma.

Table 2
Clinical Indications for Radiosurgery

Category	*Indication*
Established	Small/moderate sized, critically located AVMs
	Recurrent/residual vestibular schwannomas
	Recurrent/residual pituitary adenomas
	Multiple, critically located brain metastases
	Skull base meningiomas
Accepted	DAVFs
	Primary vestibular schwannomas
	High-grade gliomas
	Surgically resectable, solitary brain metastases
	Cavernous malformations
	Recurrent trigeminal neuralgia
	Skull base carcinomas
Proposed	Large AVMs
	Primary trigeminal neuralgia
	Movement disorders
	Mesial temporal lobe epilepsy

AVMs, arteriovenous malformations; DAVFs, dural arteriovenous fistulae.

mations (AVMs),[8,9] recurrent/residual vestibular schwannomas,[10,11] recurrent/residual pituitary adenomas,[12–14] skull base meningiomas,[15–18] and multiple or critically located brain metastases.[19–21] Radiosurgery for accepted indications is frequently performed, but the available data are not conclusive at this point as to whether patient outcomes are superior to alternative management strategies. Accepted indications for radiosurgery include dural arteriovenous fistulae (DAVF),[22,23] high-grade gliomas,[24,25] solitary brain metastasis,[26–28] cavernous malformations,[29–33] recurrent trigeminal neuralgia,[34,35] or as the primary management of patients with vestibular schwannomas.[36,37] Proposed indications are investigational procedures that are typically hypothesis-driven based on either prior clinical or basic science research, but the actual clinical usefulness has not yet been determined. The majority of such procedures involve functional neurosurgery such as movement disorder surgery and mesial temporal lobe epilepsy.[38,39] Another example of a proposed indication would be staged-volume AVM radiosurgery to manage patients with AVMs that are typically considered too large for radiosurgery.[40] It is critical that trials evaluating the safety and efficacy of radiosurgery for such proposed indications be well conceived and methodologically sound. Well-designed studies can be performed utilizing established outcome parameters and blinded assessors of patient outcomes.[19,41] Only by maintaining such high standards will radiosurgery withstand the rigors of evidence-based medicine.

Evolution of Radiosurgery Knowledge

As mentioned previously, our knowledge related to the clinical usage of radiosurgery far exceeds our understanding of the cellular and molecular mechanisms occurring after radiosurgery. It is likely that, in the near future, Phase I trials will begin investigating a variety of radiation sensitizers and protective agents to be used in conjunction with radiosurgery. Nonetheless, analysis of our clinical experience has provided answers to a wide variety of questions that significantly affect the practice of radiosurgery.

Arteriovenous malformation radiosurgery can be used as an illustration. Previously, it was unclear regarding: the radiation dose that was required to obtain complete AVM obliteration; how to predict the likelihood of developing radiation-related complications after AVM radiosurgery; and what effect radiosurgery had on the hemorrhage rate of treated AVMs. Currently, few questions related to AVM radiosurgery remain unanswered. First, we realize that obliteration correlates not with AVM volume, but rather the margin radiation dose to the malformation.[42–46] Second, radiation-related complications are predicted by the volume of tissue receiving some threshold dose of radiation (10-Gy volume, 12-Gy volume, or the mean dose to 20 cm^3),[47–49] and the location of the AVM. Third, the hemorrhage rate after radiosurgery is either unchanged until obliteration, or some protective effect is provided compared with the natural history of untreated AVMs.[50–52] Furthermore, analysis of cases that have failed to obliterate emphasizes the need for proper targeting using stereotactic MRI as an adjunct to angiography.[53] However, patients with AVMs are not the only ones to benefit from prior radiosurgical experience. Investigation of other patient groups has permitted the identification of significant factors related to improved results for a variety of disorders, including vestibular schwannomas,[54] brain metastases,[20,21] and trigeminal neuralgia.[41]

In addition to factors related to better patient outcomes after radiosurgery for specific diagnoses, two general points regarding these procedures have emerged over past years: (1) Even patients who are seemingly "cured" require diligent long-term follow-up. It has recently been reported that AVM patients can develop cysts years after angiography had confirmed complete obliteration.[55,56] Based on this information, we now recommend that AVM patients obtain additional MRI imaging 3 or more years after follow-up angiography. (2) Traditional dose prescription schemes developed from experience with fractionated radiation therapy may not apply to single-fraction, high-dose radiation delivery (radiosurgery). It is clear that commonly used dose-volume curves correlate with radiation necrosis after radiosurgery.[57,58] However, the traditional idea of increasing dose until we observe unacceptable morbidity has been gradually replaced by a different way of thinking. This new approach to radiosurgery dose prescription "turns the coin upside down" and asks the question, *"What is the lowest dose that can be used and still achieve the desired endpoint (tumor growth control, facial pain relief)?"*. For example, no significant data have been published showing a dose-response curve for tumor growth control of benign tumors such as vestibular schwannomas, meningiomas, or pituitary adenomas. Thus, because it has been well established that increasing doses does correlate with cranial nerve injury, why treat any of these lesions with margin doses above the 14- to 16-Gy range? Neurosurgeons who perform radiosurgery often disagree on this point with their colleagues in radiation oncology. Notable exceptions to such thinking include AVMs and hormone-producing pituitary adenomas, indications where data support the concept of maximizing radiation delivery whenever possible.

Impact of Radiosurgery on Neurosurgery

Radiosurgery was introduced to the Mayo Clinic in November 1989, when the Leksell Gamma Knife® (Elekta Instruments, Norcross, GA) was installed at Saint Mary's Hospital, Rochester, MN. In 1990, 57 patients underwent radiosurgery at the Mayo Clinic. That same year, 2755 patients underwent open surgical procedures by members of the Department of Neurological Surgery. Thus, radiosurgery comprised 2.0% of the neurosurgical cases during the gamma unit's first year of operation. In 1993 and 1997, radiosurgery comprised 4.3% and 7.0% of the neurosurgical practice. In 1999, 281 of 3126 neurosurgical cases (9.0%) performed were radiosurgery (Fig. 1). Overall, the annual number of radiosurgical procedures has increased almost 500% in the past 10 years. In fact, the increased number of radiosurgery cases accounts for the majority of our department's growth over the past decade.

To explain the increased number of radiosurgical procedures, several trends have occurred in the management of patients with select diagnoses. Patients who in the past underwent open surgical procedures are more frequently being managed with radiosurgery. Table 3 outlines the distribution of patients undergoing microsurgery and radiosurgery at the Mayo Clinic in 1999 for some common disorders. Since 1990 there has been a steady increase in the number of patients with vascular malfor-

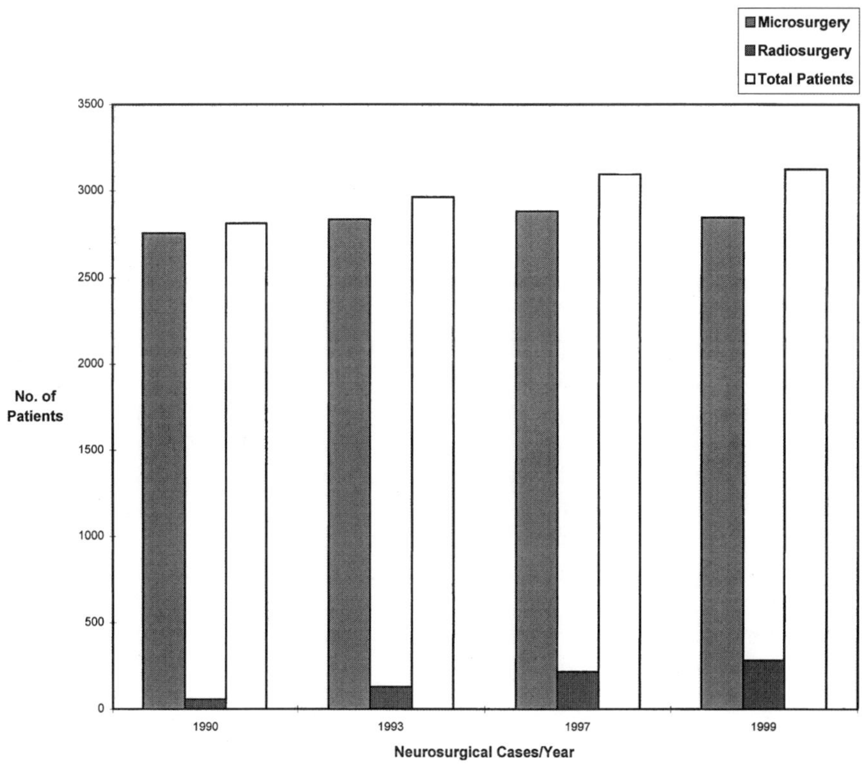

Figure 1. Graph showing the number of radiosurgery cases relative to the overall neurosurgical practice at the Mayo Clinic, Rochester, MN, from 1990 to 1999.

Table 3
Comparison of Microsurgery and Radiosurgery for Selected Indications at Mayo Clinic in 1999

Indication	*Microsurgery*	*Radiosurgery*	*Total*
AVM	13 (25%)	40 (75%)	53
DAVF	4 (20%)	16 (80%)	20
Meningioma	57 (68%)	27 (32%)	84
Pituitary adenoma	98 (85%)	17 (15%)	115
Vestibular schwannoma	36 (62%)	22 (38%)	58
Trigeminal neuralgia	30* (23%) 43† (34%)	55 (43%)	128

AVM, arteriovenous malformation; DAVF, dural arteriovenous fistulae.
*Patients having microvascular decompression.
†Patients having percutaneous surgery (radiofrequency lesion, balloon compression, glycerol rhizotomy).

mations, meningiomas, brain metastases, pituitary adenomas, and vestibular schwannomas undergoing radiosurgery. In fact, more patients with vestibular schwannomas had radiosurgery compared to surgical resection in 2001 at the Mayo Clinic (Fig. 2). Previously, only elderly patients, those with significant medical comorbidities, or patients with recurrent tumors after prior surgery were considered good candidates for vestibular schwannoma radiosurgery. Today, the indication for vestibular schwannoma radiosurgery would be an informed patient not willing to accept the risks of surgical resection. Another reason for the continued growth of radiosurgery has been its application to a number of new conditions. For example, before 1996 no patients with trigeminal neuralgia had radiosurgery. In 1999, 55 patients (20% of the radiosurgery cases) had radiosurgery for trigeminal neuralgia. In 2001, trigeminal neuralgia radiosurgery was down to 13% of our cases (35 of 270 cases) as we have gained more experience with this technique.[59] However, the majority of future radiosurgical growth will likely be the result of increased use for patients with brain metastases.[60] Even if only 20% of brain metastases patients are likely to benefit from neurosurgical intervention, then the potential number of patients undergoing radiosurgery for brain metastases would be greater than all the patients diagnosed each year with gliomas, meningiomas, schwannomas, and pituitary adenomas.

The growth of radiosurgery is not a local phenomenon. Compared to 1987, when the first gamma unit was installed in North America, there are now more than 50 Gamma Knife centers within the USA. More than 25,000 patients worldwide underwent Gamma Knife radiosurgery in 1999. Also, a large number of centers (>100) are currently performing linear accelerator (LINAC)-based radiosurgery. The number of patients

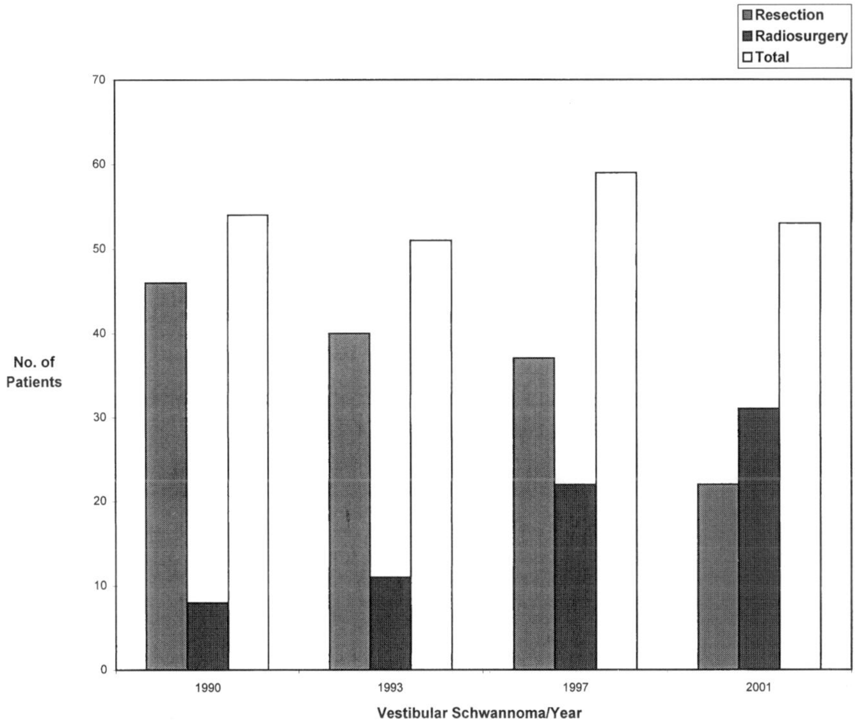

Figure 2. Graph showing the number of patients having microsurgery and radiosurgery for vestibular schwannomas at the Mayo Clinic, Rochester, MN, from 1990 to 2001.

treated annually with LINAC-based radiosurgery is more difficult to determine as there is no centralized organization to follow these patients. Proton beam radiosurgery has failed to grow because of the high cost of installation and maintenance.

It can be argued that the introduction of radiosurgery has been the most important advancement in neurosurgery over the past 20 years. The growth and utilization of radiosurgery is likely to continue as more data on the long-term results of this procedure become available. Moreover, it is likely that radiosurgery will become a mandatory part of residency training for both neurological surgery and radiation oncology.[3]

Conclusions

Radiosurgery has gained acceptance in both neurological surgery and radiation oncology as a safe and effective management strategy for a wide variety of intracranial disorders. Radiosurgery appeals to patients, their physicians, and third-party payers because of its noninvasive nature and low associated morbidity. The growth of radiosurgery should continue as more long-term follow-up data become available and as information regarding this technology reaches more patients.

References

1. Leksell L: The stereotactic method and radiosurgery of the brain. Acta Chir Scand 1951;107:316–319.
2. Larsson B: The history of radiosurgery: the early years (1950–1970). In Kondziolka D (ed): Radiosurgery. Basel, Karger, 1996, pp 1–10.
3. Niranjan A, Lunsford LD: Radiosurgery: where we were, are, and may be in the third millennium. Neurosurgery 2000;46:531–543.
4. Kondziolka D, Lunsford LD, Claassen D, et al: Radiobiology of radiosurgery: Part I. The normal rat brain model. Neurosurgery 1992;31:271–279.
5. Kondziolka D, Lunsford LD, Claassen D, et al: Radiobiology of radiosurgery: Part II. The rat C6 glioma model. Neurosurgery 1992;31:280–288.
6. Lunsford LD, Altschuler EM, Flickinger JC, et al: In vivo biological effects of stereotactic radiosurgery: a primate model. Neurosurgery 1990;27:373–382.
7. Yang T, Wu S, Liang J, et al: Time-dependent astroglial changes after gamma knife radiosurgery in the rat forebrain. Neurosurgery 2000;47:407–416.
8. Pollock BE, Flickinger JC, Lunsford LD, et al: Factors associated with successful arteriovenous malformation radiosurgery. Neurosurgery 1998;42: 1239–1247.
9. Yamamoto Y, Coffey RJ, Nichols DA, Shaw EG: Interim report on the radiosurgical treatment of cerebral arteriovenous malformations: the influence of size, dose, time, and technical factors on obliteration rate. J Neurosurg 1995; 83:832–837.
10. Kondziolka D, Lunsford LD, McLaughlin MR, Flickinger JC: Long-term outcomes after radiosurgery for acoustic neuromas. N Engl J Med 1998;339: 1426–1433.
11. Pollock BE, Lunsford LD, Flickinger JC, et al: Vestibular schwannoma management. Part I. Failed microsurgery and the role of delayed stereotactic radiosurgery. J Neurosurg 1998;89:944–948.
12. Landolt AM, Dieter H, Nicoletta L, et al: Stereotactic radiosurgery for recurrent surgically treated acromegaly: comparison with fractionated radiotherapy. J Neurosurg 1998;88:1002–1008.
13. Laws ER Jr, Vance ML: Radiosurgery for pituitary tumors and craniopharyngiomas. Neurosurg Clin N Am 1999;10:327–336.
14. Mitsumori M, Shrieve DC, Alexander E III, et al: Initial clinical results of LINAC-based stereotactic radiosurgery and stereotactic radiotherapy for pituitary adenomas. Int J Radiat Oncol Biol Phys 1998;42:573–580.
15. Chang SD, Adler JR Jr: Treatment of cranial base meningiomas with linear accelerator radiosurgery. Neurosurgery 1997;41:1019–1027.
16. Duma CM, Lunsford LD, Kondziolka D, et al: Stereotactic radiosurgery of cavernous sinus meningiomas as an addition or alternative to microsurgery. Neurosurgery 1993;32:699–705.
17. Morita A, Coffey RJ, Foote RL, et al: Risk of injury to cranial nerves after gamma knife radiosurgery for skull base meningiomas: experience in 88 patients. J Neurosurg 1998;90:42–49.
18. Subach BR, Lunsford LD, Kondziolka D, et al: Management of petroclival meningiomas by stereotactic radiosurgery. Neurosurgery 1998;42:437–443.
19. Kondziolka D, Patel A, Lunsford LD, et al: Stereotactic radiosurgery plus

whole brain radiotherapy versus radiotherapy alone for patients with multiple brain metastases. Int J Radiat Oncol Biol Phys 1999;45:427–434.
20. Sneed PK, Lamborn KR, Forstner JM, et al: Radiosurgery for brain metastases: is whole brain radiotherapy necessary? Int J Radiat Oncol Biol Phys 1999;43:549–558.
21. Weltman E, Salvajoli JV, Brandt RA, et al: Radiosurgery for brain metastases: a score index for predicting prognosis. Int J Radiat Oncol Biol Phys 2000;46:1155–1161.
22. Link MJ, Coffey, RJ, Nichols DA, Gorman DA: The role of radiosurgery and particulate embolization in the treatment of dural arteriovenous fistulas. J Neurosurg 1996;84:804–809.
23. Pollock BE, Nichols DA, Garrity JA, et al: Stereotactic radiosurgery and particulate embolization of cavernous sinus dural arteriovenous fistulae. Neurosurgery 1999;45:459–467.
24. Kondziolka D, Flickinger JC, Bissonette DJ, et al: Survival benefit of stereotactic radiosurgery for patients with malignant glial neoplasms. Neurosurgery 1997;41:776–785.
25. Shrieve DC, Alexander E, Wen PY, et al: Comparison of stereotactic radiosurgery and brachytherapy in the treatment of recurrent glioblastoma multimorme. Neurosurgery 1995;36:275–284.
26. Auchter RM, Lamond JP, Alexander E III, et al: A multiinstitutional outcome and prognostic factor analysis of radiosurgery for resectable single brain metastasis. Int J Radiat Oncol Biol Phys 1996;35:27–35.
27. Flickinger JC, Kondziolka D, Lunsford LD, et al: A multi-institutional experience with stereotactic radiosurgery for solitary brain metastasis. Int J Radiat Oncol Biol Phys 1994;28:797–802.
28. Muacevic A, Kreth FW, Horstmann GA, et al: Surgery and radiotherapy compared to gamma knife radiosurgery in the treatment of solitary cerebral metastases of small diameter. J Neurosurg 1999;91:35–43.
29. Amin-Hanjabi S, Ogilvy CS, Candia GJ, et al: Stereotactic radiosurgery for cavernous malformations: Kjellberg's experience with proton beam therapy in 98 cases at the Harvard cyclotron. Neurosurgery 1998;42:1229–1238.
30. Chang SD, Levy RP, Adler JR Jr, et al: Stereotactic radiosurgery of angiographically occult vascular malformations: 14-year experience. Neurosurgery 1998;43:213–221.
31. Karlsson B, Kihlström L, Lindquist C, et al: Radiosurgery for cavernous malformations. J Neurosurg 1998;88:293–297.
32. Kondziolka D, Lunsford D, Flickinger J, Kestle J: Reduction of hemorrhage risk after stereotactic radiosurgery for cavernous malformations. J Neurosurg 1995;83:825–831.
33. Pollock BE, Garces YI, Stafford SL, et al: Stereotactic radiosurgery of cavernous malformations. J Neurosurg 2000;93:987–991.
34. Kondziolka D, Lunsford LD, Flickinger JC, et al: Stereotactic radiosurgery for trigeminal neuralgia: a multiinstutional study using the gamma unit. J Neurosurg 1996;84:940–945.
35. Young RF, Vermeulen SS, Grimm P, et al: Gamma knife radiosurgery for treatment of trigeminal neuralgia: idiopathic and tumor related. Neurology 1997;48:608–614.
36. Pollock BE, Lunsford LD, Kondziolka D, et al: Outcome analysis of acoustic neuroma management: a comparison of microsurgery and stereotactic radiosurgery. Neurosurgery 1995;36:215–223.
37. Pollock BE, Lunsford LD, Noren G: Vestibular schwannoma management in the next century: a radiosurgical perspective. Neurosurgery 1998;43:475–483.
38. Kondziolka D: Functional radiosurgery. Neurosurgery 1999;44:12–22.

39. Régis J, Bartolomei F, Metellus P, et al. Radiosurgery for trigeminal neuralgia and epilepsy. Neurosurg Clin N Am 1999;10:359–377.
40. Pollock BE, Kline RW, Stafford SL, et al: The rationale and technique of staged-volume arteriovenous malformation radiosurgery. Int J Radiat Onc Biol Phys 2000;48:817–824.
41. Flickinger JC, Pollock BE, Kondziolka D, et al: What length should be irradiated? A randomized blinded study of radiosurgery to different lengths of trigeminal nerve for trigeminal neuralgia. Int J Radiat Oncol Biol Phys 2001; 51:449–454.
42. Flickinger JC, Pollock BE, Kondziolka D, Lunsford LD: A dose-response analysis of arteriovenous malformation obliteration by radiosurgery. Int J Radiat Onc Biol Phys 1996;36:873–879.
43. Karlsson B, Lax I, Soderman M: Can the probability for obliteration after radiosurgery for arteriovenous malformations be accurately predicted? Int J Radiat Oncol Biol Phys 1999;43:313–319.
44. Karlsson B, Lindquist C, Steiner L: Prediction of obliteration after gamma knife surgery for cerebral arteriovenous malformations. Neurosurgery 1997; 40:425–431.
45. Schwartz M, Sixel K, Young C, et al: Prediction of obliteration of arteriovenous malformations: the obliteration prediction index. Can J Neurol Sci 1997; 24:106–109.
46. Touboul E, Al-Halabi A, Buffat L, et al: Single-fraction stereotactic radiotherapy: a dose-response analysis of arteriovenous malformation obliteration. Int J Radiat Oncol Biol Phys 1998;41:855–861.
47. Flickinger JC, Kondziolka D, Lunsford LD, et al: Development of a model to predict permanent symptomatic post-radiosurgery injury for arteriovenous malformation patients. Int J Radiat Onc Biol Phys 2000;46:1143–1148.
48. Lax I, Karlsson B: Prediction of complications in gamma knife radiosurgery of arteriovenous malformations. Acta Oncologica 1996;35:49–56.
49. Voges J, Treuer H, Lehrke R, et al: Risk analysis of LINAC radiosurgery in patients with arterio-venous malformations (AVM). Acta Neurochir 1997;68: 118–123.
50. Friedman WA, Blatt DL, Bova FJ, et al: The risk of hemorrhage after radiosurgery for arteriovenous malformations. J Neurosurg 1996;84:912–919.
51. Karlsson B, Lindquist C, Steiner L: The effect of gamma knife surgery on the risk of rupture prior to AVM obliteration. Minim Invas Neurosurg 1996;39: 21–27.
52. Pollock BE, Flickinger JC, Lunsford LD, et al: Hemorrhage risk after stereotactic radiosurgery of cerebral arteriovenous malformations. Neurosurgery 1996;38:652–661.
53. Pollock BE, Kondziolka D, Lunsford LD, Flickinger JC: Repeat stereotactic radiosurgery of arteriovenous malformations: factors associated with incomplete obliteration. Neurosurgery 1996;38:318–324.
54. Flickinger JC, Kondziolka D, Pollock BE, Lunsford LD: Evolution in technique for vestibular schwannoma radiosurgery and effect on outcome. Int J Radiat Onc Biol Phys 1996;36:275–280.
55. Kihlström L, Guo W, Karlsson B, et al: Magnetic resonance imaging of obliterated arteriovenous malformations up to 23 years after radiosurgery. J Neurosurg 1997;86:589–593.
56. Yamamoto M, Jimbo M, Hara M, et al: Gamma knife radiosurgery for arteriovenous malformations: long-term follow-up results focusing on complications occurring more than 5 years after irradiation. Neurosurgery 1996;38:906–914.
57. Flickinger JC: An integrated logistic formula and prediction of complications from radiosurgery. Int J Radiat Oncol Biol Phys 1989;17:879–885.

58. Kjellberg R, Hanamura T, Davis K, et al: Bragg-peak proton-beam therapy for arteriovenous malformations of the brain. N Engl J Med 1983;309:269–273.
59. Pollock BE, Phuong LK, Foote RL, et al: High-dose trigeminal neuralgia radiosurgery associated with increased risk of trigeminal dysfunction. Neurosurgery 2001;49:58–64.
60. Pollock BE: Management of patients with multiple brain metastases. Cont Neurosurg 1999;21:1–6.

Comment
Chapter 1

L. Dade Lunsford

I first visited Japan, in 1988, a trip during which I was hosted by Kenichiro Sugita, then Professor and Chairman at Nagoya University. This consummate surgeon and elegant host remarked to me quite privately about his feelings about the last two decades and the next decade of neurological surgery. He regarded the greatest advances in neurosurgery as the reintroduction of stereotactic surgery in the 1970s (it is little known that he was a pioneer in stereotactic techniques), the advancement of microsurgery in the 1980s (he transitioned his career to become a superb microsurgeon), and his anticipation that the 1990s would see the explosion of radiosurgery. His words proved prophetic.

In this chapter, Pollock nicely outlined some seminal points about the origins of radiosurgery and its subsequent integration into a busy academic tertiary/quaternary medical center. He rightfully recalls that the origins of radiosurgery lay in the fertile mind of Professor Lars Leksell, who "grew up" in the neurosurgical development phase of the 1940s. At that time, Herbert Olivicrona was the master surgeon and Professor at the Karolinska Hospital, Stockholm, Sweden, but like all pioneers he suffered a number of untoward events in difficult clinical problems. Leksell was convinced that for many patients there had to be a better way. He was a cautious man who gave birth to the idea of radiosurgery in 1951, and nurtured it through several experimental phases using both protons from cyclotrons and photons from early generation linear accelerators. He eventually collaborated with Borje Larson to create the Gamma Knife. Leksell wanted a simple and practical tool that could be used within the context of a hospital environment. His initial interest lay in the creation of white matter lesions for chronic pain and movement disorders as well as intractable psychiatric conditions, but he facilitated the application of radiosurgery to morphologic targets beginning in approximately 1971. At that time, Steiner reported the first AVM treatment using the Gamma Knife, and cautious forays were made into the application of the Gamma Knife for acoustic neuromas (Georg Noren was the patient pioneer here). It was used to treat scattered meningiomas and pituitary tumors, but almost never for malignant neoplasms. I suspect that Leksell would be flabbergasted to see the growth of the field since his death in 1986.

Pollock has reviewed the influence of this rise of radiosurgery at the Mayo Clinic. During a decade of experience, almost 2000 patients underwent radiosurgery, primarily involving two surgeons, Dr. Robert Coffey and Dr. Pollock. Like most centers, the technology led to a combination of wonderment, excitement, competition, concerns, fear of change, bewilderment, and other anxieties. Many issues were faced: an assessment of its proper role, long-term outcome analysis for a variety of indications, risk analysis, training objectives, the influence of radiosurgery on postgraduate medical education, and cost/benefit analysis. To date, radiosurgery has not taken the role of the standard QRS complex defined by Dr. Sean Mullan at the University of Chicago. In this paradigm, an early blip of interest (the P wave) is followed by a latency period before a large spike of activity emerges (the QRS complex). This is followed by a rapid reduction in application of the technology due to recognition of complications before the appropriate role is established (T/U wave). Instead, radiosurgery has continued to experience almost an exponential rise in application. In a large part, this is related to published data, patients driving the system, third-party reimbursement, acceptance among professional societies, and increasing experience among newly trained physicians. For a number of indications (AVM, acoustic neuroma), radiosurgery has become a practice standard, based not on Class I data (there are relatively few multicenter randomized prospective trials), but strong Class II data exist. Practice guidelines exist for meningiomas, trigeminal neuralgia, and pituitary adenomas. Such guidelines are based on strong retrospective case-matched trials (Class II data). For some indications, radiosurgery remains a treatment option (based on Class III or retrospective studies). Radiosurgery requires intense commitment by its practitioners to define long-term follow-up. During the procedure itself, the patient feels nothing and the doctor sees nothing. While this has many gratifications initially, it places a burden on doctors to provide long-term outcomes analysis. In addition, such data is necessary to quell periodic anxieties related to the potential for "oncogenesis" caused by radiosurgery.

Radiosurgery continues to grow as the number of indications. Of our total patient volume at the University of Pittsburgh and its affiliated medical centers, more than 5000 brain and spine operations are performed on an annual basis. We do slightly more than 500 radiosurgical procedures per year, a figure remarkably close to the experience at the Mayo Clinic (10% at our service, 9% at Mayo). The spectrum of cases has changed considerably over the years. More than 70% of our treated patients had AVMs in 1987; currently, less than 10% are AVM patients. In our 13-year experience, more than 4000 patients have undergone radiosurgery. Brain metastasis (>800 patients treated) and trigeminal neuralgia (>350 patients treated) are now the most frequent indications. Embolization is used less frequently now than it was 13 years ago for AVMs; however, a resurgence may be seen as a result of new hypotheses that even temporary flow reduction in AVM might actually enhance delayed radiosurgical obliteration. Radiation sensitizers and brain protector trials are imminent; methods to enhance the outcomes of radiosurgery for malignant tumors using gene vector radiation sensitizers have been reported. Educational activities abound at national meetings and scientific journals increasingly feature radiosurgical reports. Radiosurgical equipment vendors are ever more active in the war for market share.

Additional data relative to the cost/benefit analysis of radiosurgery would be very worthwhile. Relatively few papers have been published related to such issues. Those that have been published show the significant superiority of radiosurgery over microsurgery for most indications. Our studies estimate that the hospital costs of radiosurgery are 40 to 70% less than the costs of conventional craniotomy (independent of back-to-work issues). Neurosurgeons must direct the field, supplemented by the knowledge base of medical physicists and radiation oncologists. Neurosurgeons must also strive to do their best in explaining the preferred treatment options to patients. Pollock is correct in being cautious about the benefits of the Internet; it is a wonderful source of information for the lay public, but such information is often distorted, biased, and unreliable. Making our peer-reviewed publications more accessible to the public may be one idea to increase our exposure to patients. [Should we have a lay translation for the public, such as we do for grant submissions?] Such an idea would not obviate our professional and academic obligations to publish reports in the standard medical vernacular.

Chapter 2

Physical Aspects of Cranial Stereotactic Radiosurgery

Michael G. Herman, Edwin C. McCullough

Introduction

Cranial stereotactic radiosurgery (CSRS) refers to the precise delivery of ionizing radiation to an imaging-defined intracranial target. The goal of CSRS is to deliver an effective dose to the planning target volume (PTV) with as little radiation as possible to adjacent tissues. As intracranial targets are often irregularly shaped, achieving precise conformation between the radiation dose and the PTV requires complex dose plans that were not possible several years ago. Several technical features are typically used in the majority of radiosurgical procedures that are currently performed. First, a coordinate system is established by application of a skeletal-fixated "frame." Second, a fiducial system attaches to the frame and has imaging elements appropriate for the image modality (computed tomography [CT]; magnetic resonance imaging [MRI]; or angiography) used for treatment planning. Third, a computer dose-planning system references the fiducial markers onto the desired images, thereby creating a stereotactic space. Current systems calculate accurate summated isodose curves showing the cumulative effect of beam isocenter placements, collimator size, beam weighting, and head angulation, and provide the treatment delivery machine "on" times. The available software also permits two- and three-dimensional analysis to determine adequacy of volume coverage and non-PTV critical structure radiation dose values. Fourth, a treatment delivery system is available with radiation beams precisely and accurately intercepting at a point in space to create a radiation isocenter. To accomplish this task, the system places the patient coordinate system-defined beam foci at the radiation isocenter of the treatment

From Pollock BE (ed). *Contemporary Stereotactic Radiosurgery: Technique and Evaluation.* Armonk, NY, Futura Publishing Company, Inc. ©2002.

delivery machinery. It is critical that treatment delivery systems provide an adequate level of interlocked performance to preclude incorrect or dangerous treatment. In addition, the delivery system must be contained in a room that adequately protects treatment personnel as well as the public. This chapter will review in detail each of the necessary components for performing CSRS, as well as a brief discussion of the features of several commercially available treatment platforms.

Stereotactic Frame and Localization Systems

Patient immobilization and target localization in CSRS is usually performed with a stereotactic frame rigidly fixated to the skull. These are available from many vendors of radiosurgical systems (e.g., Elekta, BrainLAB, Radionics, Sofamor-Danek; see later in this chapter) as well as from neurosurgical instrument suppliers. Thermoplastic immobilization systems are also used, though exclusively for fractionated treatments (so-called stereotactic radiation therapy) in recognition of the somewhat decreased precision of these systems.

The x, y, and z coordinates of intracranial structures must be precisely determined for radiosurgical applications. This is typically done through the use of add-on fiducial systems in which form and function reflect the imaging modality and image plane. Fiducial systems consist of three or more plastic plates with embedded metallic rods or strips (CT) or hollow channels filled with a copper containing liquid (MRI). Most designs use an "N" or "Z" configuration so that, on each image "slice," three sets of dots are identifiable. As one moves through an imaging set, the middle dot sequentially moves. Determination of the separation of the two fixed dots in relation to the moving middle dot makes calculation of the z coordinate for each slice a simple geometric exercise (Fig. 1).

The coordinate values within any image slice are computed from the picture element (pixel) values, which are usually included in the "header" of the scan information. All commercially available radiosurgical dose-planning software now permits some type of semi-automatic process for slice location determination as well as the ability to calculate fiducial locations from suboptimal imaging. For example, local imaging artifacts on MRI from either external or internal sources can be corrected manually if needed. Angiographic fiducial systems usually consist of two plastic plates for each view. Each plate contains four lead markers at the corner of a square. On each of the orthogonal views, the square nearest the film is inside the one next to the x-ray tube. The only remaining problem is to discern left from right and anterior from posterior. Hence, on one of the two plates for each view, a ninth marker is placed at a known location (i.e., left and anterior) (Fig. 2).

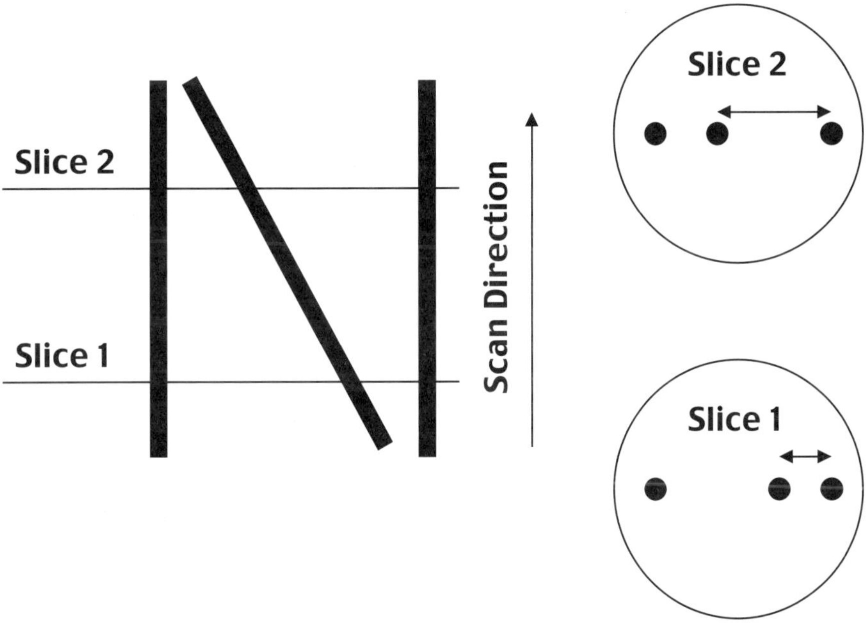

Figure 1. Computation of the coordinate value of an image slice using the distance of the diagonal fiducial mark from one of the endpoints.

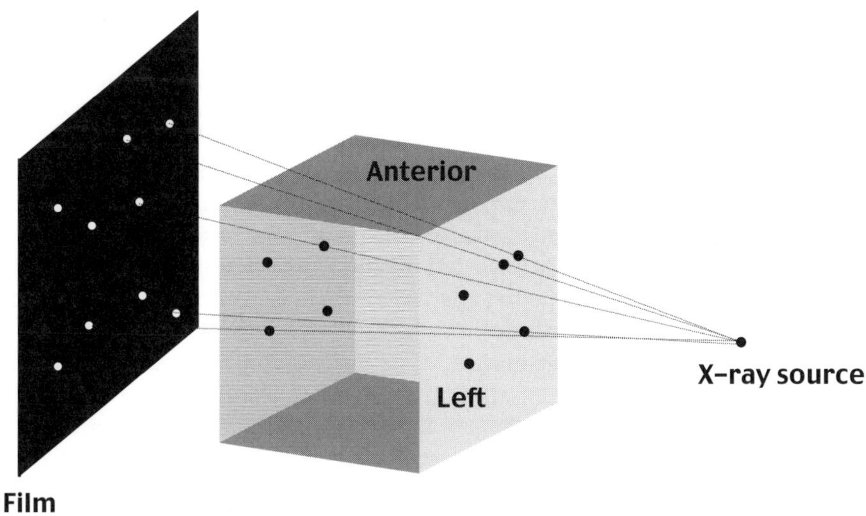

Figure 2. Generation of fiducial pattern for an angiographic view. A ninth marker defines the left anterior location.

Dose Planning

Dose-planning software must not only calculate the fiducial locations in order to create a stereotactic reference for the intracranial target, it must also permit the radiosurgical team (physicist, neurosurgeon, radiation oncologist) to develop conformal dose plans that are individualized for each patient's condition. While there are vendor-to-vendor variations, most CSRS dose-planning systems share several common features. A valuable quality is the ability to outline on two-dimensional images the desired target as well as nearby critical structures. Based on this information, the software creates three-dimensional volumes that should be adhered to in the creation of the radiosurgical dose plan. This pre-planning image segmentation is critical if the person involved in dose planning, frequently the physicist, has not had sufficient training in neuroanatomy and neuroradiology. At centers where the primary person involved in dose planning does have adequate training in these areas, usually the neurosurgeon, the usefulness and necessity of this image segmentation is reduced.

Single Isocenter Dose Distributions

The dose distributions for most CRSR treatments are the result of radiation delivered to a single point (isocenter) from multiple directions. Each isocenter isodose distribution tends to be circular or elliptical in shape. Hence, one can think of the typical CSRS treatment as trying to fill an irregular-shaped volume with "marbles" of different sizes. For example, the Leksell Gamma Knife® (Elekta Instruments, Stockholm, Sweden) can be thought of as having 4-, 8-, 14-, and 18-mm "marbles" with which dose plans can be created. Linear accelerator-based systems also use circular collimation, with the "marbles" ranging from 5 to 35 mm in diameter. However, the desire to create conformal dose plans to minimize treatment-related complications makes the use of large-diameter isocenters less frequent in the practice of modern radiosurgery.

For any single isocenter dose distribution (resulting from multiple direction treatment to that point) the dose values across the three-dimensional dose distribution can be plotted (Fig. 3). On such a plot, an effective diameter (e.g., distance between 90% or 50% of central axis [CA] value points) can be identified, as well as the fall-off at the edge. The edge fall-off, also know as the "penumbra," can be characterized in several ways; typically, most physicists regard it as the distance in which the dose profile decreases from the 80th to the 20th percentile of the CA value. In CSRS, the penumbra should be as small as possible to minimize the radiation exposure to adjacent tissues.

There is general agreement in the field among physicists that the accuracy requirement for placing the CA of the beams making up a single

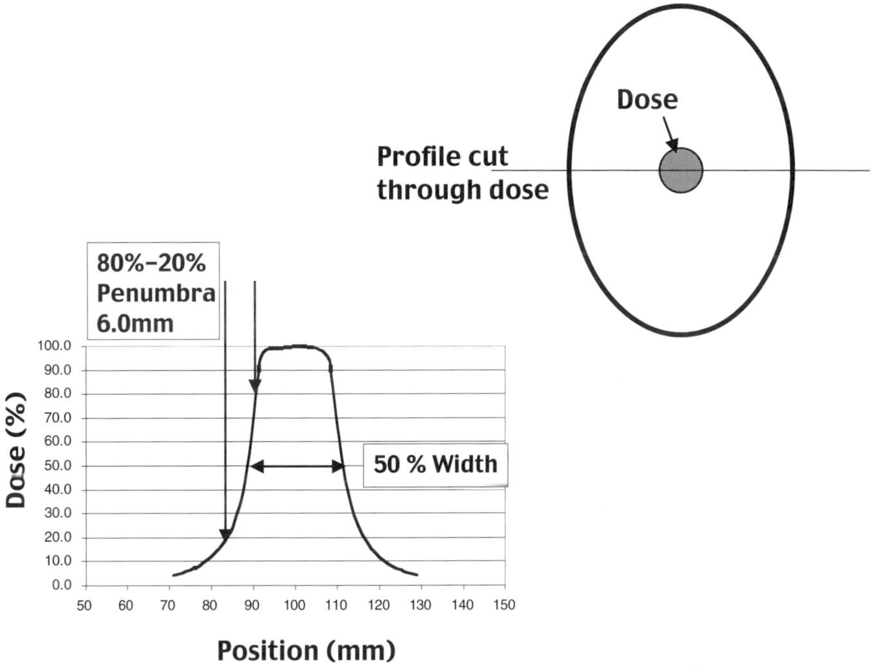

Figure 3. Beam profile from the isodose distribution for treatment with the nominal 18-mm helmet for the Leksell Gamma Knife. The points corresponding to 50% of the central axis dose are separated by 23 mm, while the penumbra (80%–20%) distance is 6.0 mm.

point dose distribution should ideally be 1 mm or less, with perhaps up to 2 mm as acceptable.[1] However, the difficulty in creating the ideal dose distribution with an abrupt edge fall-off is the need to treat from multiple directions (Fig. 4). In simple terms, a beam that irradiates at an angle away from 90 degrees will form an elliptical dose distribution with the penumbra widening in the appropriate directions. This is accounted for in the dose-planning system, and is a point checked by the physicist when commissioning the CSRS dose-planning system. The penumbra is further altered when multiple single point (multi-isocentric) distributions are summed to provide acceptable dose plans for the irregular-shaped fields almost always required in CSRS.

Multi-Isocenter Dose Distributions

With the exception of trigeminal neuralgia radiosurgery and occasional targets that are circular in shape, usually metastases, CSRS frequently involves combining multiple radiation isocenters to create acceptable dose plans that resemble the three-dimensional shape of the desired target. Each isocenter may have a different beam diameter as well as different weighting (higher or lower) relative to the other isocenters. Differential beam weighting is a very valuable tool for shaping the edge of the resultant dose distribution. Overlapping isocenters cause the location of dose maximum, the size of the radiation penumbra, and the prescription isodose shape to change with isocenter separation, beam diameter, and beam weighting (Fig. 5). Dose planning consists of changing these different variables until the dose plan adequately covers the PTV with a selected isodose line. Typical prescription isodose lines range from 40 to 90%. Treating to a higher prescription isodose line results in more dose homogeneity within the PTV, whereas prescribing to a lower prescription isodose causes more dose inhomogeneity within the dose plan.

For some patients (e.g., with multiple metastases), two or more distinct intracranial locations may need to be treated. In such cases, radiation from one treated area may overlap with other regions. At least one CSRS system has the ability to calculate multiple matrix plans and the relative influence that each matrix has on the others. This software maintains good dose point spacing in each of the dose matrices and determines the dose contributions from other dose matrix shots. It must be remembered in dose prescription that, because each dose matrix will have its

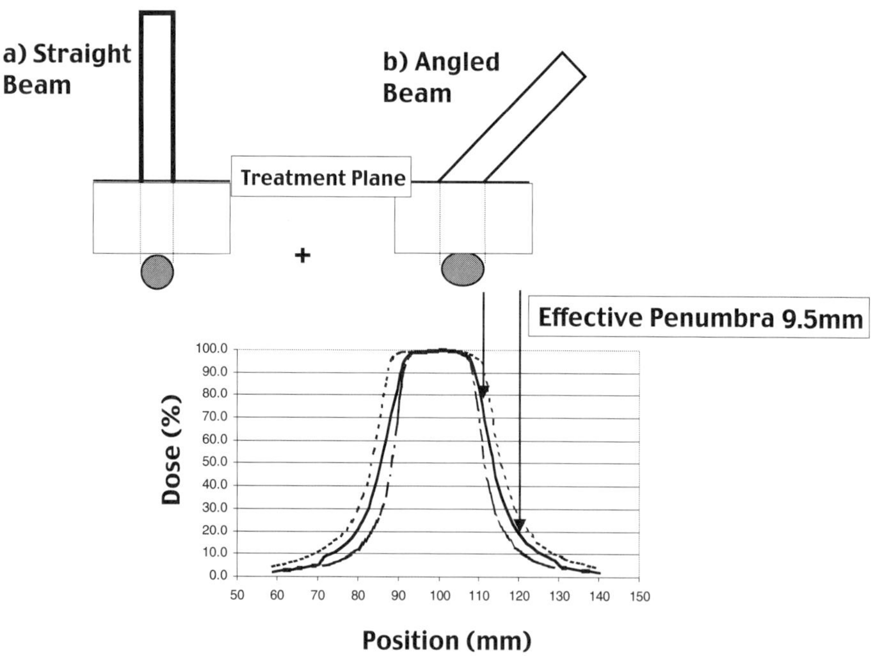

Figure 4. The effective beam penumbra of the combining multiple beams from different incident directions that contribute to the resultant dose distribution for an isocenter in cranial stereotactic radiosurgery.

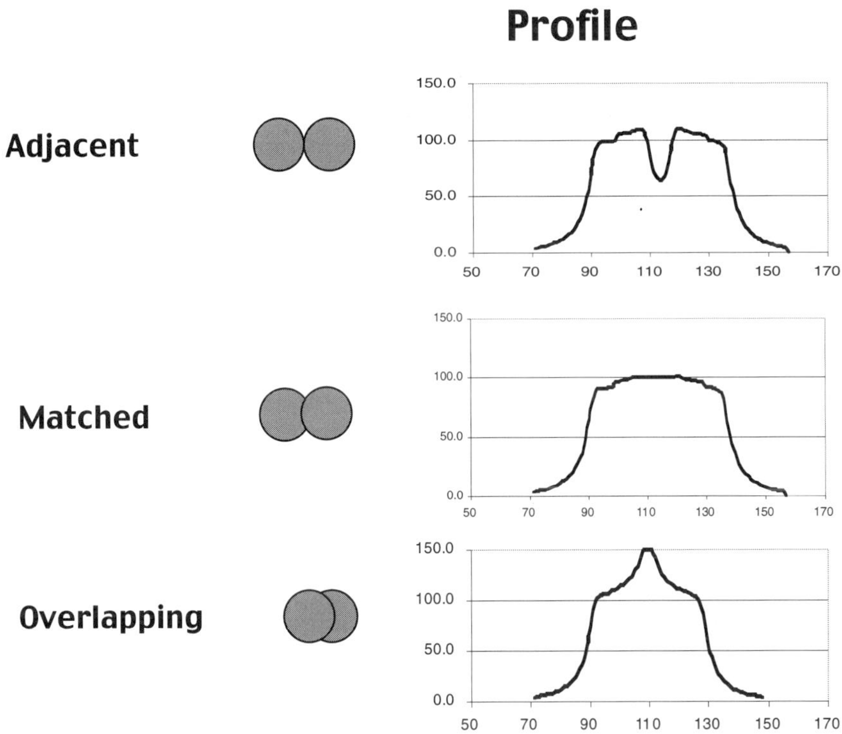

Figure 5. Effect of isocenter separation on maximum dose (location and value) and position of percent isodose lines for an 18-mm Gamma Knife collimator.

own dose maximum including contributions from other matrices, the maximum doses in the different matrices may vary widely. For example, 15 Gy to a global maximum of 30 Gy may be prescribed, with all the tumors well covered by this chosen isodose line. However, the dose maximum within each matrix may range from 18 to 30 Gy. Adjustment of the relative normalizations for each dose matrix corrects for this discrepancy; however, some further alterations of the shot configurations within individual dose matrices may be required.

Radiation Delivery Modalities and Techniques

CSRS is primarily delivered using cobalt-60 gamma rays (average energy 1.25 MeV), x-rays from linear accelerators (usually with 6 MeV maximum energy in the spectrum), and protons from a cyclotron (160 MeV). Gamma and x-ray beams are termed photonic because they behave in certain instances like packets of energy, termed photons. Protons (as opposed to photons) are particles and should be considered a form of particulate radiation.

Cobalt-60

Even though CSRS was performed more than 50 years ago using orthovoltage (≤300 kVp) x-rays, it was the packaging and commercialization of dedicated cobalt-60 units (Leksell Gamma Knife[2]) that has lead to the exponential growth of radiosurgery over the past three decades. Made in a reactor and relatively available, cobalt-60 provides a reliable source of external beam radiation for CSRS. Its 1.25 MeV energy is well suited for cranial treatment depths (5 to 8 cm) as well as allowing for unimpeded transit through the skull. However, cobalt-60 has a half-life of 5.26 years so the time required for identical treatment plans will double at this interval. There are two integrated CSRS systems commercially available that use cobalt-60 gamma rays as their radiation source: the Leksell Gamma Knife and the OUR rotating source unit from Shenzen (OUR International Technology and Science Company, Ltd., Shenzen, P.R. China).[3] A third approach using a standard isocentric cobalt unit modified to accept several sources has been patented, but to the authors' knowledge this is not available for patient use in any U.S. Food and Drug Administration-approved form.[4]

Leksell Gamma Knife

Published reports on radiosurgery performed with the Leksell Gamma Knife largely introduced CSRS to the neurosurgical community throughout the 1980s and early 1990s. Although the design of the machine has evolved over the past decades, it is still based on the principles set forth by Leksell.[2] Current machines use 201 cobalt-60 sources with an initial activity of 30 Ci (±5%) each. The earlier Model U had the sources arranged in a manner analogous to a bathing cap while the more recently marketed Models B and C have the sources arranged in a ring about the head. These later units have the secondary collimation helmets vertically aligned or perpendicular with respect to the patient and floor. This configuration makes patient positioning easier and has minimized the need for eye blocks. All models of the Gamma Knife are self-shielded with the 201 individual beams focused within the treatment housing about 40 cm from each source. Initial dose rates are in the 3 to 4 Gy/min range with the expected decay of about 1% per month. The beam placement accuracy is claimed by the manufacturer to be 0.3 mm.

The Gamma Knife is completely integrated for target localization and dose planning and the treatment system is designed for use with the Leksell stereotactic head frame and fiducial systems. During radiosurgery with the Gamma Knife, the patient needs to be released from the secondary collimation helmet and the frame coordinates are reset between each isocenter. The currently available Model C Gamma Knife has an automatic positioning system that repositions the patient's x, y, and z coordinates for different isocenters of the same collimator size. This system will minimize the chance of human error and reduce the time necessary for radiation delivery.

OUR Rotating Unit

The OUR Rotating Gamma System (RGS) is manufactured in Pleasanton, CA. It utilizes 30 cobalt-60 sources with an initial activity of 200 Ci or more, arranged symmetrically in 30 concentric circles. These concentric circles are grouped in six spirals spaced at 60-degree intervals about the axis of rotation. The sources rotate as a group in synchrony with a secondary collimator. The secondary collimator can be rotated independent of the source holder and has four sets of opening diameters allowing for collimation changes through rotation at 15-degree intervals. The stated nominal diameters at isocenter are identical to that for the Leksell Gamma Knife (4, 8, 14, and 18 mm). Newer designs permit the choice of four diameters from the following list: 3, 5, 10, 12, 16, 20, and 24 mm. An initial dose rate of nearly 3 Gy/min is achieved at the isocenter. The manufacturer claims an alignment accuracy of 0.3 mm. Performance of this unit relative to the Leksell Gamma Knife has been reported.[3]

Linear Accelerator

The linear accelerator (LINAC) uses microwave energy to accelerate electrons down a waveguide and eventually focus them onto a metal target, thereby generating high-energy x-ray beams. The x-ray beam will have photon energies ranging from the nominal accelerating potential (e.g., 6 MeV) down to a cutoff energy determined by what is contained in the path between the target and the patient (most often a thick piece of material to flatten the beam). The customary way of specifying the energy of the x-ray beam is by its peak potential, whereas single energy photon and particles have their energy specified as MeV. Table 1 outlines the classes of LINACs used for CSRS.

Standard LINAC

Since most radiation oncology departments had linear accelerators, it was only natural that these sources of radiation be investigated regarding their suitability for CSRS. The pioneering work at Harvard University's Joint Center for Radiation Therapy (JCRT) established LINACs as a viable option for CSRS. Furthermore, treatment protocols were suggested and a suitable add-on collimation system was developed.[5]

Table 1
Classes of Linear Accelerators, Collimation, and Motion Commonly Used for Cranial Stereotactic Radiosurgery

1. Classic gantry mount LINAC • Circular collimators (add-on) Non-coplanar arcs Dynamic rotation Conical rotation • Poured shaped collimators Multiple static gantry angles • Mini-multileaf collimator Multiple static gantry angles Dynamic gantry motion	2. Robotic miniature LINAC

LINAC, linear accelerator.

Circular Collimation

In LINAC-based radiosurgery only one beam is available for radiation delivery. The early set-ups used circular collimators ranging from 10 mm to over 35 mm in diameter at isocenter. This necessitated the movement of the beam about an isocenter to duplicate the highly desirable property of treating from many directions. At least three motion patterns have been promulgated in the literature.

The JCRT and a number of European centers have performed CSRS using circular collimation with a series of five or more gantry arcs combined with a large arc traverse.[5] By placing the LINAC table at a fixed position and then operating the LINAC in its arc mode while maintaining a fixed isocentric delivery point, *non-coplanar converging arcs* are created. Podgorsak et al argued that opposed beams were not desirable, and the so-called *dynamic rotation technique* of simultaneous rotation of the LINAC gantry and table was developed.[6] As major electromechanical modifications are required to the LINAC table to perform this technique, none of which are done, supported or guaranteed by the LINAC manufacturers, the dynamic rotation technique is used at a limited number of institutions. McGinley and colleagues at Emory University suggested a third approach in which the patient sits on a specially constructed chair, which is rotated with the gantry at a succession of stationary angles.[7] This technique, called *conical rotation,* may be done at up to three gantry angles.

Each of the techniques described requires movement of the radiation source about the isocenter, as well as motion of the table/chair about its axis of rotation. These axes must be stable with rotation, and coincident with each other as well as coincident with the radiation isocenter of the LINAC. Concern about reported large gantry bearing and table bearing run-outs (instability around the gantry and table axes of rotation) on many linear accelerators prompted the University of Florida group to develop a collimation system (Medtronic Sofamor-Danek, Minneapolis, MN).[8] This system does not require the run-out values to be small or require compensation.

Poured Shaped Collimation

Bourland and McCollough suggested that treating at 5 to 10 fixed gantry/table angle combinations using poured irregular filed collimator inserts could effectively carry out CSRS.[9] These collimator inserts are designed from digital radiographs created from a series of finely spaced transverse CT scan slices. The challenge of developing a treatment-planning algorithm, which accurately described the dose distributions in these fields, was never solved by these investigators. At least one commercial company (BrainLAB, Redwood City, CA) offers such a collimation system and an associated treatment-planning algorithm.

Mini-Multileaf Collimation

The irregular shape of many targets treated with CSRS has necessitated the use of multiple isocenters. This is often time consuming and results in significant dose inhomogeneities within the treated volume. These concerns have led to the development and commercialization of a miniature version of multileaf collimation (MLC). Unlike the 10-mm leaf width (at isocenter) seen on the initial MLC designs, the mini-multileaf collimators (MMLCs) have narrower leaf widths of 3 to 4 mm, either fixed in width, or rising to 5 mm near the edge of the 10×10 cm^2 field size. These units are add-on and available from several commercial vendors.

A number of integrated systems (frame/fiducial system, treatment planning, and add-on MMLC) have been commercialized in recent years. The basic principle underlying CSRS using MMLCs is that a limited number of highly conformed fields are utilized to generate a prescription isodose surface enclosing the PTV (Fig. 6). Generally, the number of fields ranges from 7 to 12 per procedure. Automation makes this a very efficient process for treating irregularly shaped lesions. Both cranial and extracranial sites can be treated. This type of equipment facilitates stereotactic radiotherapy since the daily treatment regimens are much less intensive than those using dose distributions built around combining multi-isocentric treatments. It is also possible to use an electronic record and verify system to assure quality of both CSRS and stereotactic radiotherapy treatments given with the LINAC plus MMLC technology. This technology also allows the application of intensity modulated radiosurgery in which the MLC vanes will move during treatment to provide better dose uniformity together with the inherent conformance.

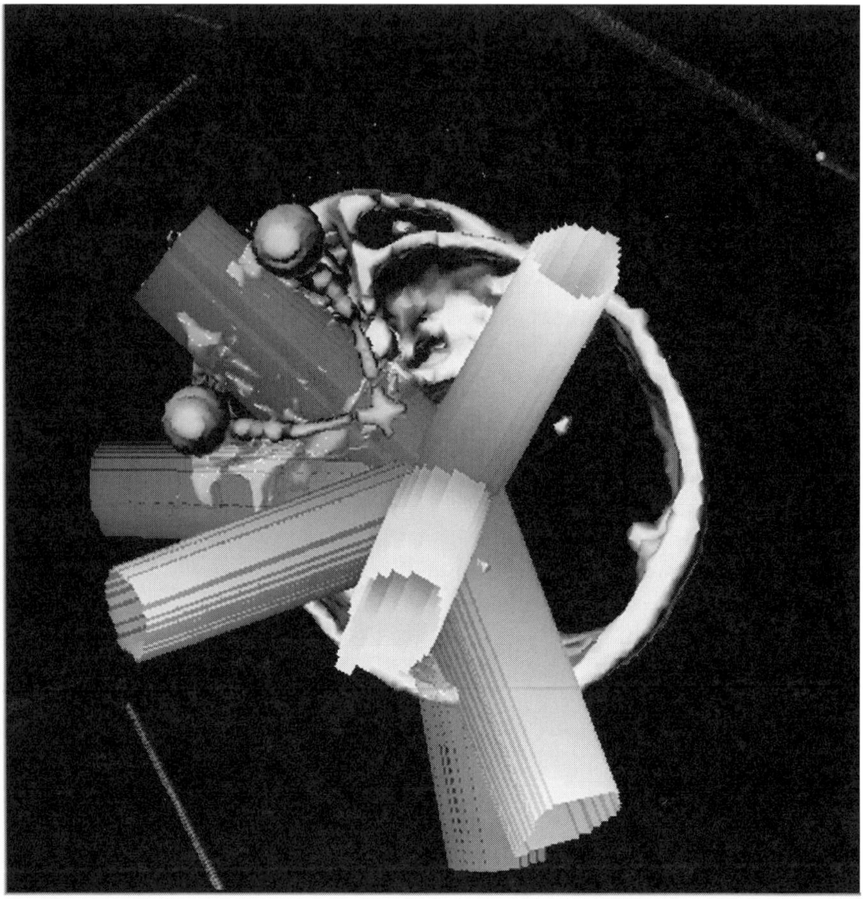

Figure 6. Principle of treatment with a number of static fields whose edge contours are defined by a mini-multileaf collimator. (Courtesy of the Charité Universitaetsklinikum Berlin, Germany.)

Robotic LINAC

The CyberKnife (Accuray, Sunnyvale, CA) is a "robotic" LINAC developed by Dr. John Adler of Stanford University as a new method to provide highly conformed fields without the use of a skeletal attached frame.[10] The treatment unit is a miniaturized LINAC capable of dose rates on the order of 3 Gy/min. The LINAC is mounted at the end of a robotic assembly capable of precise and accurate positioning. All parts of the body may be treated. During irradiation, orthogonal imaging systems measure bony landmarks and it is possible, in principle, to account for limited patient movement. Unlike conventional linear accelerators, the

CyberKnife is a dedicated device for performing both intra- and extracranial radiosurgery.

Protons

The use of protons to treat intracranial abnormalities has a long history beginning at the Gustaf-Werner Institute in Uppsala, Sweden in 1957,[11] followed by others such as Kjellberg and colleagues at the Harvard/MGH Cyclotron facility in Boston.[12] The use of protons for CSRS has created great interest because they possess the unique ability to deposit their energy at or near the end of their path. This is generally around 8 to 10 cm for 120 MeV protons. The facility size and support needed to successfully carry out proton beam treatments has limited their general applicability. There are approximately 10 to 20 proton beam facilities for radiation therapy operating at the current time.

Dose Delivery Uncertainties

Although modern CSRS integrated systems have progressed significantly over the past decade, it is important to remember that a variety of factors limit our ability to know the exact dose delivered to a particular intracranial x, y, and z position. The following factors are relevant at each stage of CSRS: imaging, fiducial localization, isodose to image registration, isodose calculation, tumor volume definition, as well as machine and patient alignment. At each of these steps, potential limitations are introduced in the treatment process.

Imaging

Imaging performed for CSRS must provide not only adequate resolution of the desired target from the surrounding tissues, but also spatial fidelity without significant distortions. The spatial resolution of CT and MRI is on the order of 1.5 times the pixel size for high contrast objects. The spatial resolution typically declines as tissue contrast is reduced. Slice thickness and the inter-image distance can significantly affect stereotactic accuracy, especially for small lesions. The greatest errors are usually in the z-plane. Most angiographic imaging performed to date has used film but this is undergoing a rapid transition to digital technology, with digitization to improve image resolution. Importantly, it introduces the possibility of image distortion from the image intensifier. Image distortion in a digital CT image is relatively rare (usually a result of an incorrect pixel size header field), whereas MRI scans are known to be prone to spatial distortions.[13] The distortions can arise from a number of sources. A frequent cause for MRI distortion is suboptimal magnet shimming, which for diagnostic applications is perfectly tolerable.

Fiducial Localization

Errors in fiducial localization result in assigning incorrect values for sectional image plane coordinates and can be due to several sources. Among these are frame shifting and image distortion. One under-suspected error results from simple distortion of the fiducial systems that are attached to the stereotactic head frame at the time of imaging. Over time, the fiducials can become bent resulting in significant fiducial localization errors. Current dose-planning software can test for this type of error. In addition, it can be simply checked at the imaging console by measuring the length of the diagonal lines connecting the four corners of the fiducial pattern. It also must be understood that there is an inherent limitation to slice localization accuracy arising from in-plane pixel size as well as the size of the fiducial markers.

Isodose Calculation

Isodose calculation algorithms may compromise some degree of accuracy for decreased computation time. This may be less so now that faster computers are commonly available. The supervising physicist should understand any compromises in the algorithm, which may affect isodose calculation accuracy. All CSRS dose algorithms sum the dose to a series of points contributed by each beam. For example, in the Gamma Knife, the contribution of the 201 beams to each of many possible isocenters is summed to each of $31 \times 31 \times 31$ points in the dose calculation matrix. The center and point spacing is usually selectable, and the smallest value consistent with obtaining dose distributions over the anatomical volume of interest should be used. Whenever multiple matrices are used, the relative contributions from each matrix on all the other matrices should be considered.

Image/Isodose Display

The conversion of a dose calculation point matrix to continuous isodose lines may introduce some uncertainties into the assessment of doses at particular anatomical locations. This is particularly true when point dose values are determined in regions of high dose gradient. However, such inaccuracies can be minimized by strict attention to detail in regard to software specification. Image distortion can cause further errors in determining the dose to specific anatomical structures.

Treatment

Following the imaging and planning phases of CSRS, the actual delivery of the radiation to the patient has the potential for introducing uncertainties or, unfortunately, absolute errors in dose delivery. The neurosurgery, radiation oncology, and physics team members need to carefully review all printed information from the treatment process. This particularly includes patient identification, anatomical site (e.g., left versus right) as well as the dose (some systems have a default). All data used to compute treatment times (e.g., skull coordinates) should be checked.

Alignment of the patient's frame needs to be assured. For dedicated units, this is done on a scheduled basis. For LINAC-based procedures, it must be assured prior to each treatment. The correct collimator must be placed in/on the equipment and its value double-checked. For multi-isocenter treatments, each isocenter must be set and double-checked followed by the proper setting of the time or monitor units (MU)/degree. All segments treated on a LINAC must be set up and checked off properly, including table and gantry settings. The completion of each isocenter treatment or segment must be unambiguously indicated in the treatment record.

Equipment Acceptance Testing and Quality Assurance

Acceptance Testing

Vendor-supplied integrated CSRS systems have their acceptance tests driven, in large part, by the vendor's acceptance test plan and a desire to stay in business. The purchasing institution needs to have a qualified person, most often a medical radiation physicist *familiar with CSRS*, review what is proposed and decide whether it meets that institution's standards prior to patient treatments; additional items may need to be added to the manufacturer's acceptance tests before clinical use is started. Generally, acceptance testing will be in the area of radiation protection, safety systems, localization/planning systems, as well as radiation profile, relative output, and calibration measurements. The American Association of Physicists in Medicine makes specific recommendations in its Report No. 54.[1]

Quality Assurance

The fact that CSRS delivers a large and potentially dangerous radiation dose in a single fraction emphasizes the necessity for quality assurance (QA) each day procedures are performed. The United States Nuclear Regulatory Commission (NRC) has specific requirements for monthly and annual checks for cobalt-60 units.[14] The American Association of Physicists in Medicine has also suggested QA programs for both Gamma Knife and LINAC-based radiosurgery programs.[1] At least one book has been dedicated to this topic by some of the world's most experienced physicists working in radiosurgery.[15]

Since LINACs with add-on collimation are routinely used for non-CSRS treatments, there needs to be a check that the center of the add-on stereotactic frame-holding system is aligned with the radiation isocenter of the treatment machine prior to each treatment session. All manufacturers of such systems provide (possibly as a purchased option) such a test tool. It should be noted that, because of pressure to compete based on price, many manufacturers of CSRS systems are breaking down systems into smaller pieces, and quality control tools which used to be prepackaged are now options to be purchased separately. This is why it is imperative that the supporting physicist completely reviews all purchases associated with the CSRS system. This person also needs to specify any dosimetry systems needed to calibrate and quality control the system to meet NRC or State Regulations.

Facilities Planning

In addition to the myriad of considerations that usually accompany the installation of major procedural equipment in a hospital environment, CSRS systems introduce the need for radiation protection. The simple addition of CSRS collimation to an existing LINAC introduces no new shielding requirements. However, it may require upgrading of the hospital type code as well as the introduction of anesthesia capabilities. Cobalt-60 units not placed in a prior shielded room will require only shielding for scattered radiation, and this is typically 18 inches of concrete (or *solid* concrete block). The robotic LINAC is capable of irradiating all walls with primary beam radiation and may require concrete shielding of 2 to 3 feet thicker than that for the self-shielded cobalt-60 units.

Summary

Intracranial stereotactic radiosurgery is capable of delivering a single high-dose fraction with high conformation to the intended treatment volume. This is a result of successfully integrating the field of stereotactic neurosurgery, specialized dose algorithms, and sophisticated treatment machinery capable of delivering small-field irradiation from multiple angles. The success in achieving this goal is clearly related to the combined expertise and skills from experts in neurological surgery, radiation oncology, and medical radiation physics.

References

1. Schell M, Bova F, Larson D, et al: Stereotactic Radiosurgery: Report of AAPM Task Group 42. 1995.
2. Leksell L: The stereotactic method and radiosurgery of the brain. Acta Chir Scand 1951;102:316–319.
3. Goetsch SJ, Murphy BD, Schmidt R, et al: Physics of rotating gamma systems for stereotactic radiosurgery. Int J Radiat Oncol Biol Phys 1999;43:689–696.
4. Shepherd JS, Rand RW: Radiation Therapy and Radiation Surgery Treatment System and Methods of Use of Same. US Patent #5748700, May 5, 1998.
5. Lutz W, Winston KR, Maleki N: A system for stereotactic radiosurgery with a linear accelerator. Int J Radiat Oncol Biol Phys 1988;14:373–381.
6. Podgorsak EB, Olivier A, Pla M, et al: Dynamic stereotactic radiosurgery. Int J Radiat Oncol Biol Phys 1988;14:115–126.
7. McGinley PH, Butker EK, Crocker IR, et al: A patient rotator for stereotactic radiosurgery. Phys Med Biol 1990;35:649–657.
8. Friedman WA, Bova FJ: The University of Florida radiosurgery system. Surg Neurol 1989;32:334–342.
9. Bourland JD, McCollough KP: Static field conformal stereotactic radiosurgery: physical techniques. Int J Radiat Oncol Biol Phys 1994;28:471–479.
10. Adler JR, Cox RS: Preliminary clinical experience with the Cyberknife: image-guided stereotactic radiosurgery. In Kondziolka D (ed): Radiosurgery. Basel, Karger, 1995, pp 317–326.
11. Larsson B, Leksell L, Rexed B: The high energy proton beam as a neurosurgical tool. Nature 1958;182:1222–1223.
12. Kjellberg RN, Shintani A, Frantz AG, et al: Proton-beam therapy in acromegaly. N Engl J Med 1968;278:689–695.
13. Sumanaweera TS, Adler JR Jr, Napel S, et al: Characterization of spatial distortion in magnetic resonance imaging and its implications for stereotactic surgery. Neurosurgery 1994;35:696–704.
14. Code of Federal Regulations, T., Chapter 1, Part 35: Medical Use of Byproduct Material. U.S. Nuclear Regulatory Commission, 1994. Washington, D.C.
15. Hartman G, Lutz W, Arndt J: Quality Assurance Program in Stereotactic Radiosurgery. Berlin, Springer-Verlag, 1995.

Comment
Chapter 2

Joseph C.T. Chen, Michael L.J. Apuzzo

The use of radiation energy for the treatment of neoplastic disease has a long history dating back to the late 19th century. As the physics and biological effects of radiation came to be better understood, technical and methodological advancements in the delivery of treatment have allowed this modality to assume a principal importance in the treatment of neoplastic diseases.

Refinements in radiation treatment have concentrated on methods for dose escalation as well as methods for more conformal treatment plans. Early efforts at achieving higher conformity of treatment have included interstitial brachytherapy and conformal external beam radiotherapy.

Radiosurgery exists as the by-product of the intersection of radiobiology with neurosurgical methods initially devised for functional procedures. We owe the concept of radiosurgery to the visionary efforts of Lars Leksell who reported the first radiosurgical system, a stereotactic frame coupled with a compact radiation source which could be moved along an arc to allow for an isocentric treatment plan. This early device served as the conceptual basis behind the development of the Gamma Knife, where cobalt radiation sources occupy fixed positions within a hemisphere allowing the generation of convergent beams of gamma radiation and precise focusing of radiation energy to a specific site within the head.

The classic implementation of radiosurgery can be defined as the single-fraction delivery of radiation energy to precisely constrained volumes of tissue. As such, the concept of radiosurgery runs directly counter to that of classic radiotherapy, which uses larger treatment volumes and dose fractionation. Because of this difference, radiosurgery has had a controversial early history. Early critics focused on poor results from initial studies where dosing and technique were likely suboptimal compared with what can be achieved currently. These concerns have been largely allayed by the burgeoning body of convincing evidence demonstrating that radiosurgery can be used for the safe and effective treatment of a wide variety of neoplastic diseases of the central nervous system. Because of these technical advancements and the consistently positive results from numerous radiosurgical centers, radiosurgery represents the current state of the art in local radiation treatment.

Regarding the choice of device for the delivery of radiosurgery for cranial treatments, gamma unit devices have been very popular because of the efficient and straightforward nature of the planning process, as well as the minimal routine maintenance and quality control requirements. LINAC-based devices, however, have been more readily available, as they are present in most radiation oncology centers. General purpose LINAC devices with moderate additional investment can easily be configured for radiosurgical treatment. LINAC-based devices using multileaf collimation and intensity modulation may offer some advantages over present gamma unit-based devices from the standpoint of improved dose homogeneity at the expense of more complex treatment planning and quality assurance measures. Particle beam radiosurgery using the Bragg-peak phenomenon has the potential advantage of higher treatment conformity than is possible with photon-based devices. These devices, however, have the disadvantage of requiring a costly cyclotron for particle generation. Furthermore, since these devices are essentially custom designed for each particular facility or site, "turn-key" implementations are uncommon, requiring on-site development of treatment planning facilities and methods.

Further advancements in radiosurgical technology will include engineering advances to maximize treatment conformity, accuracy, and efficiency of use. The role of dose fractionation in the radiosurgery setting has not been fully explored to date, and may have some role in modifying the therapeutic window of this treatment method. Last, advances in our understanding of radiobiology may allow us to predict with greater reliability the effects of radiosurgery. Targeted radiation sensitizers and protectants may also improve the therapeutic margin of these techniques.

In this chapter, Herman and McCullough have presented a concise overview of many of the fundamental technical issues of radiosurgical planning. As in all neurosurgical procedures, strict quality control and operator judgment are essential in the successful implementation of a radiosurgical program. An understanding of the immutable physical limitations of radiosurgery as it applies to control of the size of the treatment "penumbra" as well as the conformity of the treatment plan is imperative.

Radiosurgery represents a revolutionary advancement in neurosurgery and has already had a profound impact on its practice. For both malignant and benign neoplastic diseases, the recent literature provides overwhelming evidence that radiosurgery is an effective treatment modality with efficacy comparable to open surgical intervention in selected cases. In cases where tumor size or configuration may result in difficult radiosurgical treatment, a multimodal approach using sub-radical surgical extirpation combined with radiosurgery may allow for high rates of tumor control with minimization of operative morbidity.

In the realm of vascular and functional disease, it is likely that radiosurgical treatment may, for some indications, be the preferred means of definitive treatment in the near future. Presently, the utility of radiosurgery for arteriovenous malformations and trigeminal neuralgia has been established. Developing indications include treatment for movement disorders, epilepsy, and psychosurgery.

While the full extent of the role of radiosurgery in neurosurgical practice has yet to be established, it is necessarily doomed to be a stopgap measure in the treatment of neoplastic disease—inasmuch as it represents a "physical" treatment method that does not address the underlying biological cause of neoplasia or specifically take advantage of many of the unique features of tumors.

The future success of radiosurgery as a treatment modality will be based on multiple criteria including safety, efficacy, cost, availability, and patient acceptance. These criteria have largely been met by radiosurgery in its early history, and will necessarily impact on neurosurgical practice not only in academia, but also within the community setting.

Chapter 3

Radiobiological and Dosimetric Considerations in Stereotactic Radiosurgery

John C. Flickinger

Introduction

Stereotactic radiosurgery has ushered in a new era of understanding of how different approaches to radiation treatment planning and radiobiology may be modified in the clinic to achieve goals previously thought unreachable. Optimization of any clinical intervention (radiation, drug therapy, or surgery) requires equal attention to maximizing the desired outcome (tumor cure, vascular malformation obliteration, etc.) and to minimizing complications. This can be understood by the concept of paired dose-response curves for cure (tumor control or arteriovenous malformation [AVM] obliteration) and complications as shown in Figure 1. Radiosurgery exploits the radiobiological principle that small volumes of normal tissue irradiated to significant doses (such as in a radiosurgery treatment plan) can withstand much higher doses of radiation than larger volumes of normal tissue (such as when standard, nonstereotactic radiotherapy is used, where minimum margins are usually 10–15 mm). Reducing the volume of tissue irradiated can shift the complication dose-response curve down and to the right compared to treatment of a larger volume when a margin of surrounding normal tissue is included, thereby increasing the therapeutic window between cure and complications. A full understanding of radiosurgery requires knowledge of the underlying radiobiological principles affecting desired radiation effects and complications.

From Pollock BE (ed). *Contemporary Stereotactic Radiosurgery: Technique and Evaluation.* Armonk, NY, Futura Publishing Company, Inc. ©2002.

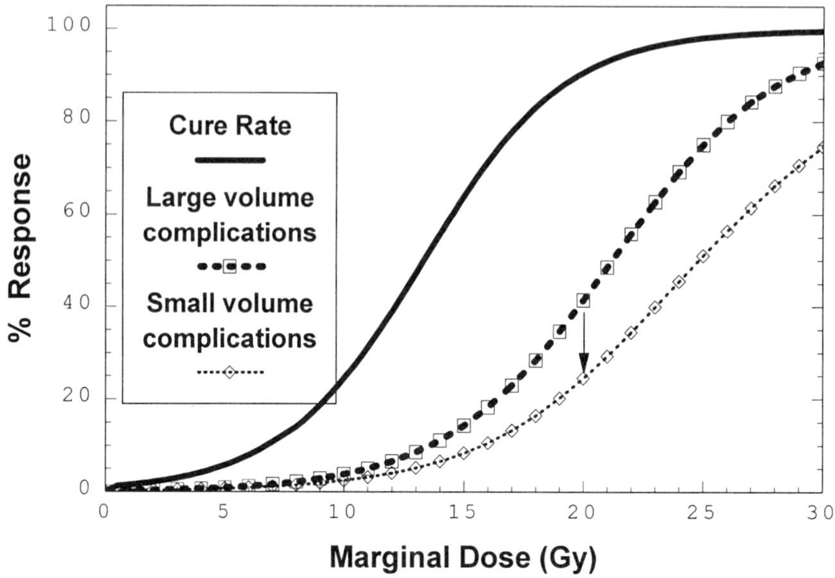

Figure 1. Typical sigmoid dose-response curves for cure and complications. Separate complication dose-response curves are shown for a larger volume and smaller volume to indicate how the risk of radiosurgery may be reduced if treatment volumes can be reduced.

The Linear-Quadratic Formula

The linear-quadratic formula is a way of representing the effect of single-fraction and fractionated radiotherapy.[1–3,7,8] It proposes that cell survival after a dose of ionizing radiation follows a combination of single-hit or linear kinetics (seemingly representing double-stranded DNA breaks) and double-hit kinetics represented by a quadratic term (seemingly representing single-stranded DNA breaks). For single-fraction irradiation, the probability of cure of a tumor or a normal tissue injury is represented by the following probabilistic double-exponential equation:

$$\text{P(cure or complication)} = \text{EXP}[-\text{K}^*\text{EXP}(-\text{alpha}^*\text{dose} - \text{beta}^*\text{dose}^2)]$$

where K = the number of clonogens, alpha and beta are coefficients for the respective single-hit and double-hit components.

This produces a sigmoid-shaped dose-response curve with the probability of cure or complication increasing from 0 to 100% as the dose is increased (Fig. 1).

The ratio of the alpha to the beta coefficients (the alpha/beta ratio or

α/β) can be used to translate the effects of fractionated radiotherapy with different doses per fraction.

Different tumors and different normal tissue reactions have different alpha/beta ratios. Studies of the effects of fractionated radiotherapy found that late-responding tissues such as brain or spinal cord have alpha/beta ratios around 2. For rapidly responding tissues such as skin or mucosal erythema reactions, alpha/beta values are usually 5 to 8, while many tumors have values closer to 10.[1,8] Low radiation dose-fractions cause proportionally less injury to tissues or tumors with a low alpha/beta ratio (a smaller alpha or single-hit component to radiation cell-kill kinetics) compared to tissues or tumors with higher alpha/beta ratios. There is a wide variation of alpha/beta ratios found in tumors. Some tumors such as melanoma or prostate cancer (or at least some strains of them) have lower alpha/beta ratios than surrounding normal tissues (skin or rectum/bladder), supporting the use of larger dose-fractions for treatment.

The normalized total dose[3] at 2 Gy per fraction, NTD_2 (the equivalent total dose if given in a course with daily 2 Gy fractions) can be given by the following simplified equation for a dose-fraction of d Gy/fraction:

$$NTD_2 = (\text{total dose given at } \mathbf{d} \text{ Gy/fraction}) * [\mathbf{d} + \alpha/\beta]/\ [2 \text{ Gy per fraction} + \alpha/\beta]$$

The above equation ignores time effects, which should be negligible for central nervous system tissue and benign tumors in normal circumstances. A time-dependent repopulation term must be added for protracted fractionated treatment of fast-growing malignant tumors. Table 1 shows the fractionated radiotherapy equivalent doses for single-fraction radiosurgery predicted using the linear-quadratic formula and older exponential formula.

Limitations of the Linear-Quadratic Formula

The linear-quadratic formula has been found to be reliable in the laboratory and the clinic for extrapolating from one treatment program to another with different sized dose-fractions, as long as the dose-fractions stay in the range of 1 to 8 Gy. Extrapolating from conventional radiotherapy with 1.8- to 2.0-Gy fractions to the high doses of single-fraction irradiation used in radiosurgery is quite another matter. Table 1 provides common single-fraction radiosurgery doses and gives the predicted equivalent doses for fractionated radiotherapy with 2-Gy fractions (NTD_2) using α/β values of 2, 5, and 10 for late-, intermediate-, and early-reacting tissues. The first column provides dose-equivalent dose calculations using an α/β value of zero (specifically, $\alpha=0$), which makes it a quadratic exponential formula rather than a true linear-quadratic formula. This is a stretch from

Table 1
Calculation of Radiobiologically Equivalent Dose (Normalized Total Dose) for Fractionated Radiotherapy with 2-Gy Fractions (NTD2) from Single-Fraction Radiosurgery, According to the Linear-Quadratic Equation Using Four Values of α/β*

Single-Fraction Dose (Gy)	*NTD_2 ($\alpha/\beta=0$) No Alpha Component*	*NTD_2 ($\alpha/\beta=2$) Late-Reacting Tissue*	*NTD_2 ($\alpha/\beta=5$) Intermediate-Reacting Tissue*	*NTD_2 ($\alpha/\beta=10$) Early-Reacting Tissue*
4	8	6	5.1	4.7
6	18	12	9.4	8.0
8	32	20	14.9	12.0
10	50	30	21.4	16.7
12	72	42	29.1	22.0
14	98	56	38.0	28.0
16	128	72	48.0	34.7
18	162	90	59.1	42.0
20	200	110	71.4	50.0
22	242	132	84.9	58.7
24	288	156	99.4	68.0

α/β, alpha/beta ratio.
*No time correction was used.

the theoretical basis of the formula, which presupposes some contribution with single-hit kinetics (the alpha component) corresponding to direct double-stranded DNA breakage. An early combined Harvard Joint Center for Radiation Therapy (JCRT)/University of Pittsburgh study of optic nerve injury after radiosurgery identified 8 Gy as the recommended safe dose-limit to the optic nerves/chiasm from single-fraction radiosurgery.[18] In that study, the lowest optic chiasm dose at which radiation-induced optic neuropathy developed was 9.7 Gy. According to Table 1, the linear-quadratic formula with values of 0 and 2 for α/β predicts that a 10-Gy single-fraction dose to the optic chiasm should have the equivalent effect of 32 or 50 Gy at 2 Gy per fraction, for $\alpha/\beta = 0$ or 2, respectively. Using an α/β value of zero, the equivalent dose at 2-Gy per fraction for the 9.7-Gy radiosurgery dose that caused optic neuropathy is only 47 Gy. From clinical experience with fractionated radiotherapy of pituitary adenomas and other parasellar tumors, the risk of optic neuropathy for 46 to 48 Gy at 2 Gy per fraction should be approximately 1/300.[6] Since the radiosurgery experience suggests that the risk for that dose is higher, the linear-quadratic formula seems to underestimate the fractionated equivalent of high-dose single fractions of radiation used in radiosurgery, even when an α/β value of zero is used (which stretches the theoretical basis of the formula).

The linear-quadratic formula also encounters problems in describing single-fraction dose-response curves. According to the theoretical basis of the formula, the values of alpha, beta, and the alpha/beta ratio can be derived from the shape of the single-fraction dose-response curve. The single-fraction dose-response curves for injury to the facial, trigeminal, and acoustic nerves after acoustic neuroma radiosurgery should allow calculation of alpha/beta ratios for radiation injury to these nerves. This was analyzed in 218 acoustic neuroma patients who underwent radiosurgery at the University of Pittsburgh from 1987 to 1997 with more than 2 years of follow-up (unpublished data). Extremely small values for beta were found with alpha/beta ratios of −61 for the facial nerve, 277 for the trigeminal nerve, and–40 for the acoustic nerve. Similar results were found in reanalyzing the linear-quadratic dose-response curve for in-field obliteration after AVM radiosurgery in 192 previously published patients, where the value of alpha/beta was −47.

Rationale for Fractionation

Eric Hall summarized the four main the radiobiological principles involved in fractionating radiotherapy as the "four R's of radiobiology."[9] These are: (1) *r*epair of sublethal damage between fractions of irradiation; (2) *r*edistribution of cells into more radiosensitive phases in the cell cycle; (3) *r*eoxygenation of relatively radioresistant hypoxic tumor cells; and (4) *r*epopulation of tumor cells. Sublethal damage repair refers to the difference between the damage caused by two fractions of radiation administered seconds apart, as opposed to 24 hours apart. Increased fractionation allows a greater degree of sublethal damage repair in the normal tissue than in tumors (resulting in a therapeutic gain) if the normal tissue's alpha/beta value is lower than the tumor's. Fractionation may redistribute tumor cells into more radiosensitive phases of the cell cycle (M, and the G1/S interphase). Increased fractionation allows relatively radioresistant hypoxic regions of a tumor to become reoxygenated after the first few fractions, thereby making them easier to kill with subsequent radiation fractions. Since normal tissue is already fully oxygenated, this also can lead to a therapeutic gain for fractionation. Malignant tumor cells are more likely to repopulate in between fractions of radiation than normal tissue, which translates to a disadvantage for fractionation in rapidly growing malignant tumors from this component of the radiobiological effect.

As discussed in the preceding paragraph, there is sufficient rationale for exploring fractionated approaches to stereotactic irradiation in malignant tumors. There is no basis for fractionating radiotherapy for functional radiosurgery or AVM. While the radiobiological response of most benign tumors seems to be similar to that of surrounding normal brain tissue, separate comparisons of radiosurgery and fractionated radiotherapy are needed for each type of benign tumor to prove any advantages with fractionation.

Dosimetric Questions

One controversial question in the early years of radiosurgery was how much inhomogeneity should be tolerated in radiosurgery treatment volumes. Gamma Knife users had historically treated with the 50% isodose as the treatment volume, preferring the steep dose fall-off outside this isodose and the ease of constructing conformal multiple isocenter treatment plans with the 50% isodose. Most linear accelerator (LINAC) users treated with the 80% isodose as the treatment volume. An early analysis of complications in LINAC radiosurgery of brain metastases and recurrent malignant primary brain tumors at the Harvard JCRT correlated complications with target dose inhomogeneity.[18] Large studies of Gamma Knife radiosurgery (with carefully tailored dose plans) have failed to identify any difference in complications in AVM or acoustic neuroma patients treated with low isodose (high target dose inhomogeneity).[4,5] The explanation for these different findings is that dose inhomogeneity ("hot spots") inside a tumor or AVM with a close-fitting treatment volume does not effect treatment complications, but inhomogeneity will increase complications when a poorly fitting treatment volume is used that contains areas of high dose or hot spots in enclosed normal tissue.

Lessons from the Radiation Therapy Oncology Group Dose-Escalation Study

The Radiation Therapy Oncology Group (RTOG) Radiosurgery Dose-Escalation Study (90–05) produced several important findings. A total of 156 patients with recurrent brain metastases or primary tumors (brainstem excluded) were treated according to a dose-escalation protocol stratified by lesion diameter.[16] After initial doses of 18, 15, and 12 Gy for diameters less than or equal to 20 mm, 21 to 30 mm, and 31 to 40 mm, respectively, doses were escalated in 3-Gy intervals until toxicity was seen in more than 30% of patients. The next lowest dose before reaching greater than 30% toxicity was defined as the maximum tolerated dose. Toxicity never exceeded 30% in the patient group with tumors less than or equal to 20 mm. Figure 2 shows plots of the reported late neurological toxicity data at each diameter that the author fitted to logistic dose-response curves. Table 2 lists the maximum-tolerated dose levels from that study and the author's estimates of the risks of acute and late toxicity at those doses derived from the preceding dose-response curves (in Fig. 2). Because tumor control seems satisfactory at lower doses and 14 to 16% risks of late toxicity seem high, the doses listed in Figure 1 as having 10% risk of late neurological sequelae were usually not exceeded.

In this study (RTOG 90-05), 125 patients underwent linear accelerator (LINAC) radiosurgery and 31 received Gamma Knife radiosurgery.

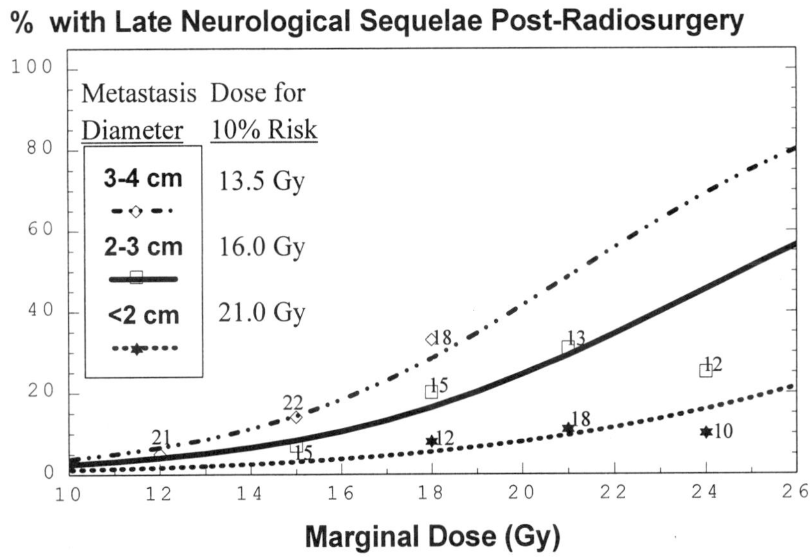

Figure 2. Logistic dose-response curves fit to the late toxicity data reported for the RTOG Radiosurgery Dose-Escalation Study. The numbers refer to the number of tumors treated at each dose level for each size category (stars, <20 mm; squares, 21–30 mm; diamonds, 31–40 mm). The doses where 10% late toxicity occurs in the fitted curves are shown next to the legend.

There were significant problems in quality control that were more frequent at the LINAC facilities compared to the Gamma Knife facilities (Mayo Clinic, Rochester, MN, and University of California-San Francisco). Postradiosurgery tumor progression occurred 2.8 times more frequently in the patients who underwent LINAC radiosurgery than in Gamma Knife patients. Although it seems reasonable to hypothesize that

Table 2

Estimation of Acute, Late, and Total (Acute + Late) Neurological Toxicity Following Radiosurgery at the RTOG Maximum-Tolerated Dose Levels*

Tumor Diameter	*Maximum Tolerated Dose*	*Acute Toxicity*	*Late Toxicity*	*Total Toxicity*
<20 mm	24 Gy	2%	16%	16%
21–30 mm	18 Gy	8%	16%	21%
31–40 mm	15 Gy	7%	14%	22%

RTOG, Radiation Therapy Oncology Group.

*Toxicity rates were estimated from fitting logistic dose-response curves to data at all dose levels tested. Since the total toxicity results were fitted separately, the acute and late toxicity estimates do not necessarily add up to make up the total toxicity risks (as in the raw data).

the higher maximum doses (greater inhomogeneity) in the Gamma Knife plans could have helped improve tumor control, the most likely explanation for this difference is incomplete tumor coverage at some of the LINAC facilities at the time of the study. It appears that quality control problems at LINAC centers have been addressed in subsequent RTOG studies.

Future Developments

Future improvements in radiosurgery are likely to come from techniques that modify the response to radiosurgery based on one of the radiobiological principles discussed in this chapter. These include fractionation strategies, radiation protectors, and radiation sensitizers. The hope with each of these approaches is to increase the separation between complications and cure as shown in Figure 1. The radiation protector amifostine looks promising outside the central nervous system but does not cross the blood brain barrier. Studies of 21-aminosteroids indicate that temporary swelling and edema in brain adjacent to a radiosurgery target can be prevented without changing tumor control or production on well-circumscribed radiation necrosis (desired in functional radiosurgery).[11] The problem of tumor hypoxia can be addressed by using fractionation to exploit reoxygenation, improving oxygen delivery, or using oxygen substitutes. The latter approach uses hypoxic radiation sensitizers, such as gadolinium texaphyrin to take the place of the oxygen missing in hypoxic zones within tumors and to fix radiation injury so that hypoxic tumor cells will be killed by the radiation.[14] RSR13 shifts hemoglobin's oxygen dissociation curve so that oxygen will only be released in areas of relative hypoxia. Because there is a slight relative reduction of oxygen delivery to previously well-oxygenated areas in the rest of the body, there is enough oxygen still adhered to the hemoglobin when it reaches highly hypoxic regions to alleviate much of the hypoxia in those regions. Initial studies with fractionated radiotherapy and RSR13 in brain metastases and high-grade gliomas appear promising.[10,17] Redistribution of cells into more sensitive portions of the cell cycle may be exploited through the use of taxanes which arrest cells in G2/M, the most sensitive part of the cell cycle. Topoisomerase I-targeting drugs interfere with topoisomerase I-mediated cleavage rejoining of DNA strands. Last, gene therapy can be used to attack tumor cells by modifying their response to radiation.

References

1. Barendsen GW: Dose fractionation, dose rate and iso-effect relationships for normal tissue responses. Int J Radiat Oncol Biol Phys 1982;8:1981–1997.
2. Dale RG: The application of the linear-quadratic dose-effect equation to fractionated and protracted radiotherapy. Br J Radiol 1985;58:515–528.

3. Flickinger JC, Kalend A: Use of normalized total dose to represent the biological effect of fractionated radiotherapy. Radiother Oncol 1990;17:339–347.
4. Flickinger JC, Kondziolka D, Lunsford LD, et al: Development of a model to predict permanent symptomatic post-radiosurgery injury for arteriovenous malformation patients. Int J Radiat Oncol Biol Phys 2000;46:1143–1148.
5. Flickinger JC, Kondziolka D, Pollock BE, Lunsford LD: Evolution in technique for vestibular schwannoma radiosurgery and effect on outcome. Int J Radiat Oncol Biol Phys 1996;36:275–280.
6. Flickinger JC, Rush SC: Linear accelerator radiotherapy of pituitary adenomas. In Landolt AM, Vance, Reilly (eds): Pituitary Adenomas: Biology, Diagnosis and Treatment. Edinburgh, UK, Churchill Livingstone, 1996, pp 475–483.
7. Fowler JF: The linear-quadratic formula and progress in fractionated radiotherapy. Br J Radiol 1989;62:679–694.
8. Hall EJ, Brenner DJ: The radiobiology of radiosurgery: rationale for different treatment regimes for AVMs and malignancies. Int J Radiat Oncol Biol Phys 1993;25:381–385.
9. Hall EJ: Radiobiology for the Radiologist. Philadelphia, JB Lippincott Company, 1988, pp 240–241.
10. Kleinberg LR, Carson K, Lesser G, et al: Survival results of a phase II trial of RSR13 and concurrent cranial RT for newly diagnosed glioblastomas multiforme. Proceedings of ASCO (abstract). 2000;19:158A.
11. Kondziolka D, Somaza S, Martinez AJ, et al: Radioprotective effects of the 21-aminosteroid U74389G for stereotactic radiosurgery. Neurosurgery 1997; 41:203–208.
12. Larson DA, Flickinger JC, Loeffler JS: The radiobiology of radiosurgery. Int J Radiat Oncol Biol Phys 1993;25:557–561.
13. Lederman G, Wronski M, Arbit E, et al: Treatment of recurrent glioblastoma multiforme using fractionated stereotactic radiosurgery and concurrent paclitaxel. Am J Clin Oncol 2000;23:155–159.
14. Miller RA, Woodburn K, Fan Q, et al: In vivo animal studies with gadolinium (III) texaphyrin as a radiation enhancer. Int J Radiat Oncol Biol Phys 1999; 45:981.
15. Nedzi LA, Kooy LI, Alexander E, et al: Variables associated with the development of complications from radiosurgery of intracranial tumors. Int J Radiat Oncol Biol Phys 1991;21:591–599.
16. Shaw E, Scott C, Souhami L, et al: Single dose radiosurgical treatment of recurrent previously irradiated primary brain tumors and brain metastases: final report of RTOG protocol 90–05. Int J Radiat Oncol Biol Phys 2000;47: 291–298.
17. Shaw E, Scott C, Stea B, et al: Survival improvement with RSR13 plus cranial radiation therapy in patients with brain metastases: comparison to the Radiation Therapy Oncology Group recursive partitioning analysis brain metastasis database. Proceedings of ASCO (abstract). 2000;19:159A.
18. Tishler RB, Loeffler JS, Lunsford LD, et al: Tolerance of cranial nerves of the cavernous sinus to radiosurgery. Int J Radiat Oncol Biol Phys 1993;27: 215–221.

Comment

Chapter 3

David W. Andrews

This chapter has considered radiobiological and dosimetric considerations in radiosurgery. It specifically addresses issues of dose equivalence between single-fraction and fractionated approaches utilizing the linear-quadratic formula and any therapeutic benefit that might accrue to either technique in various clinical scenarios. This commentary will discuss the practical limitations specifically of the linear-quadratic formula and, more generally, of theoretical radiobiological considerations as they pertain to specific intracranial targets.

The limitations of the linear-quadratic formula are acknowledged in the chapter, particularly when applying these dose calculations to achieve an acceptable therapeutic index around the optic apparatus. I would extend the concerns to include all special sensory cranial nerves, inclusive of the cochlear nerve, when considering dose and fraction selection. Based on a broad experience reflected in the literature, the optic and cochlear nerves represent a special subcategory of late-responding tissues with a greater sensitivity to radiation when compared to other cranial nerves. (It remains unclear how susceptible the olfactory nerves are to radiation.) This greater susceptibility to radiation injury is perhaps reflected in a different α/β ratio from all other central nervous system tissues, and dose extrapolations between single-fraction and 2-Gy multiple-fraction treatments when these normal structures are involved may not apply. Two examples can be considered, in which a commonly treated late-responding tumor, acoustic schwannoma and meningioma, involving, respectively, the VIII and II special sensory cranial nerves, are treated with stereotactic radiation.

Consider first meningiomas of the cavernous sinus and optic nerve sheath meningiomas (ONSM). A retrospective analysis of the tolerance of the optic apparatus to radiation by Parsons et al supports an acceptably low incidence of radiation-induced optic neuropathy when the cumulative dose does not exceed 60 Gy and the daily dose per fraction does not exceed 1.9 Gy.[1] Drawing from this experience, we treated all meningiomas involving or near the optic apparatus, including ONSM, with stereotactic radiotherapy utilizing 1.8-Gy fractions to a cumulative dose of 54 Gy. In our experience, the application of conventional-fraction stereotactic radiotherapy (CF-SRT) to cavernous sinus meningiomas has thus far resulted in no post-treatment cranial neuropathies (Fig. I), which compares favorably to single-fraction radiosurgery series reporting rates of cranial neuropathy at 12 to 13%.[2,3] We have thus far noted visual improvement in four patients, stable vision in three, and visual deterioration in two, for a 78% rate of visual preservation in patients with ONSM (Fig. I). Assuming an α/β ratio of 2 for all late-reacting cranial nerves involved, we would expect a similar outcome for all targeted cranial nerves, but this is clearly not the case when comparing outcomes as noted in Figure I. These preliminary data would support the contention that special sensory cranial nerves have a greater susceptibility to radiation injury. Based on Table 1, assuming an α/β ratio of 2 for all late-reacting cranial nerves involved, we would also expect comparable responses with a single-fraction treatment of 12 to 14 Gy. This appears thus far not to be the case for cavernous sinus meningioma by historical comparisons to series in the literature as noted above. Regarding ONSM, we know from recent radiosurgery literature cited in this chapter that the upper limit of a safe single-fraction dose to the optic chiasm is 8 Gy,[2] and this dose represents a marginal dose to the chiasm. Single-fraction radiosurgery literature does not exist for treatment of ONSM because a single-fraction dose anticipated to control meningioma (12 to 14 Gy) would represent a prohibitive risk of visual loss in patients with intact or functional vision in the affected optic nerve. This comparison does not support a dose equivalence between CF-SRT and single fraction for the treatment of ONSM. Longer follow-up will be necessary to establish both tumor control rates and rates of radiation-induced

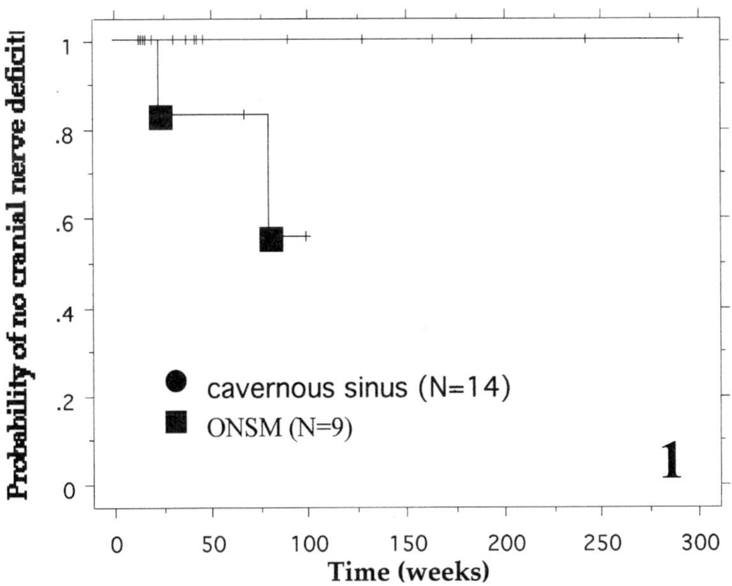

Figure I. Kaplan Meier plot for probability of no cranial nerve deficit after conventional-fraction stereotactic radiotherapy. ONSM, optic nerve sheath meningiomas.

optic neuropathy, but follow-up thus far appears to be superior to the natural history of this disease, specifically visual loss.

The same is true of acoustic schwannomas. We have compared the treatment of patients with acoustic tumors and serviceable hearing prospectively to single-fraction treatment and historically to the natural history.[4] We have obtained significantly higher rates of hearing preservation using 2-Gy fractions daily to a cumulative dose of 50 Gy when compared to high conformality/multiple shot 12-Gy single-fraction treatments. Assuming an α/β ratio of 2 for all late-reacting tissues involved, these doses fall roughly within the dose extrapolations provided in Table 1 of this chapter, yet the outcomes are significantly different and do not support a therapeutic dose equivalence (Fig. II). Follow-up thus far also supports CF-SRT over observation, as does recent literature.[5]

This chapter supports fractionation only when considering the classic radiobiological advantages it provides for high α/β ratio targets such as malignancies, notably the "four R's" achieved with fractionation. As discussed above, however, there appear to be compelling advantages to the application of stereotactic radiosurgery to low α/β ratio late-responding tissues as well. Large AVMs can be considered as an additional example. As stated in this chapter, small volumes of normal tissue can withstand much higher doses of radiation than larger volumes of normal

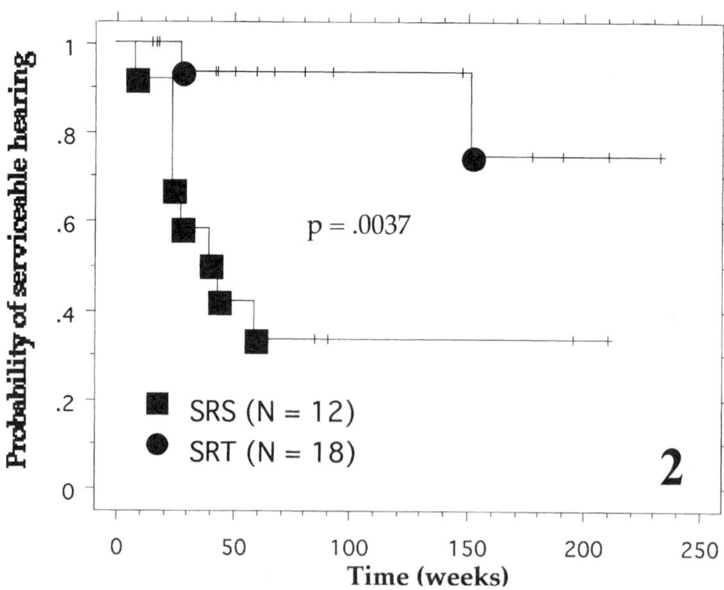

Figure II. Kaplan-Meier plot for probability of serviceable hearing for all patients with sporadic tumors. SRS, stereotactic radiosurgery; SRT stereotactic radiotherapy.

tissue (Fig. 1 in the chapter), which leaves the treatment of large AVMs a particular challenge for single-fraction radiosurgery treatments. Large inoperable AVMs of greater than or equal to 14 cm^3 have remained refractory to lower marginal dose prescription resulting in much lower obliteration rates.[6] Recent literature supports a threshold single-fraction dose of greater than or equal to 15 Gy to achieve obliteration rates in the range of greater than or equal to 80%, below which obliteration rates drop to a 20 to 30% range.[7,8] A 15-Gy dose to a large AVM volume ($\geq$14 cm^3) also represents unacceptable morbidity in recent series (see Miyawaki et al as an example[9]). More recent strategies have involved staged partial volumetric treatments over time which have proven to be thus far safe, but obliteration rates are unknown.[10] Traditional conventional fraction treatments, although safe, have been ineffective.[11]

What about hypofractionation techniques? Souhami et al described the safe application of a hypofractionation technique for a variety of low- and high-grade gliomas using a 7 Gy/fraction to 42-Gy cumulative dose technique.[12] The linear-quadratic formula as featured in this chapter only analyzes an NTD_2 (2 Gy) dose equivalence which would therefore not allow us to apply a comparable single-fraction dose to this dose-fractionation scheme for large AVMs. We treated large AVMs either previously untreated or partially obliterated by embolization with hypofractionated stereotactic radiotherapy (HF-SRT) treatments using a dedicated LINAC. Thirty patients with large AVMs were treated from January 1995 through August 1998. Our technique initially involved six 7-Gy fractions delivered on alternate days over 2 weeks to 42-Gy total dose, subsequently dropped to 5 Gy/fraction to 30-Gy total dose after late complications in one of seven patients. This patient sustained morbidity at 10 months after treatment with thrombosis of a large draining vein outside the 10% isodose line. We attribute this complication to the recently described phenomenon of occlusive hyperemia.[13] Six of the seven patients treated in this cohort had undergone prior partial embolization. Twenty-three patients were treated with 30 Gy/5 Gy fractions, with two patients lost to follow-up and three who died from unrelated causes. Of eighteen evaluable patients, eight had prior partial embolization. Mean AVM volumes at HF-SRT treatment were 14.51 ± 9.8 cm^3 and 14.54 ± 10.25 cm^3, respectively, for the 42 Gy/7 Gy fraction and 30 Gy/5 Gy fraction groups. At latest follow-up, angiographically documented AVM obliteration rates are 83% for the 42 Gy/7 Gy fraction group with a mean latency of 108 weeks (N=5) and 17% for the 30 Gy/5 Gy fraction group with an average latency of 191 weeks (N=2) (Fig. III). A cumulative hazard plot reveals a sixfold greater likelihood of obliteration with the 42 Gy /7 Gy fraction protocol (p=.0008) (Fig. IV). As with stereotactic radiosurgery, our data reflect the need for a threshold dose, in the case of hypofractionation to a marginal dose of greater than 5 Gy over six alternate day fractions to obliterate large AVMs.

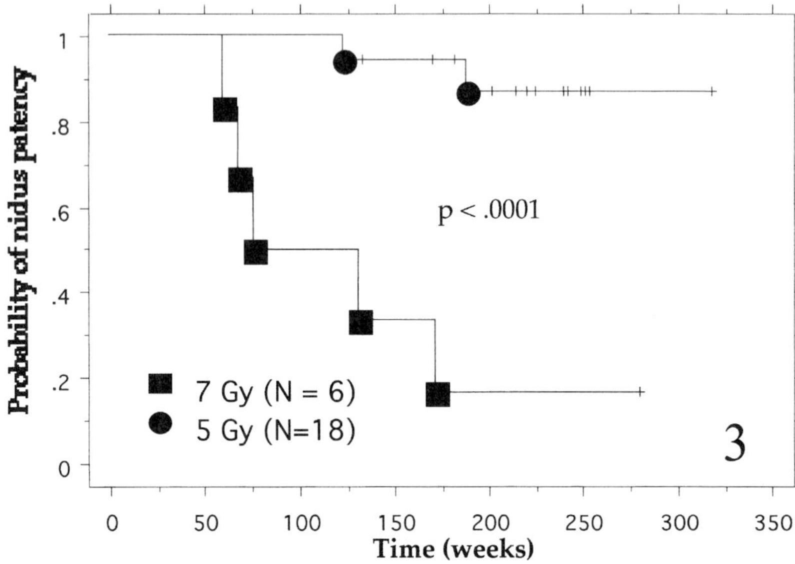

Figure III. Kaplan Meier plot for probability of nidus patency after hypofractionated stereotactic radiotherapy by treatment group.

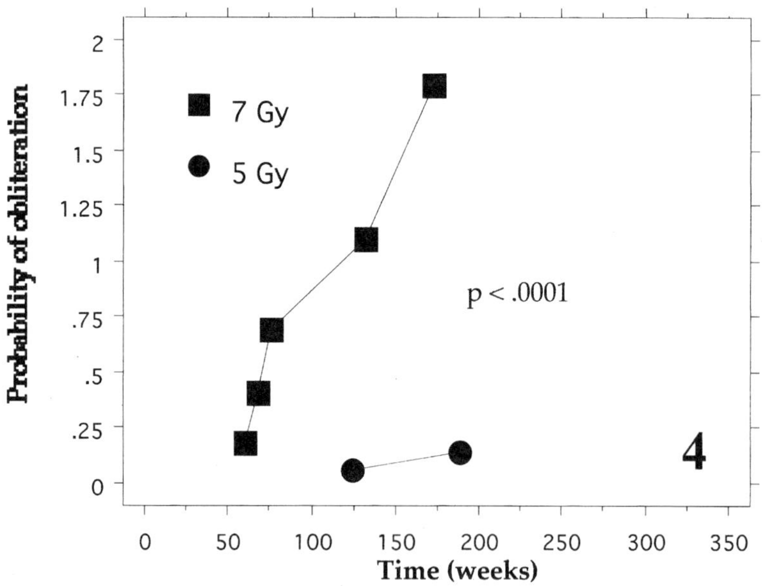

Figure IV. Kaplan-Meier cumulative hazard plot for probability of nidus obliteration.

With regard to lessons learned from RTOG 90–05, any interpretations regarding therapeutic efficacy when comparing single-fraction techniques between Gamma Knife and LINAC techniques for malignant tumors remain moot given the disparate patient groups in this study (see comments by Buatti et al[14]). We have seen no therapeutic differences in a subsequent RTOG trial involving patients with brain metastases when comparing these units (RTOG 95-08, unpublished observations).

In conclusion, theoretical considerations such as the linear-quadratic formula do not provide guidelines of dose equivalence upon which to judge what treatment might yield the highest therapeutic ratio for lesions involving or near the special sensory cranial nerves. In addition, general radiobiological principles that favor single-fraction radiosurgery for small AVMs may not necessarily apply to large AVMs. Observations regarding single-fraction techniques stratified by unit as they apply to early-responding tissues will require further experience, and ideally, prospectively designed comparisons, before any assertions of therapeutic advantage can be made.

References

1. Parsons JT, Bova FJ, Fitzgerald CR, et al: Radiation optic neuropathy after megavoltage external-beam irradiation: analysis of time-dose factors. Int J Radiat Oncol Biol Phys 1994;30:755–763.
2. Tishler RB, Loeffler JS, Lunsford LD, et al: Tolerance of cranial nerves of the cavernous sinus to radiosurgery. Int J Radiat Oncol Biol Phys 1993;27:215–221.
3. Morita A, Coffey RJ, Foote RL, et al: Risk of injury to cranial nerves after gamma knife radiosurgery for skull base meningiomas: experience in 88 patients. J Neurosurg 1999;90:42–49.
4. Andrews D, Suarez O, Goldman H, et al: Stereotactic radiosurgery and fractionated stereotactic radiotherapy for the treatment of acoustic schwannomas: comparative observations in 125 patients treated at one institution. Int J Radiat Oncol Biol Phys 2001;50:1265–1278.
5. Shirato H, Sakamoto T, Sawamura Y, et al: Comparison between observation policy and fractionated stereotactic radiotherapy (SRT) as an initial management for vestibular schwannoma. Int J Radiat Oncol Biol Phys 1999;44: 545–550.
6. Flickinger JC, Pollock BE, Kondziolka D, et al: A dose-response analysis of arteriovenous malformation obliteration after radiosurgery. Int J Radiat Oncol Biol Phys 1996;36:873–879.
7. Engenhart R, Wowra B, Debus J, et al: The role of high-dose, single-fraction irradiation in small and large intracranial arteriovenous malformations. Int J Radiat Oncol Biol Phys 1994;30:521–529.
8. Friedman WA, Bova FJ, Mendenhall WM: Linear accelerator radiosurgery for arteriovenous malformations: the relationship of size to outcome. J Neurosurg 1995;82:180–189.
9. Miyawaki L, Dowd C, Wara W, et al: Five year results of LINAC radiosurgery for arteriovenous malformations: outcome for large AVMS. Int J Radiat Oncol Biol Phys 1999;44:1089–1096.

10. Pollock BE, Kline RW, Stafford SL, et al: The rationale and technique of staged-volume arteriovenous malformation radiosurgery. Int J Radiat Oncol Biol Phys 2000;48:817–824.
11. Laing RW, Childs J, Brada M: Failure of conventionally fractionated radiotherapy to decrease the risk of hemorrhage in inoperable arteriovenous malformations. Neurosurgery 1992;30:872–875.
12. Souhami L, Olivier A, Podgorsak EB, et al: Fractionated stereotactic radiation therapy for intracranial tumors. Cancer 1991;68:2101–2108.
13. Pollock BE: Occlusive hyperemia: a radiosurgical phenomenon? Neurosurgery 2000;47:1178–1182; discussion 1182–1184.
14. Buatti JM, Friedman WA, Meeks SL, et al: RTOG 90–05: the real conclusion. Int J Radiat Oncol Biol Phys 2000;47:269–271.

Chapter 4

Dose Selection and Prediction of Stereotactic Radiosurgery Outcomes

Bengt Karlsson

Introduction

There is a close relationship between dose selection and treatment results following radiosurgery. Increased treatment doses generally correlate with a higher probability of success. However, the risk of radiation-related complications also increases with larger treatment doses. Thus, for each treatment and indication, the aim of dose selection is to treat with the dose resulting in the best risk/benefit ratio for each patient. Consequently, it is important that we to strive to report our experience as precisely and accurately as possible, to assure the reproducibility of results at other centers; accordingly, treatment parameters need to be described as unambiguously as possible. Before discussing alternatives and recommendations for describing the treatment dose, some background information is necessary.

In radiosurgery and radiotherapy, a measurement of the *absorbed dose* is used to describe the amount of radiation delivered to the target volume. In other words, radiation measurements express the amount of absorbed energy per mass unit. Formerly, the absorbed dose was expressed in radiation absorbed dose (rad), but currently, the international standard unit (SI) is the gray (Gy). The gray was chosen to honor the British physicist Louis Harold Gray. One Gy is defined as 1 J/kg, which equals 100 rads. Thus, 1 rad equals 0.01 Gy (1 cGy), which also reflects the former expression of doses in centiGray. It should be understood that the amount of energy delivered during radiosurgery is minimal. For ex-

From Pollock BE (ed). *Contemporary Stereotactic Radiosurgery: Technique and Evaluation.* Armonk, NY, Futura Publishing Company, Inc. ©2002.

ample, 10 mL of water irradiated with a dose of 20 Gy absorbs 0.2 J, which equals 0.05 calories. It takes 41.9 J (10 calories) to increase the temperature in the same amount of water 1°C. Consequently, 10 mL of water exposed to 20 Gy of radiation will increase the temperature by 0.005°. Thus, the biological effect of radiation is not due to the amount of energy absorbed, but to the way the energy is delivered.

If we were to use the definition above in everyday practice, a treatment dose of 13 Gy to a 1-cm^3 vestibular schwannoma would be interpreted as follows (assuming a density of 1 kg/dm^3): the total energy delivered to the tumor is 13 mJ. In most cases, however, this is not correct. Usually, the meaning of a treatment dose of 13 Gy is that the tumor periphery was given 13 Gy. This means that we are describing the treatment dose according to an undefined but established practice. As no definition exists for how the treatment dose should be interpreted, different individuals may have varied interpretations of the same dose plan. This may explain why different centers have varying results despite using the same treatment dose. Thus, there is an obvious need for exact definition of how to report the dose used in a specific treatment.

How should this be done? Exact definition of the treatment dose would be easy if every cell within the target volume absorbed the same dose. If so, the maximum dose would equal the minimum dose, which would equal the average dose. The integral dose would be calculated by multiplying dose with the target volume. However, in radiosurgery it is common that the dose within the target volume varies significantly. Thus, to accurately describe the dose distribution, it would be necessary to describe the dose given to each small volume element, which could be as discrete as one single cell. Obviously, this is not feasible. If we assume that the biological effect is independent of the localization of the tumor cell within the tumor, we can accurately describe the dose distribution within a target volume by using dose-volume histograms (DVHs).

There are two types of commonly used DVHs, differential and cumulative. The following example explains the information that can be extracted from a DVH. Let us assume that we treat a large arteriovenous malformation (AVM) with a lowest dose at the AVM periphery of 15 Gy. Let us further assume that the maximum dose used is 30 Gy. Thus, each small volume element within the AVM nidus will receive a dose between 15 and 30 Gy. The DVH provides detailed information regarding the doses that were received at different volumes (Fig. 1).

Although accurate, the use of DVHs when describing the dose distribution for radiosurgery is not very practical. In practice, we describe the treatment dose with one number only. Early radiosurgical procedures typically denoted only the maximum dose. During that time period, this was logical for two reasons: (1) In most procedures, only one isocenter was used. Thus, because the dose profiles were known for different isocenter

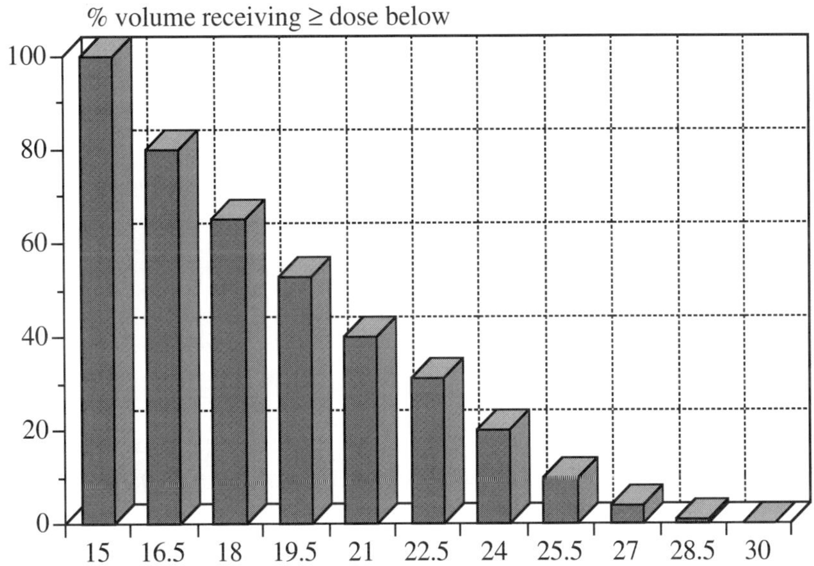

Figure 1. The dose distribution within the arteriovenous malformation nidus volume.

sizes, the DVH could be reconstructed if the maximum dose was specified. (2) The initial indications for radiosurgery were functional. Thus, no target volume could be defined, which also precluded definition of the dose to a target volume. With time, however, treatment of AVMs and tumors was increasingly based on dramatic improvements in neuroimaging–computed tomography (CT), and later, magnetic resonance imaging (MRI). It became possible to define the volume of the pathology to be treated more accurately. In addition, Steiner's early analysis of the Karolinska AVM work clearly showed that it was necessary to irradiate the whole AVM nidus volume to achieve a high chance for obliteration.[1] Consequently, it was realized that not only the maximum dose was of interest, but also the dose to the target periphery. Nonetheless, the old concept of describing the maximum dose could not be abandoned. The result was to describe the dose to the target periphery as a percentage of the maximum dose (e.g., the 50% isodose line), a practice that is still used today.

Target Volume Definition

As discussed above, the unit gray expresses the absorbed dose in a defined volume, and thus "dose" refers to an irradiated target volume. Thus, it is not possible to define a treatment dose without defining the volume receiving that dose. This may seem straightforward, but in reality it is not. The following description from a report on AVM radiosurgery illustrates the difficulty in interpreting prescription doses[2]:

> In 44 cases, an isodose of 70% of the theoretical maximum delivered dose completely covered the targeted volume of the nidus located by stereotactic angiography. In the remaining 56 cases, the 70% isodose did not encompass a part of the targeted volume of the nidus.

How should this information be interpreted? From this information, it is not possible to determine the doses that were given to the periphery of the AVM nidii. Obviously, 44% of the AVMs received 70% or higher of the maximum dose at the nidus periphery, while the other 56% received less than 70% of the maximum dose. Consequently, it is not possible to relate the outcome in the study to the dose to the AVM periphery, the decisive factor for AVM obliteration.[3,4] From the example above, it is clear that the prescription dose in some reports and treatments relates more to the features of the radiation device than to the target volume itself. Reproducibility of results is therefore not possible, as the treatments themselves cannot be replicated exactly in other centers.

Is there a difference between defining the treatment dose to a target volume as compared to defining it to a particular prescription isodose line? For example, does it matter if we define a 13 Gy dose to the 100% coverage of the tumor volume rather than 13 Gy to the 50% isodose line? In the first description, we know that all cells within the target volume receive at least 13 Gy, while in the second, we know that 26 Gy was the maximum dose used. No other information is actually given in the second description, and we have to assume that there is a reasonable conformity between the 50% isodose line and the tumor periphery. This is not always a correct assumption. Thus, there is a need for a consensus in regard to how to describe the treatment dose, and the most logical method is to relate the treatment dose to the target volume.

If one agrees with the preceding discussion, the need to define the target volume before dose planning is obvious. A counter argument is that the definition of the target volume may introduce an error, as it is sometimes difficult to exactly define the target periphery on the available images. While it may be difficult to exactly define the target periphery for some patients, it is not necessarily easier to define the target volume during, rather than before, dose planning. In addition, by defining the target volume before the treatment, one of the possible parameters that can be analyzed is the accuracy of the target definition, a factor that is impossible to analyze if the target volume is not defined. At the Karolinska, it is our standard practice to define the target volume before dose planning, and we strongly recommend that other centers to do the same.

Description of the Treatment Dose

The previous sections have proposed the concept of relating the prescription dose to the defined and treated target volume. Yet, even if there is agreement with this concept, it is not obvious how the treatment dose should be defined. Most commonly, the dose to the target periphery is reported. For instance, Kondziolka et al stated that". . . and the median radiosurgical tumor margin dose was 16 Gy (range 12–20 Gy); in most patients the 50% isodose line was selected".[5] In this study, the lowest dose to the tumor margin was 12 Gy. This could be interpreted in several different ways: that the mean dose to the tumor margin was 12 Gy; that all tumor cells at the periphery received 12 Gy, or in other words, that the tumor periphery had a 100% perfect match with the 50% isodose line, the most commonly used prescription isodose line; that no tumor cells received a dose lower than 12 Gy; or, finally, that 90% of the tumor cells received at least 12 Gy. Again, there is insufficient information to determine the exact dose that was given, and thus, it is not possible to reproduce the treatments and the results of this study at other centers. To further illustrate this problem, a dose plan for a patient having radiosurgery for a brain metastasis is shown in Figure 2. The isodose lines cover 100%, 95%, and 90% of the target volume, representing a periphery dose of 17.2, 19.9, and 21.5 Gy, respectively. Which is the correct way to describe the treatment? Actually, all of the isodose lines can be used to describe the treatment, and it is likely that different centers would consider different isodose lines to be accurate descriptions.

This underscores the need for a standardized, well-defined way to report treatment doses. In a retrospective AVM study at the Karolinska, one of the aims was to define the dose to the AVM nidus periphery.[6] We found that the estimated dose to the AVM periphery for reasonably conformal dose plans corresponded fairly well to the isodose line that covered around 90% of the target volume. We have therefore established as routine the definition of the prescription dose as the dose that covers at least 90% of the target volume. In the future, it would be valuable to define the isodose lines that cover 90%, 95%, and 100% of the target volume, and thus report three doses for each treatment instead of one. A suggestion would be to use D_{min90} to describe 90% coverage, D_{min95} to describe 95% coverage, and D_{min100} to describe 100% coverage. Future studies will show if these three numbers are effective in describing a dose plan, or if outcomes more strongly relate to one than to the others.

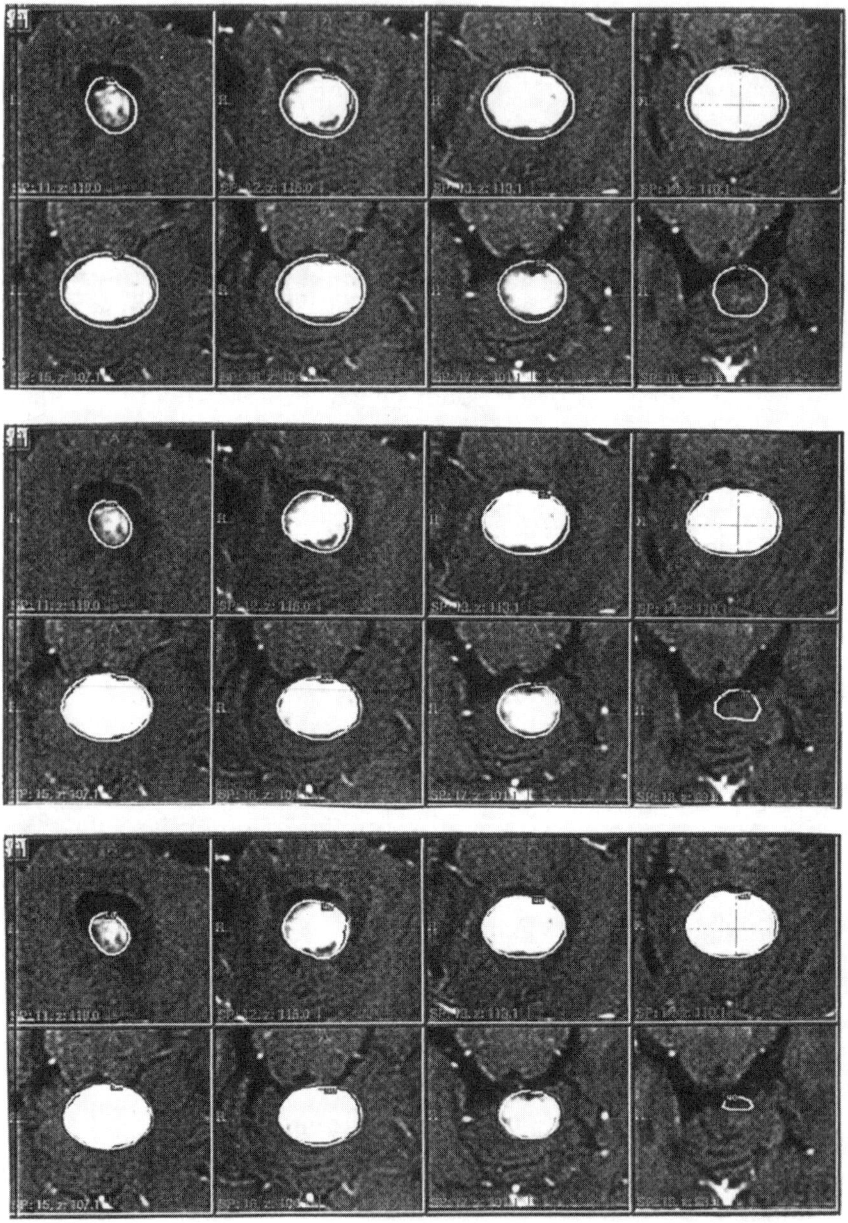

Figure 2. Dose plans from a brain metastasis treated with radiosurgery. (**Top**) The 32% isodose line covers 100% of the target volume, resulting in a conformity factor of 7.8/5.2 = 1.50. (**Middle**) The 37% isodose line covers 95% of the target volume with a conformity factor of 6.1/5.0 = 1.22. (**Bottom**) The 40% isodose line covers 90% of the target volume with a conformity factor of 5.3/4.7 = 1.13. Note that, although the dose plans are identical, the conformity factor varies with the coverage of the target volume.

What is a Good Dose Plan?

The recommendations above allow for objective reporting of the treatment dose for each radiosurgical procedure. A good dose plan is thought to be one that minimizes radiation to the surrounding normal tissue while still providing a sufficient dose to the target volume. This is achieved with a steep dose fall-off at the target periphery and a conformal dose plan. However, there are other factors that may be beneficial for a favorable treatment outcome. One strategy is to deliver the highest amount of energy as possible to the target volume without adding dose to the surrounding normal tissue; the rationale is that the tumor cells in the center may be less oxygenated and therefore more resistant to radiation. Conversely, if there is a sufficient dose of radiation and the risk of complications is related to the integral dose, then a homogenous dose to the target volume is recommended.

Unfortunately, the data needed to determine the optimal dose is lacking, except perhaps for the treatment of AVMs. Until reliable data is available, it is reasonable to aim for providong a sufficient dose to the target volume while minimizing the dose to the surrounding normal tissue. It can be shown that the most crucial factor in minimizing the dose outside the target volume is a high conformity. This means that the treatment isodose should fit as closely as possible to the target volume periphery in every dose plan, which usually can be achieved by using numerous small isocenters rather than a few large ones. Dose conformity can be measured objectively by dividing the volume within the prescription isodose line target by the target volume. Thus, for the brain metastasis in Figure 2, the conformity factors are 1.5 for 100%, 1.22 for 95%, and 1.13 for 90% coverage of the target volume.

Another important factor is to have as steep a dose fall-off at the target periphery as possible. For one isocenter, the steepest dose fall-off is around the 70% isodose line; however, for dose plans with multiple isocenters, the steepness of the dose fall-off is not directly related to the percentage of the isodose line, but instead varies from dose plan to dose plan. As a result, it is not necessarily better to use the 60% isodose line rather than the 40% isodose line when treating a lesion, especially for highly conformal dose plans. A general recommendation is to have conformity as the primary goal of dose planning, and to use the isodose line offering the best fit, independent of the number. It should also be noted that by using DVHs for the target volume and the matrix in which the dose is calculated, the amount of radiation delivered to the tissue outside the target volume can be calculated. This feature is especially important for dose planning around critical structures such as the optic nerves or chiasm.

Dose Selection for Arteriovenous Malformation Radiosurgery

AVM Obliteration

There is significant subjectivity involved in defining the volume of an AVM nidus, especially if the malformation has been embolized previously. Initially, only biplanar stereotactic angiograms were used to define the AVM nidus, but currently, source images from magnetic resonance angiography (MRA) as well as data from CT and MRI are used to delineate the actual AVM volume. The data provided in this section from the Karolinska research is derived from a retrospective analysis performed by the author on AVM cases that have been treated at the Karolinska Hospital in Stockholm, Sweden and at the University of Virginia, Charlottesville, VA, USA.

The periphery doses given are the doses estimated to cover 90 to 100% of the target volume, and the AVM nidus volume is defined as the volume within the best fit isodose line.[4] A complication is defined as an event in which new, or aggravating old clinical symptoms, transient or permanent, appear together with evidence of radiation-induced edema or radionecrosis on neuroimaging. Finally, a hemorrhage is defined as an event with immediate evidence of elevated intracranial symptoms and/or neurological deficits that appear together with evidence of a fresh intracranial hemorrhage on neuroimaging or lumbar puncture.

A successful radiosurgical treatment of an AVM will result in a total obliteration of the AVM nidus without causing undue effects of the radiation, and without occurrence of intracranial hemorrhage in the latency period between the treatment and its final result. To achieve this, it is necessary to define the different parameters related to the chance of cure and the risk of complications. In addition, the dose plan must be designed to maximize the relation between the probability of obliteration and the risk of complications.

Several factors are thought to correlate with the probability of total AVM obliteration following radiosurgery, including the dose to the AVM periphery,[3,4,6,7] the AVM size,[8,9] and the age of the patient.[8,10] No study has clearly related the maximum dose and the incidence of AVM obliteration. Actually, the latest studies with the largest patient data bases have concluded that the only proven factor related to the probability of AVM obliteration is the dose to the AVM periphery.[3,4] Figure 3 shows the relation between the periphery dose and incidence of AVM obliteration in these two studies. In the author's opinion, the curves should be interpreted as follows: there is a limit around 30 Gy or above at which the chance for obliteration no longer increases. Better results with even higher doses, shown by the logarithmic curve below, may be due to a larger volume receiving 25 to 30 Gy, compensating for potential errors in outlining the AVM nidus.

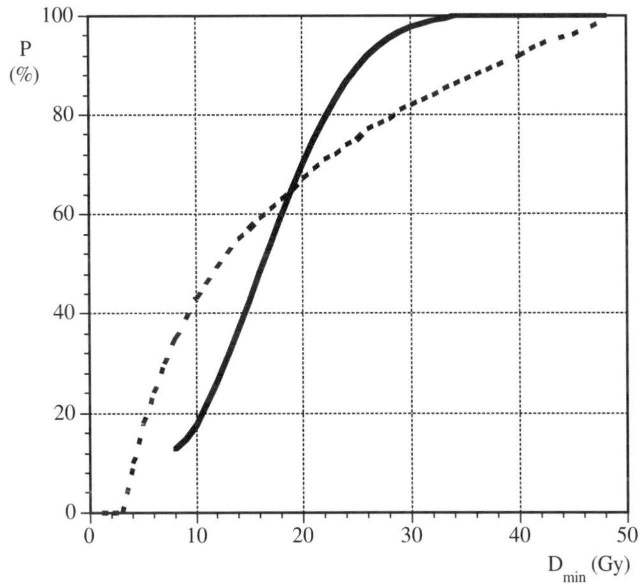

Figure 3. The relation between the periphery dose and incidence of arteriovenous malformation (AVM) obliteration in the studies of Flickinger[11] and Karlsson et al.[6] Note that the curves are similar throughout the dose range typically prescribed to the AVM periphery in actual treatments.

The obliteration rate (x) can be expressed as:

$$f(x) = 35.68 * \ln(x) - 39.66 \quad (1)$$

where $x = D_{min90}$.

Another finding, which may be of importance when interpreting treatment results, is the observation of the linear relation between the average dose to the AVM nidus and the time between treatment and complete AVM obliteration.[6] Thus, the higher the dose the more rapid the obliteration process. Accordingly, when treating larger malformations and using lower radiation doses, a longer time between the treatment and cure must be accepted.

In conclusion, the single most important factor relating to total obliteration is the dose to the AVM nidus periphery. Based on the available data, a dose of 25 to 30 Gy to the AVM periphery should be given whenever possible to maximize the probability of total obliteration.

AVM Risk Management

The management of risk following AVM radiosurgery involves two potentialities: the risk of a radiation-related complication, which hereafter will be denoted as radionecrosis, and the risk of hemorrhage in the latency period between the treatment and obliteration. Two types of radionecrosis are possible, depending on the affected tissue. One is caused by a general reaction in the brain parenchyma surrounding the AVM. The other relates to injury of some radiation-sensitive structure (e.g., cranial nerves). This section will address the first type only.

The mechanism behind radiation-related complications observed following AVM radiosurgery is complex and depends on multiple factors. However, for the development of a risk estimation model, a hypothesis is necessary regarding the relevant part of the irradiated volume for potential complications. Three possibilities can be considered. First, all of the irradiated volume, including that of the AVM, is of importance for the genesis of complications (hypothesis A). Second, only the irradiated volume outside the AVM is of relevance in this context (hypothesis B). Third, all of the volume outside the AVM plus a fraction of the AVM volume (representing normal brain tissue within the AVM volume) is of relevance (hypothesis C).

The first published model by Flickinger predicted the risk of complications following radiosurgery without having access to solid clinical data.[11] In this landmark paper, hypothesis B was used and it was assumed that the target volume was equal to the volume within the 70% isodose line. The first study that showed a dose-volume relationship following radiosurgery was presented by the present author in 1989, at a meeting entitled "Radiosurgery: A Neurosurgical Approach to Intracranial Lesions," in Charlottesville, VA, USA. However, the first risk estimation analysis based on a large radiosurgical AVM patient group was not published until 1996.[12] In this analysis, we used hypothesis A and clearly showed that the incidence of radionecrosis was directly correlated to the average dose in the 20-cm^3 volume which received the most radiation. In our AVM patient group, the average dose given to this 20-cm^3 volume was 12 Gy. Thus, we could have chosen to relate the incidence of complications to the volume receiving greater than or equal to 12 Gy. The later work of Flickinger et al supported our findings.[13]

It was initially considered that a risk estimation model could be developed that also is accurate and reliable when treating other diagnoses, but this idea has largely been abandoned.[14] On the contrary, further research concluded that one risk estimation model is not sufficient when predicting the risk for radionecrosis following AVM radiosurgery. Our most recent publication also takes into consideration the AVM location and the absence or presence of a pretreatment hemorrhage and how each relates to the risk of radionecrosis.[15] To summarize, the risk of radionecrosis increases with the amount of radiation delivered to the AVM volume and the surrounding brain tissue. A central AVM location and no history of a prior hemorrhage also increase the risk of radionecrosis. The formulas below can be used to calculate the risk of radionecrosis for individual patients:

For centrally located AVMs:	$f(y) = 1.446 * \exp(0.1114*y)$	(2)
For peripheral AVMs without hemorrhage:	$f(y) = 1.0854 * \exp(0.1076*y)$	(3)
For peripheral AMVs with hemorrhage:	$f(y) = 0.4032*y + -2.871$	(4)

where y = the average dose given to the 20-cm^3 volume which received the most radiation.

A study by Pollock et al related the clinical outcomes after AVM radiosurgery both to obliteration rate and radionecrosis.[16] In this report, several AVM factors including volume, the number of draining veins, younger patient age, and hemispheric AVM location related to excellent patient outcomes. Conversely, previous embolization was a negative predictor for outcomes. However, the impact of the dose to the AVM was not analyzed in this study.

The issue of whether the risk of hemorrhage is different in the latency time period after radiosurgery compared with the natural history of untreated AVMs is more complex. This can partly be ascribed to different opinions regarding the natural course of AVM. Varying reports have stated the annual risk of rupture of an untreated AVM as ranging from 1 to 33%.[17,18] It is therefore not surprising that authors have concluded that the risk of post-treatment hemorrhage is increased,[19,20] unchanged,[21,22] or decreased as compared with untreated AVMs.[23,24] However, if the question is rephrased from "Does radiosurgery change the risk of hemorrhage in the latency period?" to "How high is the risk of hemorrhage in the latency period?" a consensus may be reached without the need to agree on the natural course of the disease. We therefore related the incidence of hemorrhage in the latency period to a number of AVM and treatment parameters.[23] It was concluded that the risk of hemorrhage increased with increasing patient age and AVM volume, and decreased with higher radiation doses to the AVM. A subsequent effort was made to quantify the risk of hemorrhage within the first 2 years after radiosurgery,[25] resulting in the following formula:

$$P(\%) = \frac{7.29*\exp(-0.00226*[Dmin]^2)*f(age)}{(1.28-0.204*\ln[v])} \qquad (5)$$

where the AVM volume (in cm^3) $v \geq 1$ and f(age) can be estimated to f(age) = 0.025*age + 0.049. (For further detail, see Karlsson et al.[25])

Therefore, it is currently possible to predict patient outcomes after AVM radiosurgery with reasonable accuracy, if the AVM nidus volume is accurately defined, by using the aforementioned formulas (1) to (5).

Benign Tumors

As discussed in the previous sections on AVM radiosurgery, there are two types of radiation injury; one is expressed as a contrast enhancement at the site of the lesion and/or edema in the surrounding brain tissue, whereas the other is damage to cranial nerves. There is little published data on the dose-volume effects when treating benign tumors. Thus, caution must be exercised in using risk estimation models based on AVM data to determine the risk of complications when treating benign tumors, though in the past this may have been considered accurate.[14] Although radiation-induced edema in the surrounding brain tissue is rarely seen with the doses currently used (12 to 14 Gy) and the volumes (seldom >10 mL) treated, we must not assume that the risk of radiation-induced edema is lower with benign tumors as compared to AVMs. In our early experience, we saw the development of devastating edema and radionecrosis when larger volumes were treated with higher doses. In the author's opinion, the risk of complications is actually much higher when treating meningiomas as compared to treatment of AVMs with the same dose, as supported by an early study of Engenhart et al.[26]

Several reports have reached different conclusions regarding cranial nerve complications. This may be due to the fact that the nerves are often not visible on the stereotactic images, rendering it difficult to estimate the dose that the nerve has actually received. Most would agree that the visual pathways, including the optic tracts, can tolerate a dose less than 8 Gy, even though a dose of 10 Gy had earlier been considered safe. Tischler et al found that 4 of 17 patients (24%), in whom the optic apparatus received a dose greater than 8 Gy, developed a complication; however, none of 35 patients who received a dose less than 8 Gy developed any visual complications.[27] Motor nerves are considered more radioresistant than sensory nerves, although little hard data is available to quantify this statement. With our present treatment strategy, we typically prescribe 12 to 14 Gy to the tumor periphery for patients with meningiomas. Patients rarely develop complications to cranial nerves III, IV, or VI, and it is more common that cranial nerve function improves after radiosurgery. Based on published data, the trigeminal nerve appears to be more radiosensitive than the oculomotor nerves.[27] The author has treated a patient with a brain metastasis compressing the gasserian ganglion, who developed devastating trigeminal pain 8 hours after the treatment, which later improved but never disappeared.

The most common complication of treating acoustic neuromas (vestibular schwannomas) with radiosurgery is the development of facial weakness or numbness. In the first report by Norén et al in 1983,[28] facial weakness was observed in 5 of 13 patients (39%) and trigeminal dysfunction in 2 patients (15%). In the initial Pittsburgh series, an unacceptably high incidence of cranial nerve deficits occurred with 20 Gy as the periphery dose; the investigators consequently lowered the dose to the periphery to 16 to 18 Gy.[29] In this study, the actuarial rate of preserved nerve function was only 60 to 70%. Another study based on this early experience found no relation between dose (>17 Gy vs. ≤17 Gy) and incidence of facial or trigeminal neuropathies, which was instead related to the tumor size.[30] This led to the later hypothesis that the risk of facial neuropathy is nerve length-dependent.[31] A more recent study from this group, however, found that the dose to the tumor periphery was related to the incidence of neuropathy.[32] None of 22 patients treated with a periphery dose of less than or equal to 13 Gy developed a neuropathy. For hearing preservation, their experience was similar, with a strong relation to dose but also to tumor size, with an actuarial rate of hearing preservation of 55%.

Consistent with the aforementioned data, the dose used to treat acoustic neuromas has decreased with time. Regarding the effect of decreased doses on the tumor control rate, the Pittsburgh group reported an 89% tumor control rate in 1993,[30] a 91% tumor control rate in 1996,[33] and an increase to 98% in 1998.[5] The current treatment strategy at the Karolinska Hospital is to treat acoustic neuromas with a prescription dose of 13 Gy. The ongoing study at this institution shows a tumor control rate of 85%, based on Kaplan-Meier analysis. Among the 90 most recently treated patients, we have observed one transient facial weakness, one transient facial spasm, and one transient facial numbness. When comparing our experience with the published reports, it seems that we use slightly lower doses, resulting in a small decrease in tumor control and a lower incidence of cranial neuropathies.

For meningiomas, the results are more difficult to interpret because tumor control and tumor cure are not necessarily the same. For example, even following radical tumor removal (Simpson Grade I), the tumor may recur.[34] In addition, the tumor may invade the bone and other surrounding structure, a feature not seen in acoustic neuromas. This makes tumor volume definition more difficult, and the risk of leaving tumor cells outside the target volume higher. Furthermore, fewer reports regarding treatment results are available as compared to published results for acoustic neuromas. Thus, some of the following information is based on the author's personal experience only.

At the Thai Neurosurgical Society meeting in Thailand in 1994, we reported the long-term results of 38 meningiomas, with a follow-up period of more than 10 years. A treatment success was defined as a tumor decrease after 5 years or more, or an unchanged tumor size after 10 years or more. Overall, the treatment success rate was 80%. In recent papers with shorter follow-up periods, tumor control rates of 89 to 100% have been reported.[35–39] It is also interesting to note that two studies of low-dose radiosurgery had similar results.[40,41] Considering that we have seen tumor growth many years after radiosurgery, and that long-term recurrences can be seen even after complete microsurgical tumor removal, it must be expected that the long-term tumor control rates will decrease, most likely to 80 to 90%. Therefore, short-term tumor control rates of 90 to 100% appear possible even with low-dose radiosurgery. In addition, because of the devastating complications that we have experienced with higher prescription doses, our present treatment strategy at the Karolinska is to use a prescription dose of 12 to 15 Gy for these patients.

Malignant Tumors

The analysis of the optimal dose for treating malignant tumors is even more complex than for benign tumors. This complexity relates to the infiltrative nature of gliomas, the additive effect of radiotherapy and/or chemotherapy, difficulties in differentiating between radionecrosis and tumor recurrence, and the use of patient survival as an outcome parameter. For brain metastases, patient survival is more dependent on tumor control elsewhere in the body than on local control following radiosurgery.[42] Most patients with malignant tumors do not survive long enough for radionecrosis to develop, which must also be taken into consideration. Treatment for malignant tumors should be more aggressive than for benign tumors, and thus higher doses may be necessary to control malignant tumors as compared to benign neoplasms.

The published reports provide varying information regarding the doses needed to achieve tumor control, undoubtedly related to different definitions of the treatment dose at different centers. Another factor is the impact that fractionated radiotherapy will have on both tumor control and radiation injury. When radiotherapy is added, the cumulative dose to the tumor will be higher. The dose recommendation for brain metastases will therefore be based on our experience at the Karolinska, where we do not add radiotherapy after the radiosurgical treatment; data for gliomas will be derived from the literature, due to our lack of experience.

The present treatment strategy at the Karolinska for brain metastases is a prescription dose of 20 to 25 Gy to cover 90 to 95% of the target volume. Some preliminary data is available from the evaluation of a patient group currently under study. The local cure rate is around 90% and approximately 5% of tumors have increased in size; in 5% of the patients, the survival time is too short to allow any meaningful follow-up examinations to be performed. The increased tumor size, based on positron emission tomography, appears to be due to radionecrosis in two-thirds of the cases, and to tumor recurrence in one-third. However, it must be kept in mind that most patients do not survive long enough to actually develop radionecrosis. In summary, with a prescription dose of 20 to 25 Gy, the incidence of complications is less than 5% and the tumor control rate is approximatley 90%.

For primary tumors, radiosurgery can be considered as an adjunct to other treatments. Some centers report that a radiosurgical boost provides survival benefit to properly selected patients. Loeffler et al reported significantly longer survival times when a radiosurgical boost with a marginal dose of 10 to 20 Gy was given.[43] Other opinions are also represented in the literature. For example, Shenouda et al did not find any advantage, but they did find more late complications, with the addition of a 20-Gy radiosurgical boost for patients with high-grade gliomas.[44] The author's opinion is that a well-conducted, randomized prospective study is needed before the role of radiosurgery can be defined for this indication, primarily because patient selection is so strongly related to the expected survival time.

References

1. Steiner L: Radiosurgery in cerebral arteriovenous malformations. In Fein JF (ed): Cerebrovascular Surgery. New York, Springer-Verlag, 1984, pp 1161–1215.
2. Touboul E, Al Halabi A, Buffat L, et al: Single-fraction stereotactic radiotherapy: a dose-response analysis of arteriovenous malformation obliteration. Int J Radiat Oncol Biol Phys 1998;41:855–861.
3. Flickinger JC, Pollock BE, Kondziolka D, Lunsford LD: A dose-response analysis of arteriovenous malformation obliteration after radiosurgery. Int J Radiat Oncol Biol Phys 1996;36:873–879.
4. Karlsson B, Lax I, Söderman M: Can the probability for obliteration after radiosurgery for arteriovenous malformations be accurately predicted? Int J Radiat Oncol Biol Phys 1999;43:313–319.
5. Kondziolka D, Lunsford LD, McLaughlin M, Flickinger J: Long-term outcomes after radiosurgery for acoustic neuromas. N Engl J Med 1998;339: 1426–1433.
6. Karlsson B, Lindquist C, Steiner L: Prediction of obliteration after Gamma Knife surgery for cerebral arteriovenous malformations. Neurosurgery 1997;40:425–431.
7. Colombo F, Pozza F, Chierego G, et al: Linear accelerator radiosurgery of cerebral arteriovenous malformations: an update. Neurosurgery 1994;34:14–20.
8. Lunsford LD, Kondziolka D, Flickinger JC, et al: Stereotactic radiosurgery for arteriovenous malformations of the brain. J Neurosurg 1991;75:512–524.
9. Schwartz M, Sixel K, Young C, et al: Prediction of obliteration of arteriovenous malformations after radiosurgery: the obliteration prediction index. Can J Neurol Sci 1997;24:106–109.
10. Altschuler EM, Lunsford LD, Coffey RJ, et al: Gamma knife radiosurgery for intracranial arteriovenous malformations in childhood and adolescence. Pediatr Neurosci 1989;15:53–61.
11. Flickinger JC: An integrated logistic formula for prediction of complications from radiosurgery. Int J Radiat Oncol Biol Phys 1989;17:879–885.
12. Lax I, Karlsson B: Prediction of complications in gamma knife radiosurgery of arteriovenous malformation. Acta Oncol 1996;35:49–55.
13. Flickinger JC, Kondziolka D, Pollock B, et al: Complications from arteriovenous malformation radiosurgery: multivariate analysis and risk modeling. Int J Radiat Oncol Biol Phys 1997;38:485–490.

14. Flickinger JC, Lunsford LD, Kondziolka D: Dose prescription and dose-volume effects in radiosurgery. Neurosurg Clin N Am 1992;3:51–59.
15. Karlsson B, Lax I, Söderman M: Factors influencing the risk for complications following Gamma Knife radiosurgery for cerebral arteriovenous malformations. Radiother Oncol 1997;43:275–280.
16. Pollock BE, Flickinger JC, Lunsford LD, et al: Factors associated with successful arteriovenous malformation radiosurgery. Neurosurgery 1998;42: 1239–1244.
17. Itoyama Y, Uemura S, Ushio Y, et al: Natural course of unoperated intracranial arteriovenous malformations: study of 50 cases. J Neurosurg 1989;71: 805–809.
18. Mast H, Young W, Koennecke HC, et al: Risk of spontaneous hemorrhage after diagnosis of cerebral arteriovenous malformation. Lancet 1997;350: 1065–1068.
19. Fabrikant JI, Levy RP, Steinberg GK, et al: Charged-particle radiosurgery for intracranial vascular malformations. Neurosurg Clin N Am 1992;3:99–139.
20. Steinberg GK, Fabrikant JI, Marks MP, et al: Stereotactic heavy-charged-particle Bragg-peak radiation for intracranial arteriovenous malformations. N Engl J Med 1990;323:96–101.
21. Friedman W, Blatt D, Bova F, et al: The risk of hemorrhage after radiosurgery for arteriovenous malformations. J Neurosurg 1996;84:912–919.
22. Pollock BE, Flickinger JC, Lunsford LD, et al: Hemorrhage risk after stereotactic radiosurgery of cerebral arteriovenous malformations. Neurosurgery 1996;38:652–659.
23. Karlsson B, Lindquist C, Steiner L: Effect of Gamma Knife surgery on the risk of rupture prior to AVM obliteration. Min Invas Neurosurg 1996;39:21–27.
24. Levy RP, Fabrikant JI, Frankel KA, et al: Stereotactic heavy-charged-particle Bragg peak radiosurgery for the treatment of intracranial arteriovenous malformations in childhood and adolescence. Neurosurgery 1989;24:841–852.
25. Karlsson B, Lax I, Söderman M: Risk for hemorrhage during the 2–year latency period following gamma knife radiosurgery for arteriovenous malformations. Int J Radiat Oncol Biol Phys 2001;49:1045–1051.
26. Engenhart R, Kimmig BN, Hover KH, et al: Stereotactic single high dose radiation therapy of benign intracranial meningiomas. Int J Radiat Oncol Biol Phys 1990;19:1021–1026.
27. Tischler RB, Loeffler JS, Lunsford LD, et al: Tolerance of cranial nerves of the cavernous sinus to radiosurgery. Int J Rad Oncol Biol Phys 1993;27:215–221.
28. Norén G, Arndt J, Hindmarsh T: Stereotactic radiosurgery in cases of acoustic neurinoma: further experience. Neurosurgery 1983;13:12–22.
29. Flickinger JC, Lunsford LD, Coffey RJ, et al: Radiosurgery of acoustic neurinomas. Cancer 1991;67:345–353.
30. Flickinger JC, Lunsford LD, Linskey M, et al: Gamma Knife radiosurgery for acoustic tumors: multivariant analysis of four years results. Radiother Oncol 1993;27:91–98.
31. Linskey ME, Flickinger JC, Lunsford LD: Cranial nerve length predicts the risk of delayed facial and trigeminal neuropathies after acoustic tumor stereotactic radiosurgery. Int J Radiat Oncol Biol Phys 1993;25:227–333.
32. Flickinger JC, Kondziolka D, Lunsford LD: Dose and diameter relationship for facial, trigeminal and acoustic neuropathies following acoustic neuroma radiosurgery. Radiother Oncol 1996;41:215–219.
33. Flickinger J, Kondziolka D, Pollock B, Lunsford L: Evolution in technique for vestibular schwannoma radiosurgery and effect on outcome. Int J Radiat Oncol Biol Phys 1996;36:275–280.

34. Mathiesen T, Lindquist C, Kihlström L, Karlsson B: Recurrence of cranial base meningiomas. Neurosurgery 1996;39:2–9.
35. Hakim R, Alexander E III, Loeffler J, et al: Results of linear accelerator-based radiosurgery for intracranial meningiomas. Neurosurgery 1998;42:446–453.
36. Muthukumar N, Kondziolka D, Lunsford L, Flickinger J: Stereotactic radiosurgery for tentorial meningiomas. Acta Neurochir 1998;140:315–321.
37. Shafron D, Friedman W, Buatti J, et al: Linac radiosurgery for benign meningiomas. Int J Radiat Oncol Biol Phys 1999;43:321–327.
38. Subach B, Lunsford L, Kondziolka D, et al: Management of petroclival meningiomas by stereotactic radiosurgery. Neurosurgery 1998;42:437–445.
39. Vermeulen S, Young R, Li F, et al: A comparison of single fraction radiosurgery tumor control and toxicity in the treatment of basal and nonbasal meningiomas. Stereotact Funct Neurosurg 1998;72:60–66.
40. Iwai Y, Yamanakn K, Yasui T, et al: Gamma knife surgery for skull base meningiomas: the effectiveness of low-dose treatment. Surg Neurol 1999; 52:40–45.
41. Nakaya K, Hayashi M, Atsuchi S, et al: Low-dose radiosurgery for meningiomas. Stereotact Funct Neurosurg 1999;72:67–72.
42. Huang CF, Kondziolka D, Flickinger JC, Lunsford LD: Stereotactic radiosurgery for brainstem metastases. J Neurosurg 1999;91:563–568.
43. Loeffler J, Alexander E III, Shea M, et al: Radiosurgery as part of the initial mangement of patients with malignant gliomas. J Clin Oncol 1992;10: 1379–1385.
44. Shenouda G, Souhami L, Podgorsak E, et al: Radiosurgery and accelerated radiotherapy for patients with glioblastoma. Can J Neurol Sci 1997;24:110–115.

Comment

Chapter 4

David M.C. Forster

The advent of digital subtraction angiography, MRI, and image fusion combined with more sophisticated dose planning has led to improved outcomes with reduced side effects in the radiosurgery of AVMs as well as of tumors. Nevertheless, the rate of thrombo-obliteration, which correlates well with the radiation delivered to the nidus, will be lower if, in the interests of safety, there is any reduction in the recommended marginal dose of 25 Gy. The author describes well what is known about the relationship between the dose, the AVM volume, and the eloquence of the location in light of the patient's age and expectations.

The task of writing a chapter on radiation dose selection would have been simpler if it was only necessary to determine the dose of radiation to obtain a required effect. However, as is admirably argued, even a universally accepted definition of radiation dose cannot be assumed; difficulties exist first in establishing and then in delineating the targets, as well as in finding satisfactory ways to express how tightly the distribution of dose delivered conforms to the targets chosen. Even knowing the dose to obtain the desired pathological effect in a particular patient is not sufficient–the patient will want to know not only the likely clinical outcome, but also the size of the risk of transient or permanent ill effects, as well as the possible nature and severity of those effects.

No matter how large the available data bank or the duration of follow-up, there will be no certainty of the therapeutic effect or the risk of complications in an individual patient until there is a clearer understanding of the mechanisms by which the radiation exerts its effect on the pathological tissues. In addition, the risk may be affected by the actual functions in the individual patient of the adjacent brain from which the ill effects may be derived. The latter may be easier to assess when the vulnerable structure is a lower cranial nerve conveying hearing, sensation, or facial movement, as in the treatment of a vestibular neuroma, than with an AVM in the depths of a parietal lobe. Although it is convenient to attribute certain functions to particular anatomical areas of the brain, there remains considerable individual variation and uncertainty. In the future, improved functional mapping of the brain may help reduce these difficulties.

Unfortunately, as the author points out, there is a shortfall in many areas of data recording and in the nature of the information obtained. Often, the length of follow-up is inadequate for a condition whose threat may remain dormant for long periods. Furthermore, the process by which radiation leads to thrombo-obliteration of some small arterial vessels, reduction of neuronal function, nerve conduction, or brain edema, and ultimately to recovery, permanent dysfunction, or necrosis is far from completely understood. The same dose of radiation delivered accurately and conformally to two apparently similar AVMs can lead to complete obliteration in one and to no visible response in the other. While analysis of large series can offer a statistically valid incidence of obliteration with different doses and target volumes, it cannot answer the need for outcome prediction in a particular individual. The absence of a good animal model for cerebral AVM makes it difficult to increase understanding of the mechanisms of radiation-induced obliteration. As with tumors, there is much variation and the responses of vessels in vitro are not necessarily representative of human vessel responses in vivo.

Few statements about cerebral AVMs are supported by strong evidence and can be made without fear of contradiction. AVMs do not appear to be congenital in the sense of being fully developed at birth, although the defect necessary for their development may already be present.[1] The development of new AVMs has seldom been reported in children[2–5] and has been seen even more rarely in adults.[6,7]

In addition, the factors that lead an AVM to rupture and bleed are also not well understood. An AVM nidus is a dynamic lesion that is associated with progressive vessel changes, some of which can be mimicked in experimental vascular models.[8] Although it is not thought to grow, there may be some angiogenesis and increases in volume related to changes in blood flow. In endothelial cells grown in tissue culture there appears to be defective growth regulation.[9] AVMs can also spontaneously regress or disappear, possibly by spontaneous thrombosis.[5,9,10]

Reports concerning hemorrhage risk factors are also contradictory. Most find a higher risk with larger AVMs[11] (contradiction[12]), during pregnancy[13–16] (contradiction[17]), after previous hemorrhage[13,18,19] (contradiction[15,20]), with increasing age,[15] a central location,[15,21–23] and in the presence of venous stasis.[22]

The therapeutic goal in the treatment of AVM, unlike the total or partial inhibition of the neoplastic tendency in a tumor, is to prevent future hemorrhage, which may or may not have happened in the past and which may or may not occur again—in some ways like vaccination against a possible infection. Thus, there cannot be too much information gleaned about the risks of bleeding both before and after irradiation, the significant risk factors, or the outcomes of the alternative therapies of surgical excision or endovascular occlusion.

The clinician must offer advice based on the evidence available at the time and cannot expect patients to await the outcome of some future, more scientifically valid, trial. In addition, such trials are difficult to set up and execute and slow to mature, even if the necessary ethical approval can be obtained. Despite these difficulties, there is an overwhelming need for the continued careful accumulation of data on obliteration rates, incidence of complications, and the adoption of internationally recognized ways of recording target volumes, radiation doses actually delivered, and the degree of conformality. In addition, improvement is necessary in the existing predictive models. The Gamma Knife, with its common delivery system and standardized dose planning, lends itself to such uniform data collection, and LINAC or other system users should also strive as much as possible to adopt a common nomenclature and meet similar standards.

References

1. Sonstein WJ, Kader A, Michelson WJ, et al: Expression of vascular endothelial growth factor in pediatric and adult arteriovenous malformations: an immunocytochemical study. J Neurosurg 1996;85:838–845.
2. Kader A, Goodrich JT, Sonstein WJ, et al: Recurrent cerebral arteriovenous malformations after negative postoperative angiograms. J Neurosurg 1996; 85:14–18.
3. Lax I, Karlsson B: Prediction of complications in gamma knife radiosurgery of malformations. Acta Oncol 1996;35:49–55.
4. Lindqvist M, Karlsson B, Guo WY,et al: Angiographic long-term follow-up data for arteriovenous malformations previously proven to be obliterated after gamma knife radiosurgery. Neurosurgery 2000;46:803–810.
5. Yasargil M: Enlargement, Growth and Regrowth of AVMs. Microneurosurgery. Stuttgart, Georg Thieme Verlag, (IIIA), 1987, pp 138–160.
6. Gabriel EM, Sampson JH, Wilkins RH, et al: Recurrence of cerebral arteriovenous malformation after surgical excision. J Neurosurg 1996;84:879–882.
7. Hino A, Fujimoto M, Iwamoto Y, et al: An adult case of recurrent arteriovenous malformation after "complete" surgical excision: a case report. Surg Neurol 1999;52:156–159.
8. Greenhill N, Stehbens WE: Scanning electron microscopic investigation of the afferent arteries of experimental femoral arteriovenous fistulae in rabbits. Pathology 1987;19:22–27.
9. Waltimo O: The change in size of intracranial arteriovenous malformations. J Neurol Sci 1973;19:511–520.
10. Wautier MP, Boval B, Chappey O, et al: Cultured endothelial cells from human arteriovenous malformations have defective growth regulation. Blood 1999;154:2020–2028.
11. Pollock BE, Flickinger JC, Lunsford LD, et al: Factors that predict the bleeding risk of cerebral arteriovenous malformations. Stroke 1996:27:1–6.
12. Spetzler RF, Hargraves RW, McCormick PW, et al: Relationship of perfusion pressure and size to risk of hemorrhage from arteriovenous malformations. J Neurosurg 1992;76:918–923.
13. Crawford P, West CR, Chardwick DW, Shaw MD: Arteriovenous malformations of the brain: natural history in unoperated patients. J Neurol Neurosurg Psychiatry 1986;49:1–10.
14. Forster DMC, Kunkler IH, Hartland P, et al: Risk of cerebral bleeding from arteriovenous malformations in pregnancy. Ster Func Neurosurg 1993;61 (suppl 1):20–22.
15. Karlsson B, Lindquist C, Johansson A, Steiner L: Annual risk for the first hemorrhage from untreated cerebral arteriovenous malformations. Min Invas Neurosurg 1997;40:40–46.

16. Robinson JH, Hall CS, Sedzimir CB, et al: Arteriovenous malformations, aneurysms, and pregnancy. J Neurosurg 1974;41:63–70.
17. Horton JC, Chambers WA, Lyons SL, et al: Pregnancy and the risk of hemorrhage from cerebral arteriovenous malformations. Neurosurgery 1990;27: 867–871.
18. Forster DMC, Steiner L, Hakanson S, et al: Arteriovenous malformations of the brain: a long term clinical study. J Neurosurg 1972;37:562–570.
19. Mast H, Young WL, Koennecke HC, et al: Risk of spontaneous haemorrhage after diagnosis of cerebral arteriovenous malformation. Lancet 1997;350: 1065–1068.
20. Ondra SL, Troupp H, George ED, Schwab K: The natural history of symptomatic arteriovenous malformations of the brain. J Neurosurg 1990;73: 387–391.
21. Duong DH, Young WL, Vang MC, et al: Feeding artery pressure and venous drainage pattern are primary determinants of hemorrhage from cerebral arteriovenous malformations. Stroke 1998;29:1167–1176.
22. Mansmann U, Meisel J, Brock M, et al: Factors associated with intracranial hemorrhage in cases of cerebral arteriovenous malformation. Neurosurgery 2000;4:272–279.
23. Nataf F, Meder JF, Roux FX, et al: Angioarchitecture associated with hemorrhage in cerebral arteriovenous malformations: a prognostic statistical model. Neuroradiology 1997;39:52–58.

Chapter 5

Stereotactic Radiosurgery for Arteriovenous Malformations

Masaaki Yamamoto

Introduction

Cerebral arteriovenous malformations (AVMs) are generally understood to be a congenital maldevelopment of blood vessels with one or more primitive direct communications between arteries and veins. Although the incidence of AVMs is low (estimated at 0.14% per year),[1] AVMs constitute a very important neurosurgical indication as these lesions are benign but carry significant risk to a patient over a lifetime. While some AVMs are diagnosed in patients with headaches or seizures, the majority of AVMs are determined only after the patient has sustained an intracranial hemorrhage (ICH). According to analyses of the natural history of untreated AVMs by Graf et al[2] and Ondra et al,[3] the annual incidence of bleeding ranged from 2 to 4%, with significant morbidity and mortality rates. Although Hartmann et al recently reported that the morbidity associated with hemorrhage from cerebral AVMs is lower than currently thought, their findings appear unrealistic to most experienced cerebrovascular neurosurgeons.[4] It has also been reported that the annual rate of rebleeding is increased for ruptured AVMs during the first post-ictal year compared to subsequent years.[5] Kondziolka et al reported that a 35-year-old patient diagnosed with an AVM has between a 58 and 83% chance of sustaining an ICH within his or her lifetime.[6] Therefore, the goal of AVM management is to eliminate the risk of future bleeding with minimal morbidity.

Three treatment modalities (microsurgery, embolization, and radiosurgery) are available for patients with AVMs. Advances in neuroimaging and microsurgical techniques permits experienced cerebrovascular neu-

From Pollock BE (ed). *Contemporary Stereotactic Radiosurgery: Technique and Evaluation.* Armonk, NY, Futura Publishing Company, Inc. ©2002.

rosurgeons to resect many AVMs completely with a low morbidity rate. When possible, this strategy is unquestionably ideal. Nevertheless, some AVMs cannot be resected safely even by the most experienced neurosurgeon because of their location in or near a critical brain structure, or because the patient has contraindications for general anesthesia. The role of embolization alone is considered to be relatively small in the management of AVM patients because only 10 to 20% of AVMs are completely curable using this technique.[7,8] In contrast, radiosurgery is widely accepted as an alternative to microsurgery in the treatment of AVMs, particularly, in deep brain locations (brainstem, basal ganglia, or thalamus) or critical lobar areas (sensorimotor, speech, or visual cortex). It is clear that complete nidus obliteration, which eliminates the risk of hemorrhage, can be achieved in 80 to 90% of cases within several years for small AVMs (<2 cm^3) treated with an optimal irradiation dose (>20 Gy) at the nidus margin.[9–27] For such patients, the risk of irradiation-related complications is low ($<3.0\%$).

The availability of three different treatment modalities renders decision making for individual patients often complex. Jokura and Yoshimoto recommended that all untreated AVM patients be referred to three specialists, a vascular neurosurgeon, an endovascular therapist, and a radiosurgeon.[28] In their facility, the AVM Treatment Board, consisting of experienced neurosurgeons individually specialized in the three modalities, was established with the initial installation of a Gamma Knife (GK). Every AVM patient is referred to the Board and an individual treatment strategy is then designed. Of 86 patients reviewed by the Board during a 1.5-year period after January of 1995, 59 (69%) underwent GK radiosurgery. This illustrates the increasing role that radiosurgery now plays in the management of patients with AVMs. Worldwide, more than 20,000 patients have undergone AVM radiosurgery since the 1960s. It should be emphasized that whatever management strategy is used, the goal should be complete elimination of the AVM. Palliative treatment cannot prevent bleeding and may actually increase the hemorrhage risk when compared with the natural history of untreated AVMs, as recently reported by Miyamoto et al.[29]

History of Arteriovenous Malformation Radiosurgery

The GK was initially designed to perform functional neurosurgical cases by the late Professor Lars Leksell.[30] However, cerebral AVMs quickly became the most common indication for radiosurgery over the next three decades, since the early 1970s.[31] Most notably, after the redesigned second GK gained routine clinical acceptance in 1975 at the Karolinska Hospital, Stockholm, Sweden, Steiner and his colleagues, particularly Lindquist and Karlsson, greatly expanded the role of GK radiosurgery in the treatment of AVMs. As of June 1992, they had treated more than 1600 AVM patients. During this same period, radiosurgery using a particle beam system was also applied for AVM patients. However, this type of system has not been in general use because of management complexity and extremely expensive equipment.[12,13,17,24] Still, installation of the first North American GK at the University of Pittsburgh in 1987 opened a great epoch in GK radiosurgery. Lunsford and his co-workers, particularly Kondziolka, Flickinger, and Pollock, expanded GK radiosurgery not only to the neurosurgical community in the USA, but also to the rest of the world. There has been an explosive increase in the number of GK sites worldwide since the early 1990s after the initial 20-year period, primarily attributable to the long-term efforts of the Karolinska group. However, the contributions of the Pittsburgh group must be recognized when discussing the remarkable expansion of GK radiosurgery realized in the late 1990s.

Success in radiosurgery using a GK has prompted many investigators to modify existing linear accelerator (LINAC) systems to deliver higher doses of radiation to small target volumes in a single session. Colombo and colleagues, and Friedman and colleagues, were truly innovative pioneers in LINAC-based stereotactic radiosurgery for AVMs. They proved, based on their relatively large series of patients and sufficiently long follow-up results, that their systems had essentially the same abilities for AVM radiosurgery as GKs.[10,11,14,15] This form of radiosurgery has recently developed into quite a novel frameless system using robotic techniques, the "CyberKnife."[32] The present author, however, considers it crucial to delay final evaluation of this system until sufficiently long-term follow-up results have been accumulated.

Histopathology of Arteriovenous Malformations After Radiosurgery

Radiosurgery results in AVM obliteration, after a 1- to 3-year latency period, in most cases. The changes induced by radiosurgery within an AVM are considered to occur as follows: ionizing radiation initially injures the endothelial cells of vessels, which causes a reparative process of gradual thickening of connective tissue (myofibroblasts, histiocytes, collagen, and fibrin) within the vessel wall. This process gradually obstructs the lumina of the AVM vessels, resulting in AVM obliteration (Fig. 1).[25,33–36] However, little information has become available on the connective tissue stroma that may play an important role in the obliterative process occurring within irradiated AVMs. Szeifert et al reported that the immunohistochemical reactions of these stromal cells demonstrated marked positivity for smooth muscle actin (SMA) while being somewhat less positive for vimentin and desmin.[35] They concluded, based in part on electron microscopic observations, that the contractile activity of myofibroblasts could be relevant to the process of shrinkage and eventual occlusion of AVMs after radiosurgery. However, the present author and colleagues found that, despite the remarkable positivity for SMA demonstrated immunohistochemically in patent vessels, completely obliterated vessels within the treated nidus showed no SMA staining whatsoever (Fig. 2). Consequently, we consider the role of myofibroblasts a major contributor in postradio-

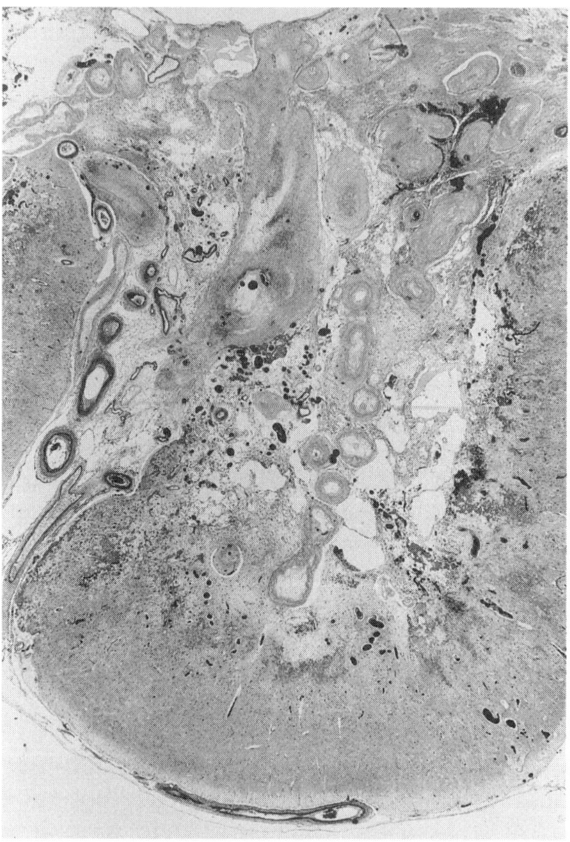

A

Figure 1. Pathological studies of angiographically confirmed nidus obliteration after Gamma Knife radiosurgery. (**A**) Masson-trichrome, (**B**) Elastica van Gieson, and (**C**) Elastica hematoxylin-eosin. The majority of vessels were obliterated by intimal hypertropy (A and B). Lymphocytic aggregation (short arrows in B) and recanalizing vessels (long arrows in B) were seen in the obliterated vessel wall. Although recanalization is observable, these vessels are located within the thickened vessel wall and have no potential to bleed. Some of the vessels had patent lumina (C); however, they were considered to be part of the venous component of the arteriovenous malformation (AVM); most arterial vessels were completely obliterated. There were areas with exudation of albuminous fluid (star in C). *(Continued.)*

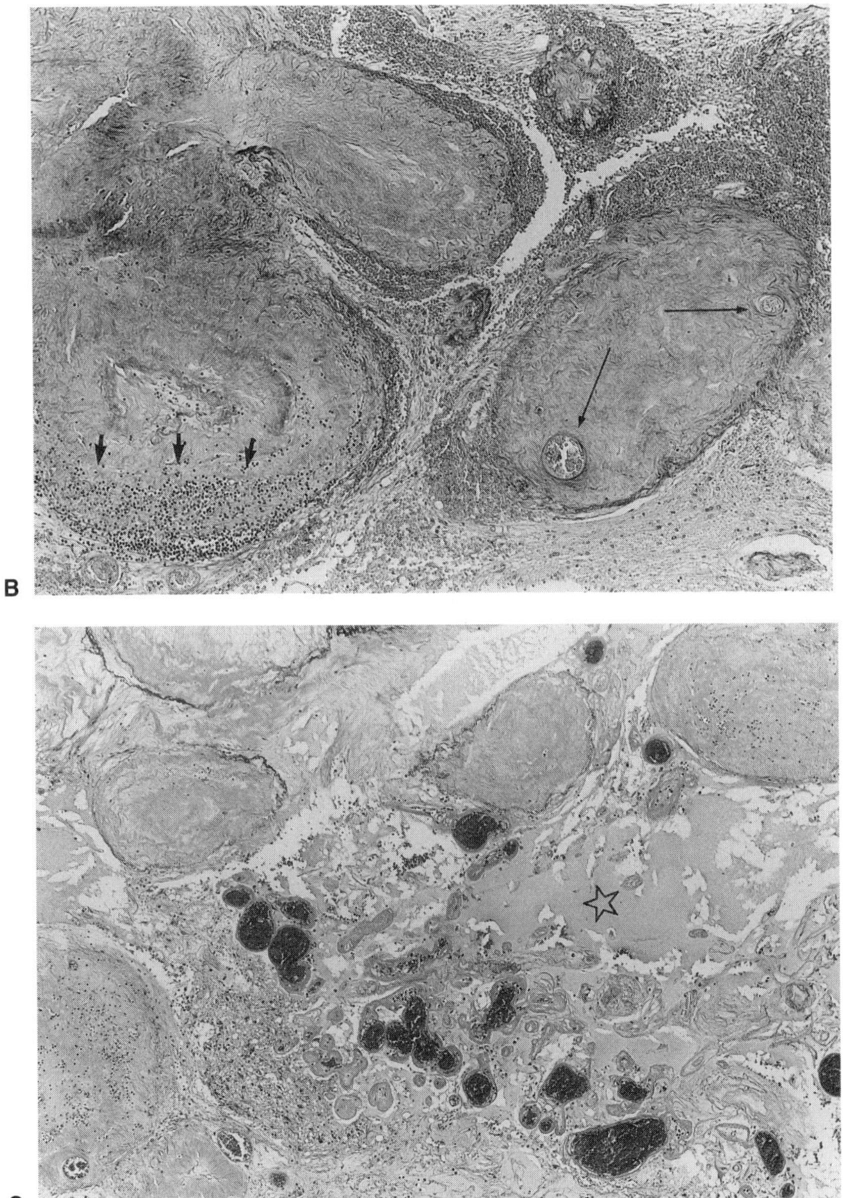

Figure 1.

surgical nidus obliteration, but limited to the early stages of AVM obliteration.

Schneider et al recently categorized the obliteration process of radiosurgically treated AVMs into three stages: (1) endothelial or subendothelial damage; (2) proliferation of intimal smooth muscle cells; and (3) cellular degeneration and increased matrix.[34] The first stage was evidenced by a denuded endothelium or by disruption and separation of the endothelial lining from the underlying vessel walls. In the second stage, proliferation of smooth muscle cells around most or the entire wall circumference produced concentric or eccentric narrowing of the vessel lumina. The proliferative zone was immunohistochemically positive for SMA and collagen type IV while being negative for collagen types I and III. In the third stage, cellular degeneration was evidenced by nuclear pyknosis and decreased cell number, most vessels had undergone obliteration of the entire vascular structure, with more or less uniformly dense hyalinization, and these changes were accompanied by loss of SMA and collagen type IV.

A

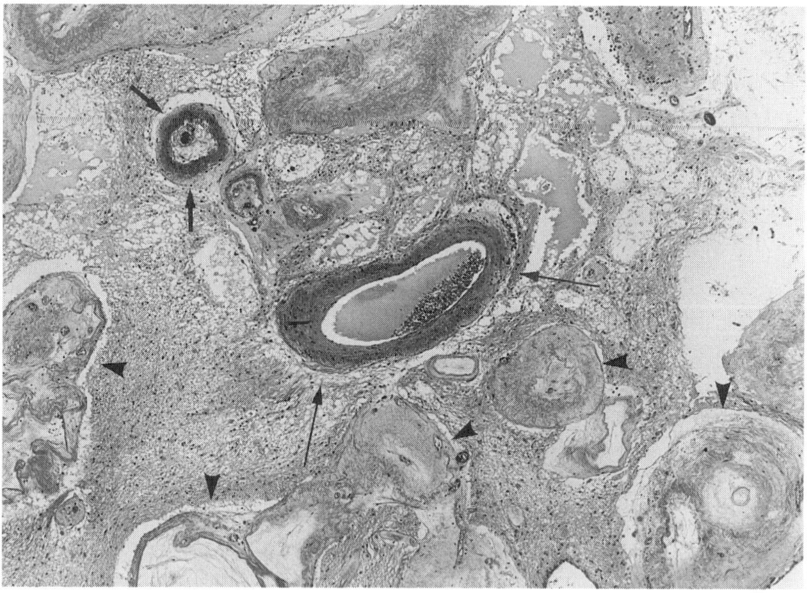

Figure 2. Immunohistochemical studies of an obliterated AVM. (**A**) The irradiated AVM vessels had extremely variable morphologic features; although most vessels were completely occluded (arrow heads), there was a considerable number of patent vessels, some of which showed only partial obliteration (short arrows) while others were patent (long arrows) (hematoxylin-eosin). (**B**) Smooth muscle actin positivity is seen only in the patent or partially obliterated vessels. (**C**) Collagen type I positivity is demonstrated in the completely obliterated vessels. (**D**) Collagen type III positivity is demonstrated in the completely obliterated vessels. (**E**) Collagen type IV positivity is demonstrated in the patent or partially obliterated vessels. *(Continued.)*

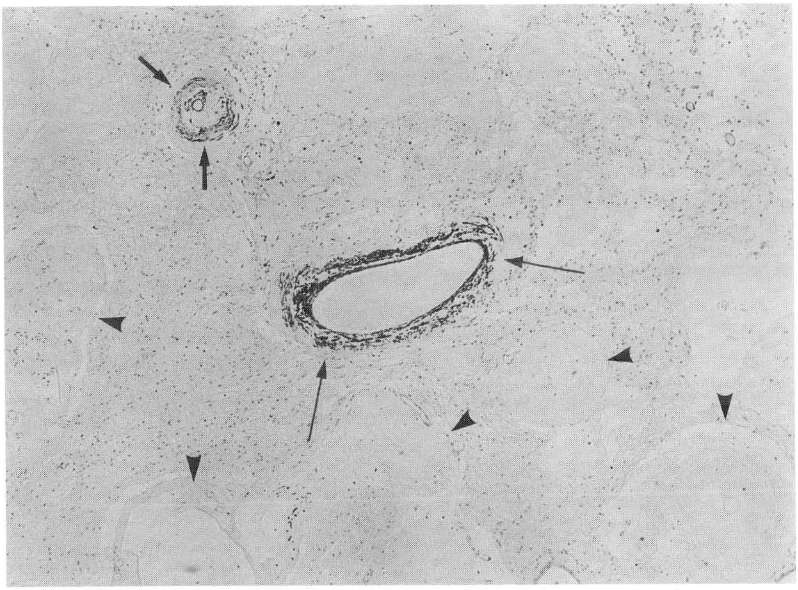

B

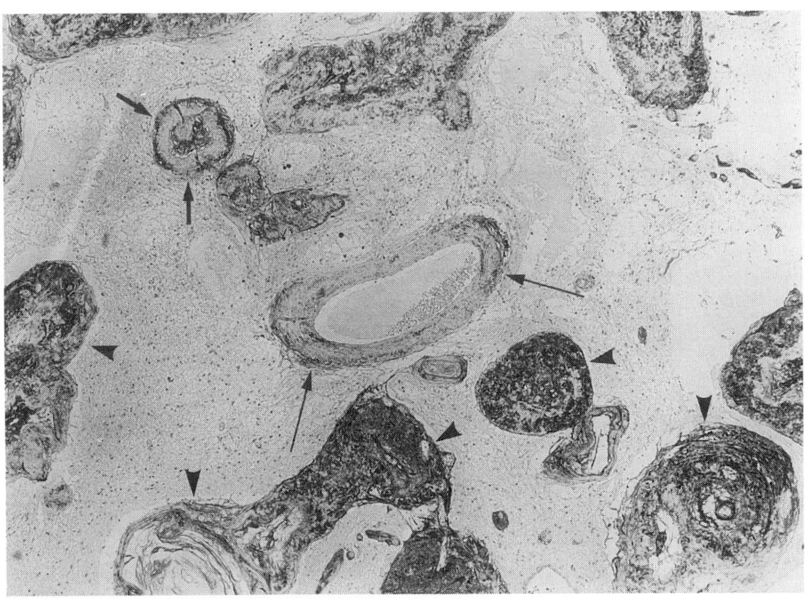

C

Figure 2.

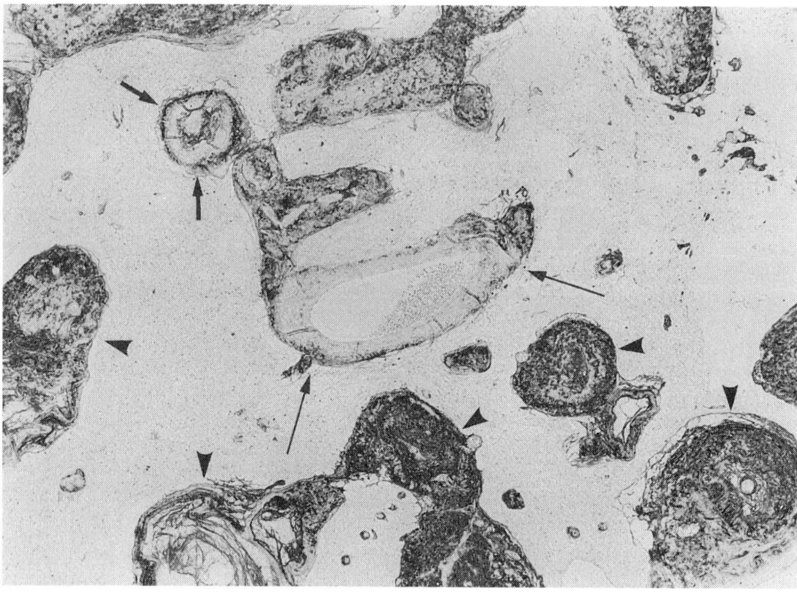

D

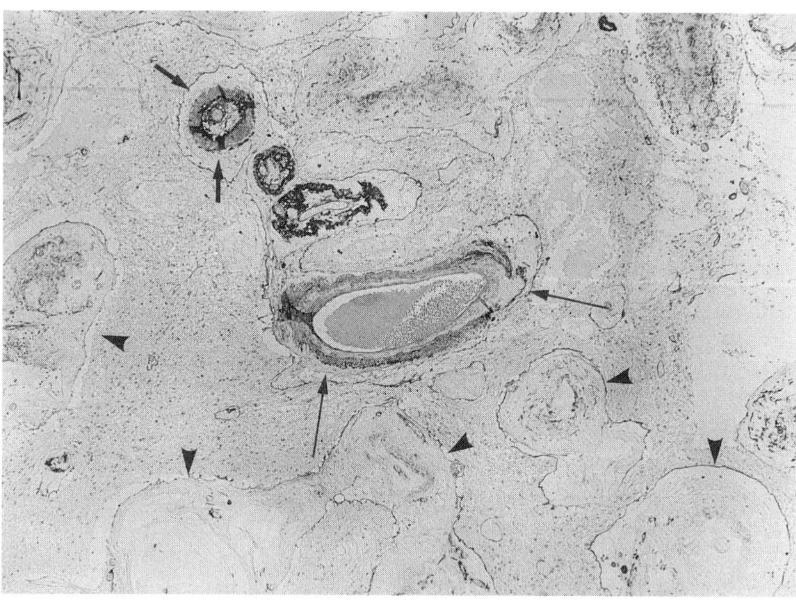

E

Figure 2.

Observations made at the author's facility support their results as we have noted similar findings, especially in the second and third stages. Furthermore, although the pathological significance is uncertain, the herein-reported investigations revealed SMA and collagen type IV (basement membrane type) replaced by collagen types I and III (fibrillary structure type) as vessels progress to occlusion.

Stereotactic Localization and Dose Planning

Although the GK has been modified and upgraded since the mid-1970s, the overall concept and design has remained unchanged. There are three GK models currently in clinical use, Models U, B, and C. All are referred to as the GK and have 201 ^{60}Co sources and four collimator sizes, 4, 8, 14, and 18 mm (Leksell Gamma Unit, Elekta Instruments AB, Stockholm, Sweden). The latest model (Model C) became available recently. In contrast to earlier versions, the Model C moves the patient through target points by means of an automatic positioning system. The Model C reduces the probability of human error, increases comfort for both the patient, and reduces treatment time. However, there is a slight chance that such a mechanical treatment procedure would depersonalize the relationship between the patient and doctor.

Several points regarding stereotactic head frame placement should be noted. As we now rely more on magnetic resonance imaging (MRI) and digital subtraction angiography (DSA), instead of computed tomography (CT) and cut-film angiography, factors that can cause image distortion must be considered. For this reason, the target should be placed as near to the center of the frame (x-, y-, and z-coordinate values of 100) as possible. In most cases, the author performs this procedure with the patient in the supine position using a specially designed adapter firmly fixed to the operating table, as described in detail elsewhere.[37] With the use of this technique, the unpleasant surprise of the coordinate box not fitting on the frame is avoided. As compared with the sitting position, this method has several advantages: (1) Patient condition, including emotion (anxiety), headache, nausea and vomiting, dizziness, unstable blood pressure, and so on, can be controlled more easily. (2) Relatively deep sedation or general anesthesia can be applied without complex procedures. This point is crucial for AVM patients. Although it is very rare, bleeding can occur just as the frame is placed. Inoue et al reported one patient who hemorrhaged during this procedure.[37a] (3) Adequate head positioning within the frame can be attained with either earplugs or an experienced assistant who, in the case of the sitting position, would be needed to support the frame during the procedure. (4) This also allows the patient to maintain a comfortable neck position during imaging examinations. (5) Precise pin positions can be selected, particularly in a patient who has previously undergone craniotomy.

As mentioned earlier, imaging for AVM radiosurgery dose planning typically uses two or three imaging modalities (DSA, CT scans, and/or MRI) without exception. Excluding some cases in which the MRI is contraindicated for various reasons or a patient is allergic to contrast material, both CT scanning and MRI should be performed. Although anatomical and pathological resolution is much better with MRI than CT, there may be a degree of distortion in the MR images. Therefore, if the CT and MR images are not congruent, which is not uncommonly encountered, the CT images are most likely to be accurate. For AVM radiosurgery, T1-weighted sequences without gadolinium are important for ascertaining the anatomical structures; T2-weighted images or three-dimensional time-of-flight MR angiograms are absolutely crucial for outlining the

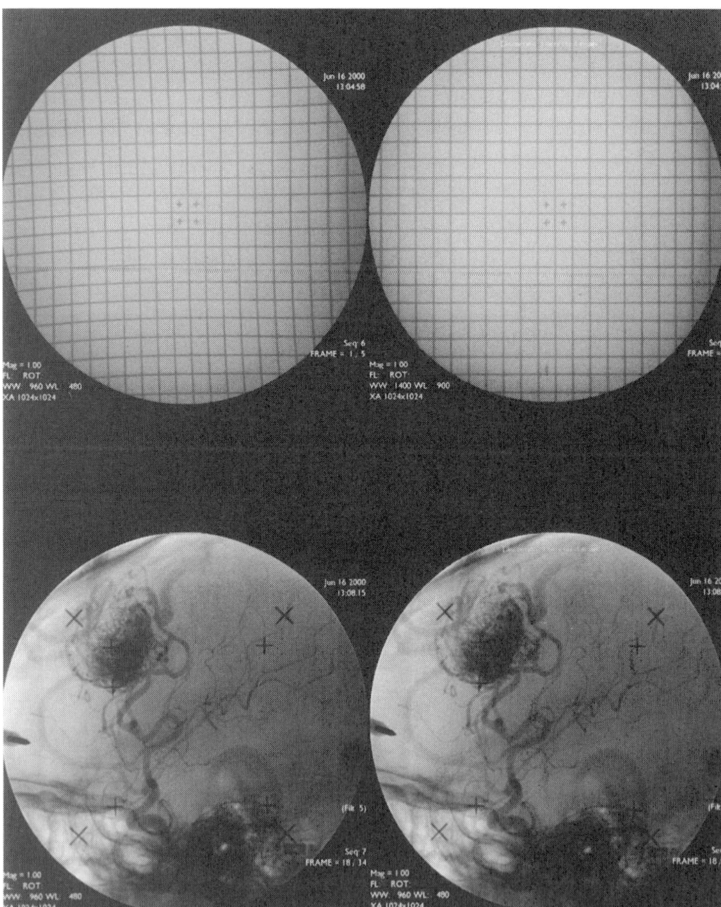

Figure 3. Stereotactic digital subtraction angiogram, before (left) and after (right) correction of distortion.

AVM nidus. Magnetic resonance angiography, in particular, has come into routine use over the past 6 to 7 years. Current dose-planning software allows simultaneous visualization of the CT, MRI, and DSA images.

The most remarkable change that has occurred in AVM radiosurgery over the last several years is improved dose planning. Although conventional angiography, or stereotactic DSA with distortion correction programs (Fig. 3), remain important for delineating nidus configuration and angioarchitecture, angiography provides two-dimensional information only. Thus, dose planning for AVMs is performed primarily based on CT scans and/or MR images, with DSA used only to outline the maximal dimension of the nidus. The defined area on DSA provides the maximum extent of the nidus as a hexahedral configuration (Fig. 4). This is projected onto the axial CT or MR images as a tetragonal area in each slice. The region of interest (ROI) is defined by delineating the "true" AVM nidus only within the tetragonal area, excluding all normal brain tissue. Magnetic resonance imaging not only provides three-dimensional information of the AVM, but also delineates critical anatomical structures not demonstrated by angiography. Multiple isocenter treatments using smaller collimators allow better conformity between the size and shape of the lesion

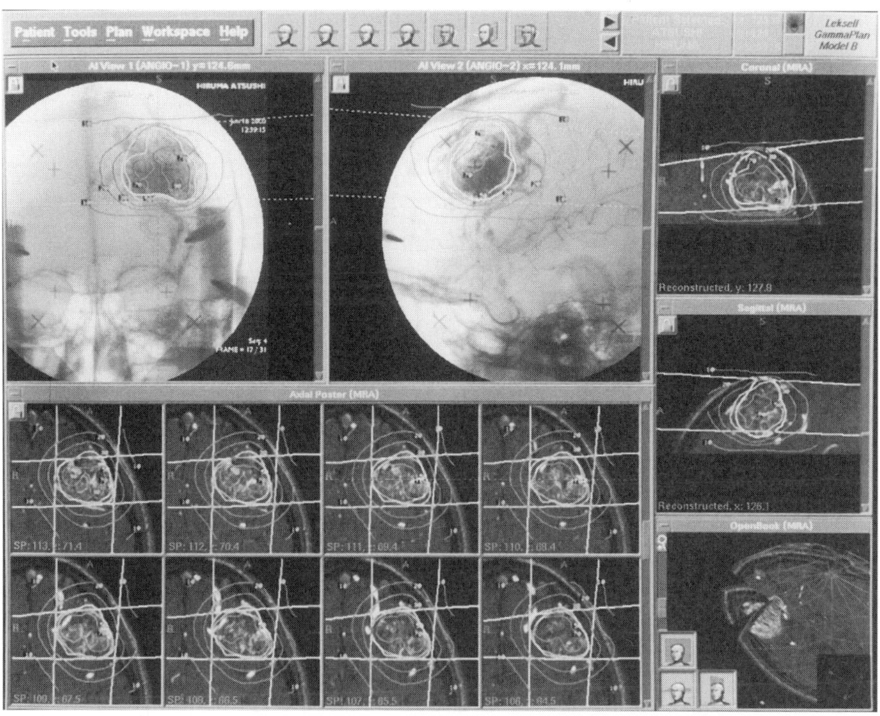

Figure 4. Dose planning for an AVM using the Leksell GammaPlan.

and the dose distribution. Although the total procedure time is considerably prolonged with this technique, better conformity can be achieved and the integrated dose to the critical brain structures can be markedly decreased despite selection of the same marginal dose. Thus, we can anticipate more precise and safer treatment using these techniques, thereby lowering morbidity and possibly improving results.

Dose Selection

Although optimal doses for AVM obliteration are widely considered to be between 18 and 25 Gy at the nidus periphery, the treatment dose for each patient is decided based on the nidus volume and neighboring brain structures. It is well known that the higher doses to the AVM periphery increase the chance for total obliteration. Also, a higher dose can be expected to shorten the latency period to AVM obliteration. However, the higher doses directly correlate with the incidence of post-treatment complications. Thus, using the dose-volume curve proposed by Flickinger et al,[38] we should first consider minimizing the complication risk so as to not exceed an incidence of 3%. Furthermore, if the nidus is located in or close to critical brain structures, a further decrease in the dose may be required to limit for risks of complications in each structure.

In a case where, for some reason, the nidus cannot be treated with the optimal peripheral dose, staged radiosurgery with an interval between the two procedures of 2 or 3 years is recommended (Fig. 5). The author has abandoned volume-fractionated radiosurgery (the nidus is divided into two or three compartments, with each compartment being irradiated over some interval). This type of treatment can be regarded as risky in terms of (re-)bleeding because the partial obliteration within the nidus can increase hemodynamic stress in the remaining patent part, ultimately resulting in hemorrhage. The author had a patient with fatal rebleeding 27 months after volume-fractionated radiosurgery. Therefore, instead of a volume-fractionated technique, dose-fractionated radiosurgery can be recommended for patients with relatively large AVMs. In this technique, the entire nidus is treated with a relatively low dose (12–16 Gy at the nidus periphery) during the first procedure, followed by a second procedure for the residual nidus 2 to 3 years later, if needed.

Recently, Schwartz et al reported the obliteration prediction index to determine the probability of postradiosurgical nidus obliteration for individual patients.[39] Expressed as the peripheral dose (Gy) divided by the largest nidus diameter (cm), the authors found that this method was applicable to both GK and LINAC-based AVM radiosurgery. Likewise, Karlsson et al proposed the K index.[40] The K index is defined as the product of the peripheral dose (Gy) multiplied by the cube root of the nidus volume (cm^3). According to their retrospective analyses of 945 AVMs treated

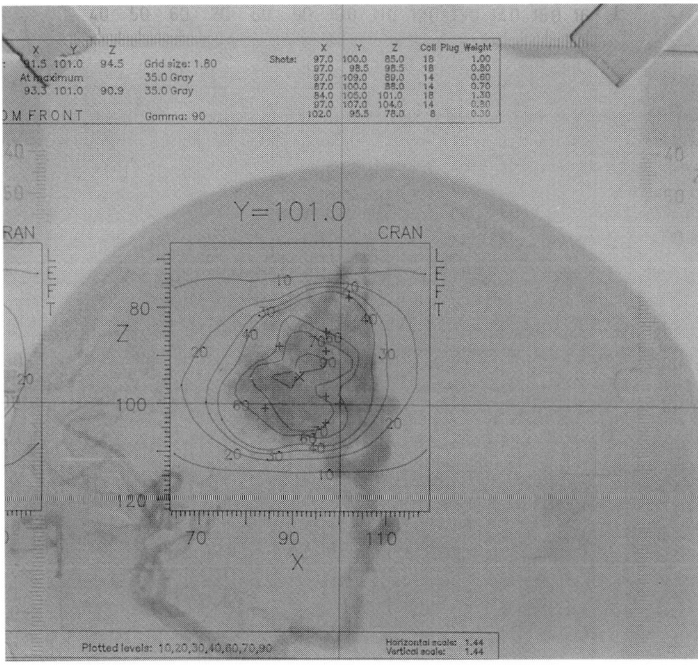

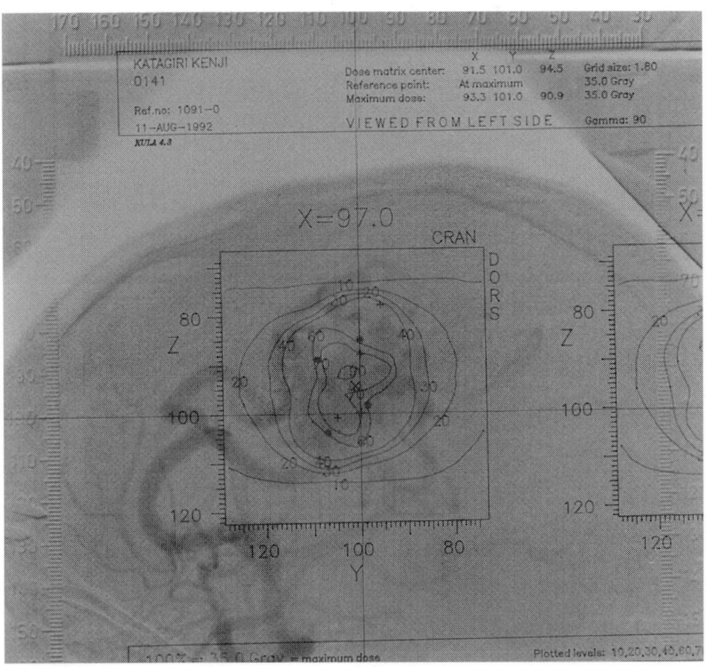

Figure 5A. Anterior-posterior (**top**) and lateral (**bottom**) right carotid angiograms of a frontal AVM at first radiosurgery. *(Continued.)*

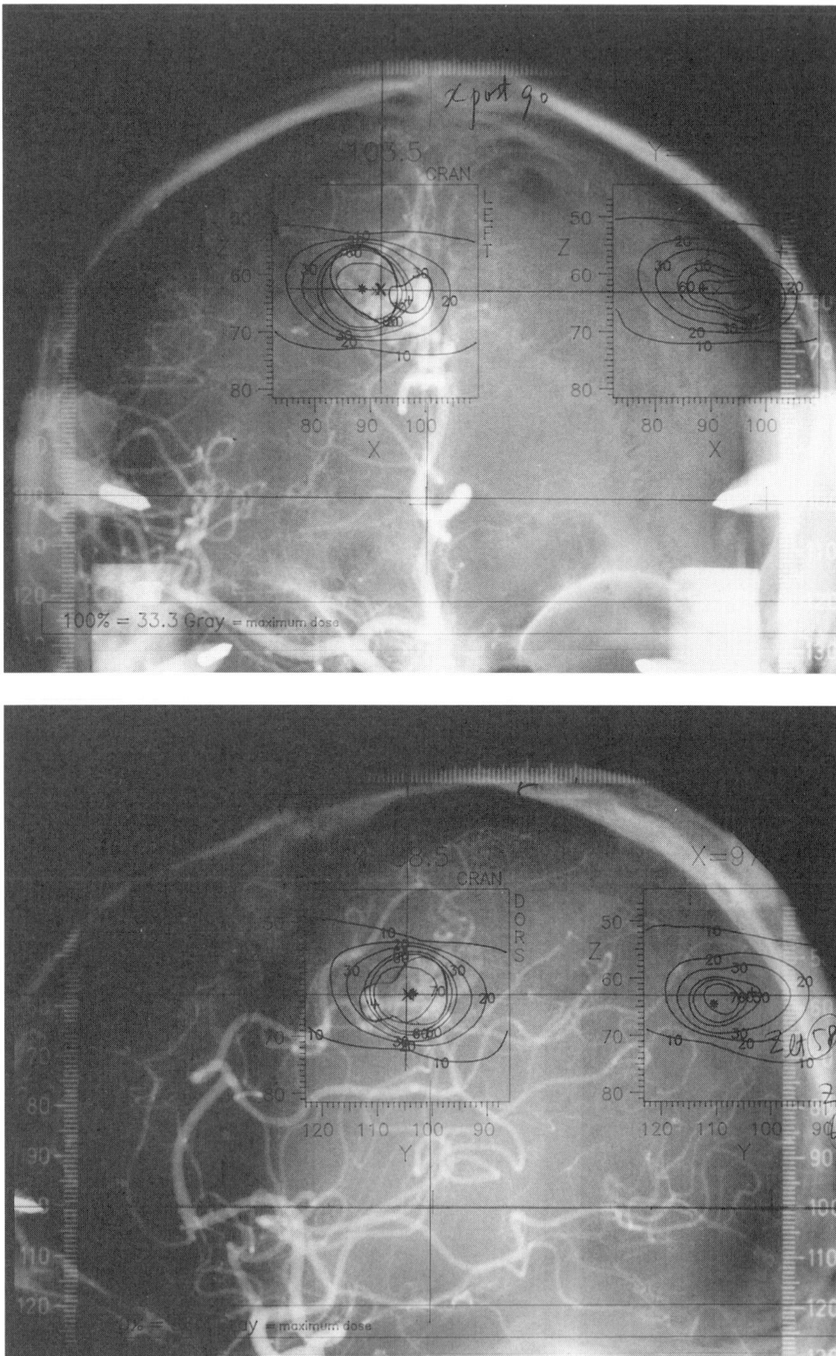

Figure 5B. Anterior-posterior (**top**) and lateral (**bottom**) right carotid angiograms of a frontal AVM 36 months later at the second radiosurgery. *(Continued.)*

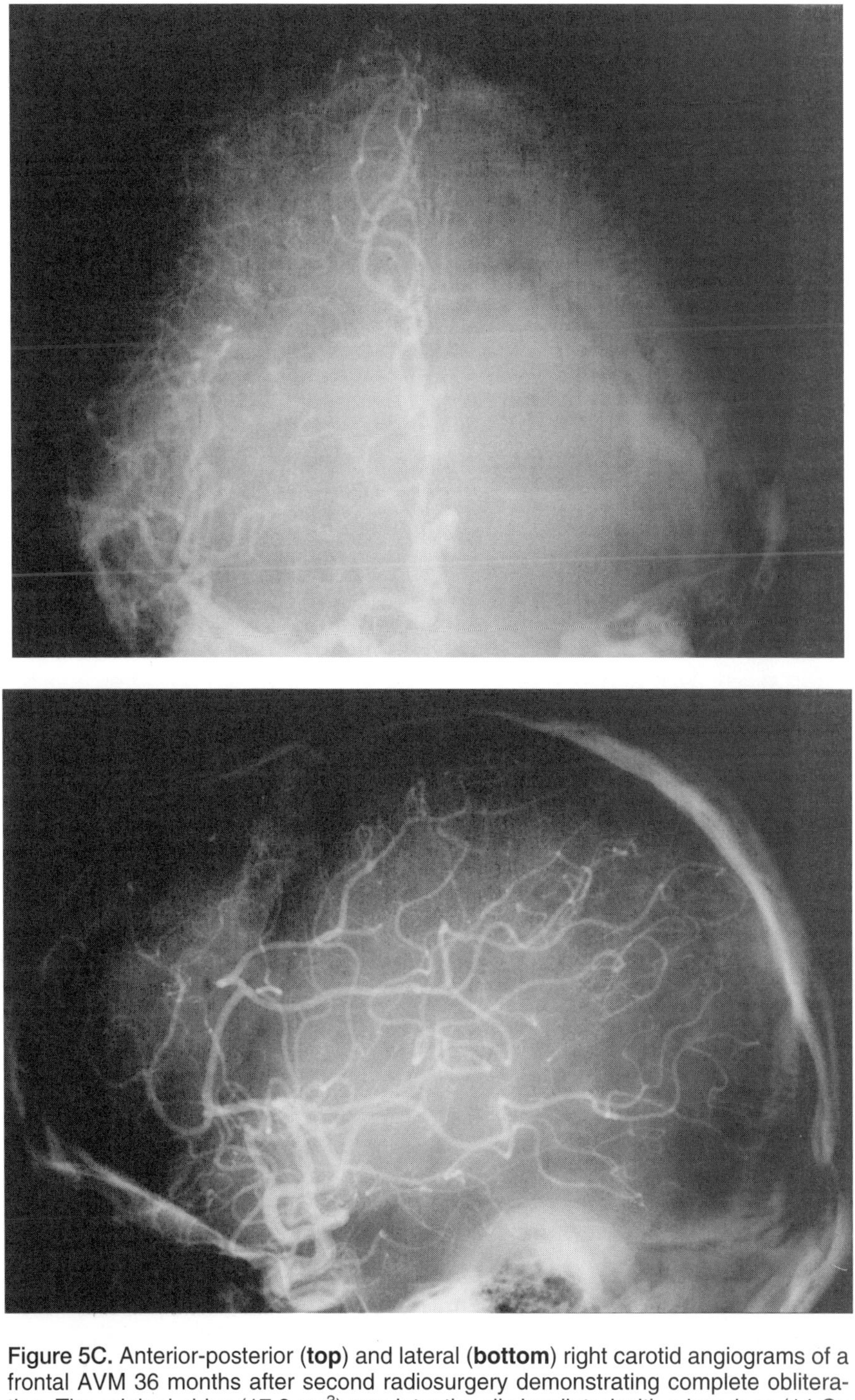

Figure 5C. Anterior-posterior (**top**) and lateral (**bottom**) right carotid angiograms of a frontal AVM 36 months after second radiosurgery demonstrating complete obliteration. The original nidus (17.8 cm^3) was intentionally irradiated with a low dose (14 Gy at the periphery) at the time of the first treatment. Three-year postradiosurgical angiography demonstrated remarkable nidus shrinkage but there was a small residual nidus. This residual AVM was reirradiated with a margin dose of 20 Gy.

with GK radiosurgery, the obliteration rate increased linearly with the K index up to a value of approximately 27, and for higher K values, the obliteration rate had a constant value of approximately 80%.

Treatment Results

Rates of Angiographically Confirmed Obliteration

Angiographically confirmed nidus obliteration is achieved in 70 to 80% of AVM patients undergoing radiosurgery using a GK, a LINAC-based system, or a particle beam system.[9–27] However, as Friedman et al pointed out, the reported percentages of angiograms showing complete thrombosis do not give a complete picture of outcomes for the entire group of radiosurgically treated AVM patients.[15] Steiner and colleagues have published numerous reports on GK radiosurgery for AVMs. In one report, they stated "of 880 patients with the AVM considered as optimally treated, 461 had an appropriate angiographic follow-up. . . of the 461 AVMs with satisfactory angiographic follow-up, 369 (80%) were totally obliterated within two years following the treatment."[40] The reported thrombosis rate in this report applied only to these 461 patients (52%); therefore, 42% (369 of 880 patients) is the real AVM obliteration rate for the entire group of patients. Lunsford et al stated in their report "among the 75 patients who were potentially evaluable two years or more after radiosurgery, two-year angiography was performed in 46. Complete obliteration was confirmed in 37 patients (80%)."[19] Thus, the real obliteration rate is 61% (46 of 75 patients). Similarly, according to a report by the same group, the thrombosis rate was not 84% (27 of the 32 patients evaluated by postradiosurgical angiography) but rather 42% (27 of the entire group of 65 patients who had Spetzler-Martin Grade I-II AVMs).[20] Yamamoto et al stated in their report, based on a total of 121 AVM patients treated at the Mayo Clinic, that complete nidus obliteration was angiographically confirmed in 32 (74.4%) of the 51 patients who underwent angiography.[27] Unfortunately, no data was presented regarding the number of subjects eligible for follow-up angiography among the 70 remaining patients.

As described herein, as well as by Heffez et al,[41] the lack of data on all treated patients is a major criticism of AVM radiosurgery. Therefore, the author has described all obliteration rates based on the entire group of treated patients. In one of the author's reports, the overall obliteration rate was regarded as approximately 65% for the entire group of patients in whom meticulous follow-up was possible.[42] In another publication, based on a total of 885 AVM patients treated at the 11 GK facilities in Japan, the overall obliteration rate of 50% after a single course of irradiation seems low.[43] This is due to the rate being based on the entire group of patients; the obliteration rate for the 681 patients having angiography was 65%. If our results were based only on the group of patients who underwent angiography, 83% of AVMs with volumes of 2.0 cm^3 or less, as well as 82% of AVMs irradiated with 25 Gy or more, have demonstrated complete nidus obliteration. Such obliteration rates are essentially the same as those reported by other investigators, for angiographically confirmed AVM obliteration after a 2- or 3-year latency period following radiosurgery.

Whether obliteration of a radiosurgically treated AVM is permanent has long been a central question. Lindquist et al recently reported 48 patients who underwent angiography 5 to 24 years after GK radiosurgery, and 4 to 17 years after the AVMs was shown to be obliterated.[44] Recanalization was demonstrated in four patients: there was evidence of AVM nidus at the sites of previously occluded AVMs in two patients and adjacent to the previously irradiated sites in the remaining two patients. The recurrent AVMs manifested with hemorrhage in three of the four patients; all three of these patients were 14 years of age or younger at the time of radiosurgery. These results show that there is a small possibility of AVMs reappearing after having been completely occluded after radiosurgery, especially in pediatric patients. Interestingly, AVM recurrence has also been reported in pediatric patients in whom microsurgical resection of AVMs had been successful.[45]

Treatment Failure and Retreatment

Pollock et al reported four factors associated with successful AVM radiosurgery: smaller AVM volume, number of draining veins, younger patient age, and hemispheric AVM location.[46] As Pollock et al[47] and Gallina et al[48] reported, there are five primary causes of treatment failure: (1) inadequate nidus visualization at the time of radiosurgery; (2) recanalization of a previously embolized AVM; (3) improper assessment of the three-dimensional AVM shape; (4) delivery of an insufficient radiation dose; and (5) radiobiological resistance of the AVM, which is only speculative.

A second course of radiosurgery is required for patients in whom complete nidus obliteration is not attained after the initial treatment, because even a very small residual nidus has the potential to bleed. A second radiosurgery is usually performed more than 3 years after the first procedure. Karlsson et al reported that the obliteration rate after the second course of radiosurgery was similar to that after primary treatment, but there was a significantly higher risk for complications.[49] Fourteen radiation-induced complications occurred, while the expected number of complications, calculated using a risk estimation model for single-session radiosurgery, was five. The author has seen severe complications in two patients after two courses of GK radiosurgery (Figs. 6 and 7).

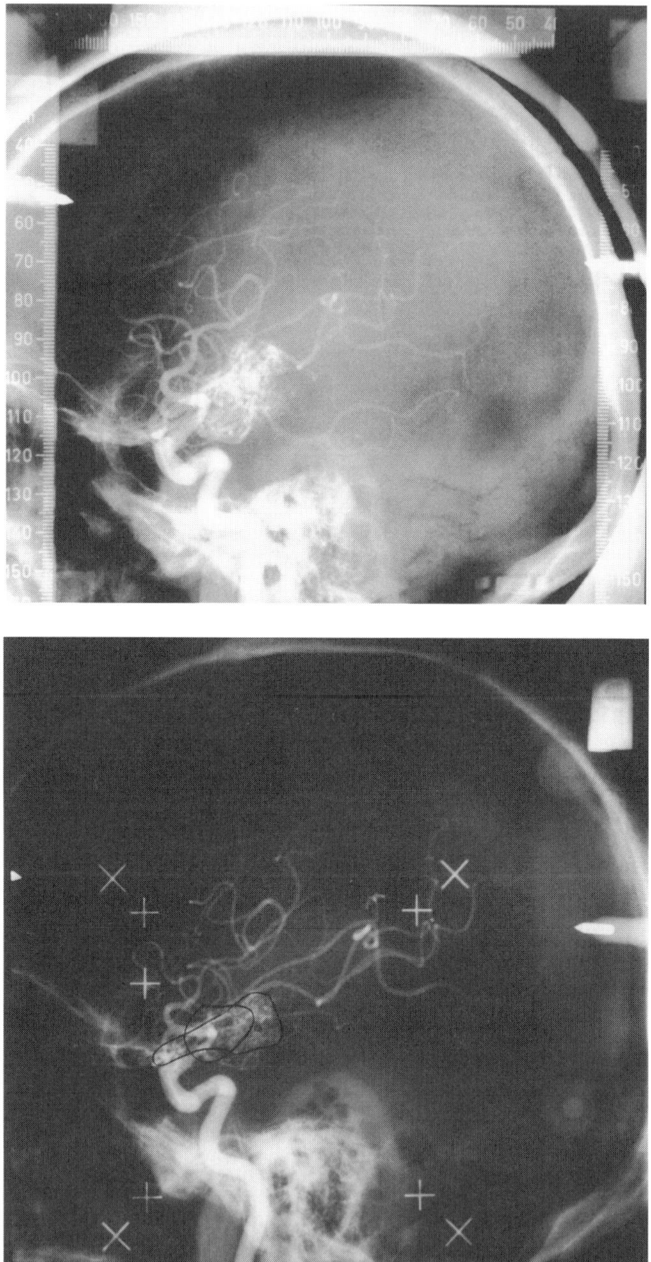

A

B

Figure 6. (A and B) Right lateral carotid angiograms of a patient with a hypothalamic AVM. (**A**) At the first radiosurgery; margin dose, 16.7 Gy. (**B**) At the second radiosurgery 43 months later; margin dose, 14 Gy. (**C**) Post gadolinium MRI 12 months after second radiosurgery demonstrates enhancement of the right optic tract (arrow). The patient suffered a left homonymous hemianopsia. *(Continued.)*

C

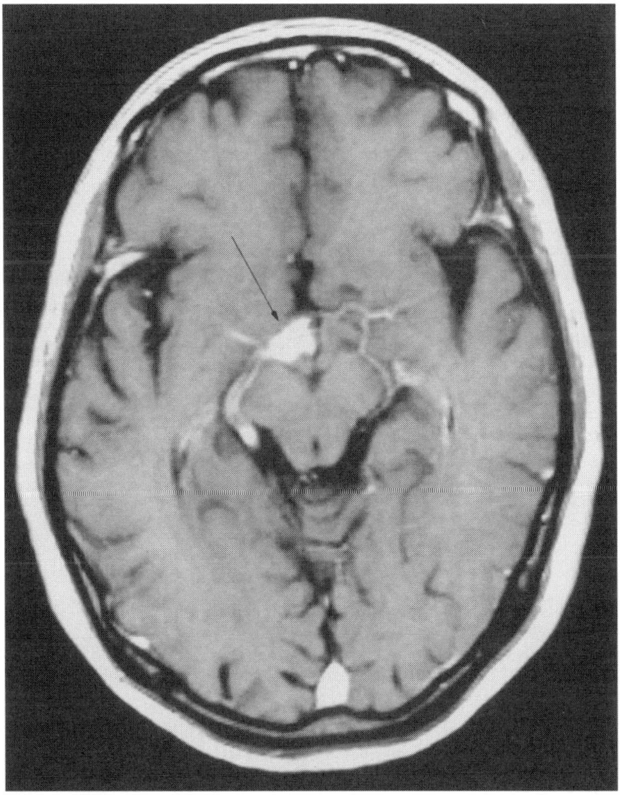

Figure 6.

Seizure and Headache Control

Although the most common manifestation of cerebral AVMs is ICH, the second most common presentation is seizures. Steiner et al reported that 41 (69.4%) of 59 AVM patients with seizures became seizure free or were significantly improved after GK radiosurgery.[50] Kurita et al reported similar results.[51] Twenty-eight of 35 patients with unruptured epileptogenic AVMs remained seizure free at a mean of 43 months after GK radiosurgery. They described a decreasing frequency of seizures several months before neuroimaging demonstrated changes in the nidus.

Headache is the third most common symptom of cerebral AVMs. Steiner et al reported that of 98 AVM patients with chronic headache, this symptom disappeared entirely or improved significantly in 74 (75.5%) after GK radiosurgery.[50] Recently, Kurita et al[52] analyzed 37 patients with migraine-like headache who underwent GK radiosurgery for occipital AVMs. According to their results, headache resolved in 70.6% of patients and amelioration correlated closely with nidus obliteration.

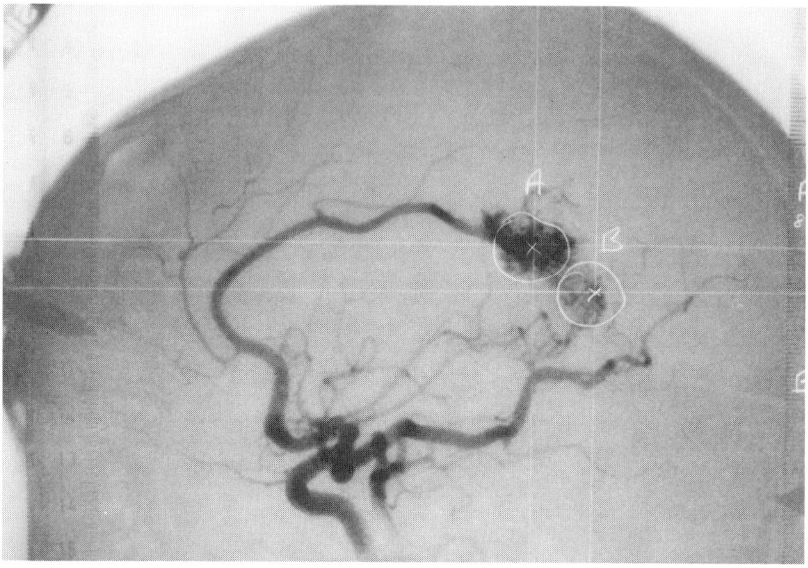

A

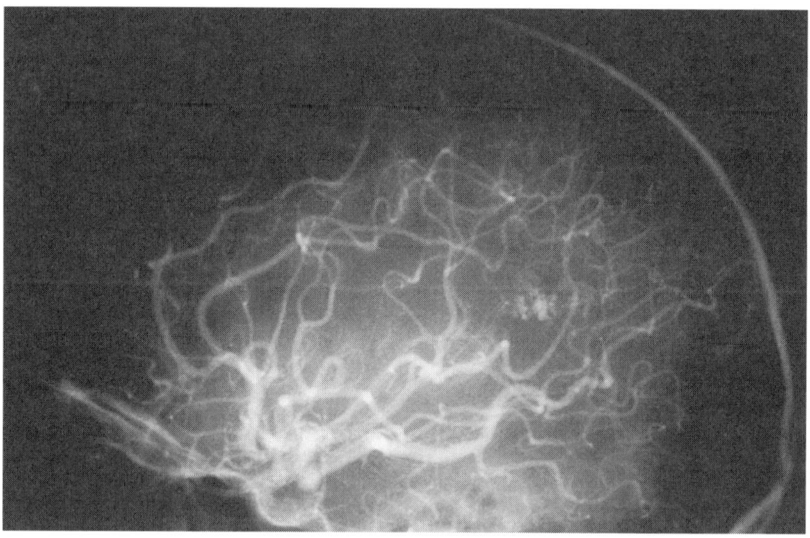

B

Figure 7. (A, B, D, E) Left lateral carotid angiograms of a patient with a corpus callosum/medial left parietal AVM. (**A**) At the first radiosurgery; margin dose, 25 Gy. (**B**) At the second radiosurgery 72 months later; margin dose, 22 Gy. (**C**) MRI obtained 85 months after the second radiosurgery when the patient developed headaches, nausea, vomiting, and right hemiparesis. Note abnormal enhancement, cyst formation, and diffuse white matter edema. (**D, E**) Angiograms at that time demonstrated no arteriovenous shunt in the arterial phase but dysgenetic vessels (arrow) in the venous phase. *(Continued.)*

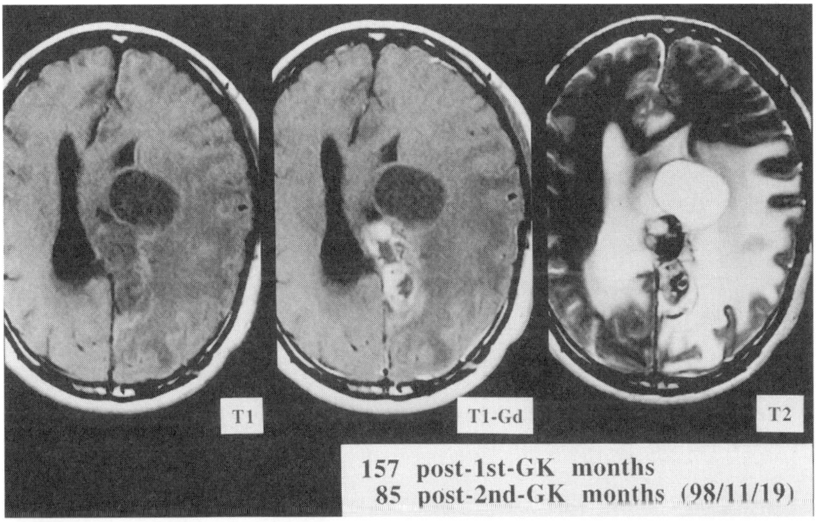

C

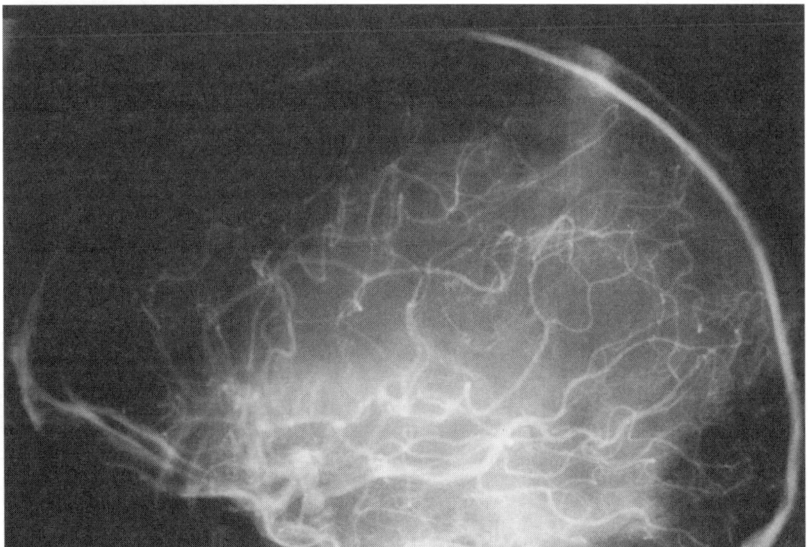

D

Figure 7.

E

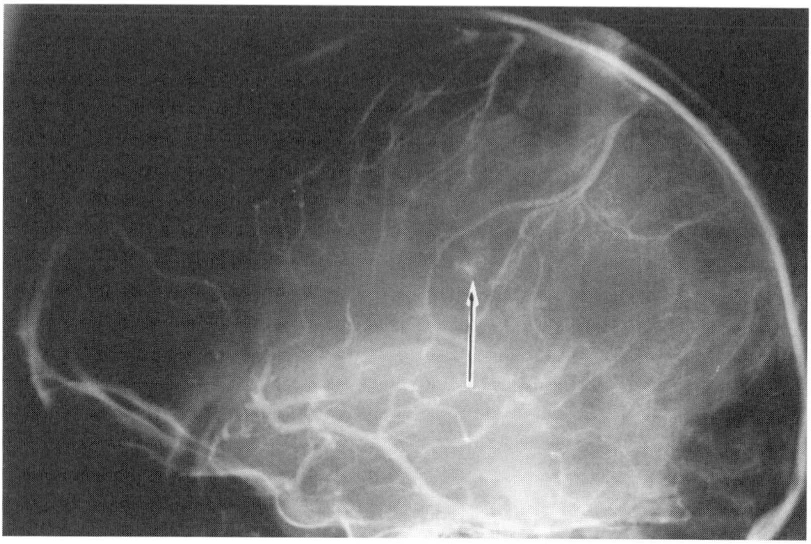

Figure 7.

Riva et al reported that radiosurgical treatment for AVMs did not influence postradiosurgical neurobehavioral outcomes in pediatric patients.[53] Rather, the less invasive nature of this treatment appeared to have contributed to the patients' good physical, mental, and emotional outcomes.

Hemorrhage After Arteriovenous Malformation Radiosurgery

As shown in Table 1, AVM bleeding during the latency period prior to obliteration has been recognized in major reported series on radiosurgery using a GK, a LINAC system, or a particle beam system. The incidence ranges from 2.7 to 11.6%; Steiner reported the overall risk of this complication to be 3.4% at 36 months after radiosurgery.[25] Karlsson et al found that during the first 2 years after radiosurgery, 49 of 1604 AVM patients (3.1%) suffered an ICH.[54] An additional 41 patients experienced hemorrhage more than 2 years after treatment. Mortality rates of approximately 30% have been reported for AVM hemorrhage after radiosurgery.

Pollock et al reported that radiosurgery conferred no protective benefit on patients in whom nidus obliteration was incomplete.[55] However, Karlsson et al[54] found that the calculated incidence of bleeding was roughly half that predicted for a similar group of untreated AVM patients.[54] Thus, it remains unclear whether radiosurgical treatment can prevent AVM rupture even if the treated nidus is not completely obliterated. Based on the current evidence, however, the author is confident that stereotactic radiosurgery does not increase the risk of AVM hemorrhage

Table 1
Incidences and Latency Periods of Hemorrhage After Radiosurgery

Authors/Ref.	*No. of Patients*	*No. of Patients with Bleeding*	*No. of Patients with Fatal Bleeding*	*Latency Period (months)*
Linear accelerator system				
Colombo et al[11]	180	15 (8.3%)	5 (2.7%)	6–24
Friedman et al[14]	158	6 (3.8%)	1 (0.6%)	2–11
Particle beam system				
Kjellberg et al[17]	75	2 (2.7%)	2 (2.7%)	< 12
Steinberg et al[24]	86	10 (11.6%)	2 (2.3%)	4–34
Gamma Knife				
Lunsford et al[19]	227	10 (4.4%)	2 (0.9%)	< 23
Yamamoto et al[27]	121	7 (5.8%)	3 (2.5%)	3–30
Yamamoto et al[43]	858	41 (4.6%)	13 (1.5%)	1–48
Karlsson et al[54]	1604	90 (5.6%)	14 (0.9%)	< 24, 49 patients > 24, 41 patients

during the latency period preceding obliteration. As the incidence of this complication after GK radiosurgery is fortunately, low, it is difficult to assess quantitatively the influence of various factors on the risk of hemorrhage.

It is clear that angiographically demonstrated nidus obliteration eliminates the risk of hemorrhage in the vast majority of patients. However, as reported previously, the author experienced one patient who likely suffered a symptomatic hemorrhagic stroke 5 years after 2-year postradiosurgical angiography had demonstrated complete obliteration.[43] Furthermore, the author recently experienced an additional patient who sustained an intracerebral hematoma that developed 15 years after 1-year postradiosurgical angiography had demonstrated complete obliteration (Fig. 8). Surgical removal of the hematoma was required.

Delayed Radiation-Induced Complications

Delayed radiation-induced complications reportedly occur in 3.2 to 12.5% of patients after AVM radiosurgery (Table 2). It is widely accepted that the dose-volume relation is the most important factor influencing the risk for delayed complications after radiosurgery. As nidus volume increases or higher radiation doses are used, the greater the risk of radiation-induced complications. Flickinger et al reported that of 30 patients who developed radiation-related complications, symptoms resolved in 58% within 27 months.[56] Patients receiving less than 20 Gy at the nidus periphery were more likely to improve than were patients treated with

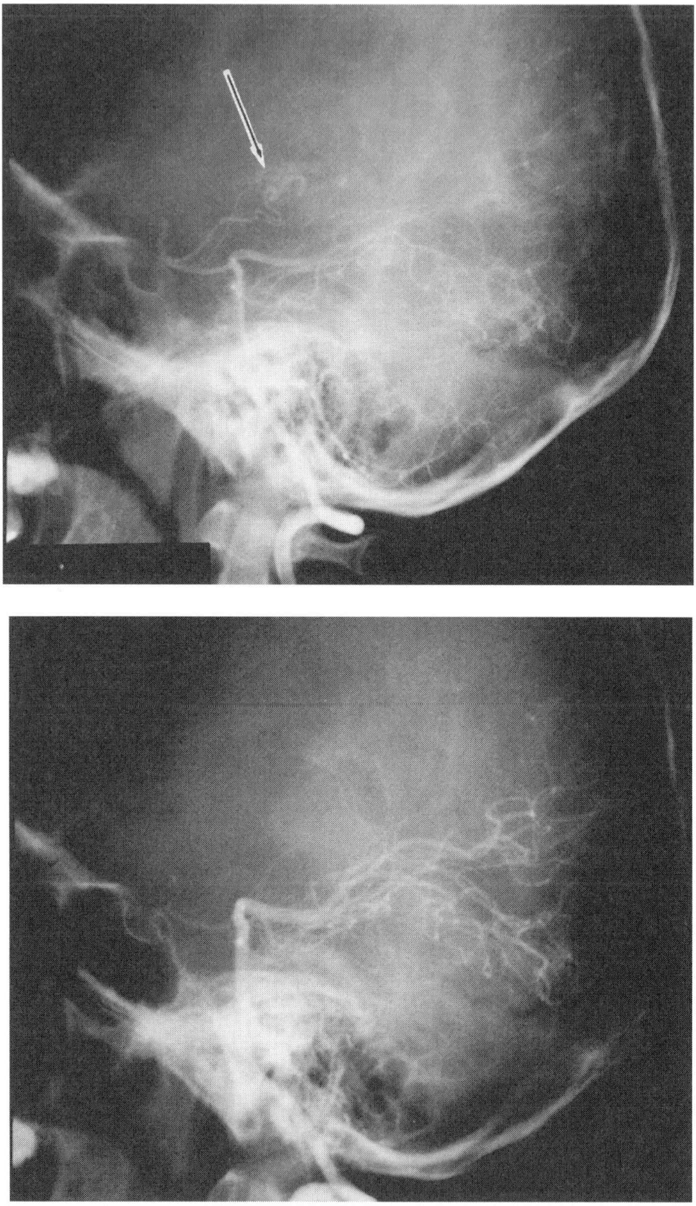

A

B

Figure 8. (A, B, D) Lateral vertebral angiograms of a patient with a basal ganglia AVM. (**A**) At the time of radiosurgery. (**B**) 12 months after radiosurgery showing complete obliteration. (**C**) CT 191 months after radiosurgery showing left temporal hematoma requiring surgical removal. (**D**) Angiography at the time of surgery demonstrated no vascular abnormalities. *(Continued.)*

C

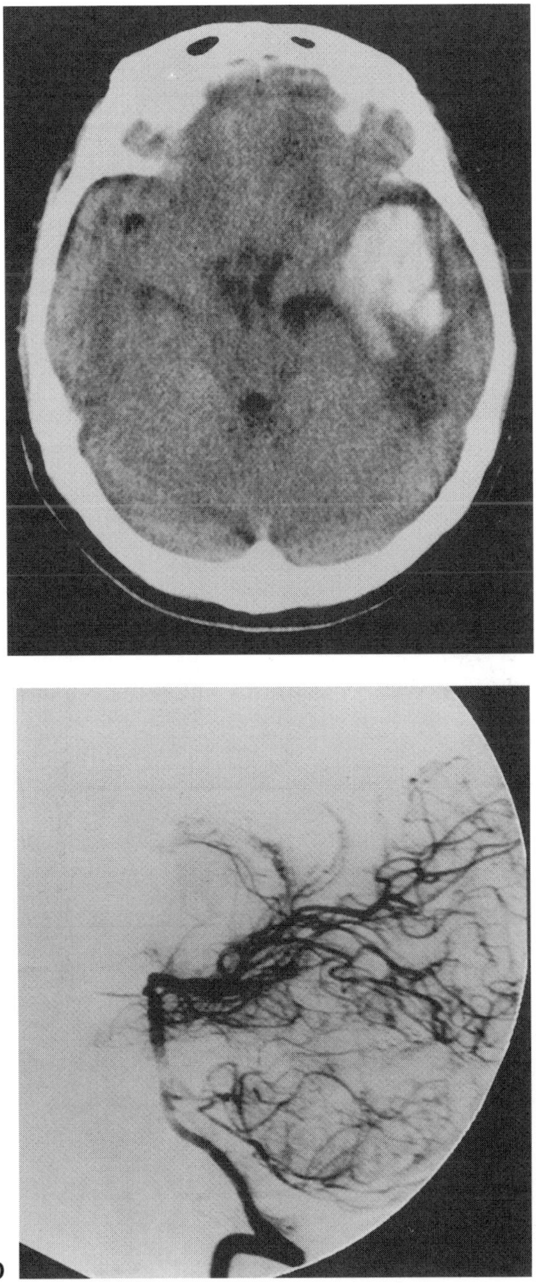

D

Figure 8.

Table 2
Incidences and Latency Periods of Radiation-Related Complications

Authors/Ref. No.	*No. of Patients*	*No. of Patients with Complications*	*Latency Period (months)*
Linear accelerator system			
Colombo et al[11]	180	9 (5.0%)	2–18
Friedman et al[14]	158	5 (3.2%)	11–15
Souhami et al[23]	33	3 (10.0%)	6–9
Particle beam system			
Kjellberg et al[17]	75	8 (10.7%)	?
Steinberg et al[24]	86	17 (19.8%)	3–33
Gamma Knife			
Lunsford et al[19]	227	10 (4.4%)	4–18
Steiner et al[26]	1000	35 (3.5%)	4–56
Yamamoto et al[27]	121	6 (5.0%)	?
Yamamoto et al[43]	858	24 (2.7%)	4–24
Present study	58	7 (12.1%)	9–146

more than 20 Gy (89% vs. 36%, p=0.006). Another important factor related to radiation-induced complications after AVM radiosurgery is the volume of normal brain volume included within the target volume. As described above, recent dose-planning techniques allow the avoidance of excess irradiation to the normal brain, which can be expected to significantly reduce the risks for delayed complications. Karlsson et al,[57] using their own risk estimation model,[58] found that centrally located AVMs had a higher incidence of complications. Also, a previous hemorrhage reduced the risk, as compared with estimates made with their model. According to a multi-institutional analysis of complication outcomes reported by Flickinger et al, significantly greater symptom resolution was observed in patients with no prior history of hemorrhage and in those with symptoms of minimal severity.[56]

The majority of radiation-induced complications occur by the third year after radiosurgery. However, the author and colleagues previously reported two patients who experienced symptomatic complications developing more than 5 years after irradiation.[42] Recent analysis of the author's personal series of 58 AVM patients who have been followed from 5 to 21.7 years (mean, 10.2 years) after GK radiosurgery disclosed seven radiation-related morbidities (12.1%), five of which manifested 5 years or more after radiosurgery. One patient, who experienced radiation-induced injury of the pons 19 months after radiosurgery, had a second ictus occurring at 81 post-GK months. Five patients also experienced asymptomatic radiation-related adverse effects.[59] These included cyst formation (n=3), stenosis of a major artery (n=1), and appearance of dural arteriovenous fistula (n=1). Furthermore, Sakaki et al recently presented an AVM patient who died due to glioblastoma multiforme that developed within the target area several years after irradiation.[60]

Conclusions

The following discussion is based on personal experiences. Although radiosurgery is undoubtedly an alternative to microsurgical resection for appropriately selected AVMs, the treatment result should be weighed against cumulative management risks, which are not negligibly low. Follow-up data from my consecutive series of 58 patients with AVMs who underwent GK radiosurgery during the period between 1978 and 1995 were reviewed. With a mean follow-up of 10.2 years, there were two mortalities (3.4%), one AVM-related (massive rebleeding) and the other angiography-related, at 26 and 27 post-GK months, respectively. Seven patients had radiation-related morbidities (12.1%) which manifested at 9, 19, 54, 66, 84, 91, and 146 post-GK months. One patient sustained an ICH 188 months after radiosurgery. Using the Kaplan-Meier method, actuarial rates for total management complications were 8.9%, 15.3%, and 20.6% at the 5th, 10th, and 15th post-GK years, respectively (Fig. 9). However, the incidences at more than 10 years after radiosurgery are obviously overes-

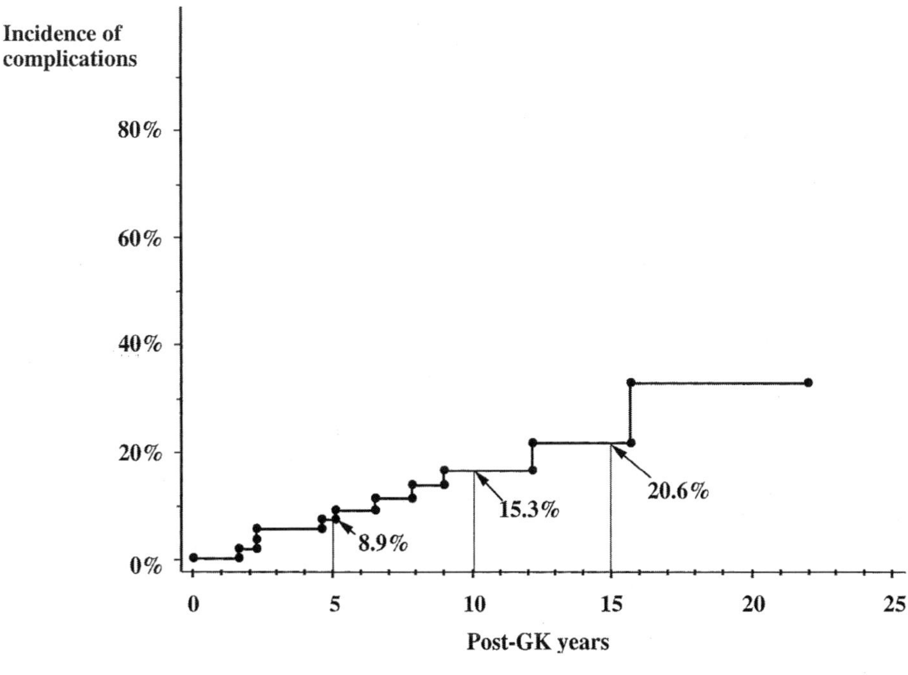

Figure 9. Cumulative incidence of postradiosurgical complications.

timated because of the small sample size for this period. Moreover, it should be noted that approximately two-thirds of the patients described herein had radiosurgery early in the "learning curve." Because there is still some anxiety stemming from the use of radiation in young patients with benign lesions such as AVMs, it is essential for radiosurgeons to determine, based on very large patient series with 10- to 20-year follow-up, the actual incidences of very rare postradiosurgical complications like tumor neogenesis, cyst formation, and major vessel obliteration.[42,59–61]

Acknowledgment: The author would like to thank Bierta E. Barfod, MD, University of Michigan, School of Public Health, for her assistance in the preparation of this manuscript. The author is also very grateful to Makio Mukai, MD, Department of Pathology, Keio University School of Medicine, for his novel work in immunohistochmical analyses.

References

1. Garretson HD: Intracranial arteriovenous malformations. In Wilkins RH, Rengachary SS (eds): Neurosurgery. 2nd Edition. New York, McGraw-Hill, 1996, pp 2433–2442.
2. Graf CJ, Perret GE, Torner JC: Bleeding from cerebral arteriovenous malformations as part of their natural history. J Neurosurg 1983;58:331–337.
3. Ondra SL, Troupp H, George ED, et al: The natural history of symptomatic arteriovenous malformations of the brain: a 24-year follow-up assessment. J Neurosurg 1990;73:387–391.
4. Hartmann A, Mast H, Mohr JP, et al: Morbidity of intracranial hemorrhage in patients with cerebral arteriovenous malformation. Stroke; 1998;29: 931–934.
5. Mast H, Young WL, Koennecke HC, et al: Risk of spontaneous haemorrhage after diagnosis of cerebral arteriovenous malformation. Lancet 1997;350: 1065–1068.
6. Kondziolka D, McLaughlin MR, Kestle JRW, et al: Simple risk predictions for arteriovenous malformation hemorrhage. Neurosurgery 1995;37:851–855.
7. Wikholm G, Lundqvist C, Svendsen P: Embolization of cerebral arteriovenous malformations: Part I. Technique, morphology, and complications. Neurosurgery 1996;39:448–459.
8. Lundqvist C, Wikholm G, Svendsen P: Embolization of cerebral arteriovenous malformations: Part II. Aspects of complications and late outcome. Neurosurgery 1996;39:460–469.
9. Betti OO, Munari C, Rosler R: Stereotactic radiosurgery with the linear accelerator: treatment of arteriovenous malformations. Neurosurgery 1989;24: 311–321.
10. Colombo F, Benedetti A, Pozza F, et al: Linear accelerator radiosurgery of cerebral arteriovenous malformations. Neurosurgery 1989;24:833–840.
11. Colombo F, Pozza F, Chierego G, et al: Linear accelerator radiosurgery of cerebral arteriovenous malformations: an update. Neurosurgery 1994;34:14–21.
12. Fabrikant JI, Frankel KA, Phillips MH, et al: Stereotactic heavy charged-particle Bragg peak radiosurgery for intracranial arteriovenous malformations. In Edwards MSB, Hoffman HJ (eds): Cerebral Vascular Diseases in Children and Adolescents. Baltimore, Williams & Wilkins, 1989, pp 389–409.
13. Fabrikant JI, Lyman JT, Hosobuchi Y: Stereotactic heavy-ion Bragg peak radiosurgery for intracranial vascular disorders: method for treatment of deep arteriovenous malformations. Br J Radiol 1984;57:479–490.

14. Friedman WA, Bova FJ: Linear accelerator radiosurgery for arteriovenous malformations. J Neurosurg 1992;77:832–841.
15. Friedman WA, Bova FJ, Mendenhall WM: Linear accelerator radiosurgery for arteriovenous malformations: the relationship of size to outcome. J Neurosurg 1995;82:180–189.
16. Kawamoto S: Radiosurgery of arteriovenous malformations. No-Shinkei-Geka (Neurol Surg, Tokyo) 1994;22:403–420 (in Japanese).
17. Kjellberg RN, Hanamura T, Davis KR, et al: Bragg-peak proton-beam therapy for arteriovenous malformations of the brain. N Engl J Med 1983;309:269–274.
18. Loeffler JS, Alexander E III, Sidden RL, et al: Stereotactic radiosurgery for intracranial arteriovenous malformations using a standard linear accelerator. Int J Radiat Oncol Biol Phys 1989;17:673–677.
19. Lunsford LD, Kondziolka D, Flickinger JC, et al: Stereotactic radiosurgery for arteriovenous malformations of the brain. J Neurosurg 1991;75:512–524.
20. Pollock BE, Lunsford LD, Kondziolka D, et al: Patient outcomes after stereotactic radiosurgery for "operable" arteriovenous malformations. Neurosurgery 1994;35:1–8.
21. Pollock BE, Lunsford LD, Kondziolka D, et al: Stereotactic radiosurgery for postgeniculate visual pathway arteriovenous malformations. J Neurosurg 1996;84:437–441.
22. Sasaki T, Kurita H, Saito I, et al: Arteriovenous malformations in the basal ganglia and thalamus: management and results in 101 cases. J Neurosurg 1998;88:285–292.
23. Souhami L, Olivier A, Podgorsak EB, et al: Radiosurgery of cerebral arteriovenous malformations with the dynamic stereotactic irradiation. Int J Radiat Oncol Biol Phys 1990;19:775–782.
24. Steinberg GK, Fabrikant JI, Marks MP, et al: Stereotactic heavy-charged particle Bragg peak radiation for intracranial arteriovenous malformations. N Engl J Med 1990;323:96–101.
25. Steiner L: Treatment of arteriovenous malformation by radiosurgery. In Wilson CB, Stein BM (eds): Intracranial Arteriovenous Malformations. Baltimore, Williams & Wilkins, 1984, pp 295–313.
26. Steiner L, Lindquist C, Steiner M: Radiosurgery. In Symon L (ed): Advances and Technical Standards in Neurosurgery. Wien, Springer-Verlag, 1992, pp 19–102.
27. Yamamoto Y, Coffey RJ, Nichols DA, et al: Interim report on the radiosurgical treatment of cerebral arteriovenous malformations: the influence of size, dose, time and technical factors on obliteration rate. J Neurosurg 1995;83:832–837.
28. Jokura H, Yoshimoto T: Decision making in treatment strategy of AVMs: Treatment Board system at Tohoku University. No-Socchu-No-Geka (Surgery for Cerebral Stroke) 1999;27:343–349 (in Japanese, English abstract).
29. Miyamoto S, Hashimoto N, Nagata I, et al: Posttreatment sequelae of plaintively treated cerebral arteriovenous malformations. Neurosurgery 2000;46:589–595.
30. Leksell L: The stereotaxic method and radiosurgery of the brain. Acta Chir Scand 1951;102:316–319.
31. Steiner L, Leksell L, Greitz T, et al: Stereotaxic radiosurgery for cerebral arteriovenous malformations: report of a case. Acta Chir Scand 1972;138:459–462.
32. Adler JR, Murphy MJ, Chang SD, Hancock SL: Image-guided robotic radiosurgery. Neurosurgery 1999;44:1299–1307.
33. Chang SD, Shuster DL, Steinberg GK, et al: Stereotactic radiosurgery of ar-

teriovenous malformations: pathologic changes in resected tissue. Clin Neuropathol 1997;16:111–116.
34. Schneider BF, Eberhard DA, Steiner LE: Histopathology of arteriovenous malformations after gamma knife radiosurgery. J Neurosurg 1997;87:352–357.
35. Szeifert GT, Kemedy AA, Timperley WR, et al: The potential role of myofibroblasts in the obliteration of arteriovenous malformations after radiosurgery. Neurosurgery 1997;40:61–77.
36. Yamamoto M, Jimbo M, Kobayashi M, et al: Long-term results of radiosurgery for arteriovenous malformation: neurodiagnostic imaging and histological studies of angiographically-confirmed nidus obliteration. Surg Neurol 1992;37:219–230.
37. Yamamoto M: Gamma knife radiosurgery: technology, applications, and future directions. Neurosurg Clin N Am 1999;10:181–202.
37a. Inoue HK, Nakamura M, Hirato M, et al: Approaches for arteriovenous malformation management: how to combine intravascular, radio, and direct surgery. No-Socchu-No-Geka (Surgery for Cerebral Stroke) 1992;20:359–364. (In English.)
38. Flickinger JC, Lunsford LD, Kondziolka D: Dose prescription and dose-volume effects in radiosurgery. Neurosurg Clin N Am 1992;3:51–60.
39. Schwartz M, Sixel K, Young C, et al: Prediction of obliteration of arteriovenous malformations after radiosurgery: the obliteration prediction index. Can J Neurol Sci 1997;24:106–109.
40. Karlsson B, Lindquist C, Steiner L: Prediction of obliteration after gamma knife surgery for cerebral arteriovenous malformations. Neurosurgery 1997; 40:425–431.
41. Heffez DS, Osterdock RJ, Alderete L, et al: The effect of incomplete patient follow-up on the reported results of AVM radiosurgery. Surg Neurol 1998;49: 373–384.
42. Yamamoto M, Jimbo M, Hara M, et al: Gamma knife radiosurgery for cerebral arteriovenous malformations: long-term follow-up results focusing on complications occurring more than 5 years after irradiation. Neurosurgery 1996;38: 906–914.
43. Yamamoto M, Tanaka T, Boku N, et al: Gamma knife radiosurgery for cerebral arteriovenous malformations: a multi-institutional study in Japan. In Kondziolka D (ed): Radiosurgery 1997. Vol 2. Basel, Karger, 1998, pp 147–156.
44. Lindqvist M, Karlsson B, Guo WY, et al: Angiographic long-term follow-up data for arteriovenous malformations previouly proven to be obliterated after gamma knife radiosurgery. Neurosurgery 2000;46:803–810.
45. Kader A, Goodrich JT, Sonstein WJ, et al: Recurrent arteriovenous malformations after negative postoperative angiograms. J Neurosurg 1996;85: 14–18.
46. Pollock BE, Flickinger JC, Lunsford LD, et al: Factors associated with successful arteriovenous malformation radiosurgery. Neurosurgery 1998;42: 1239–1247.
47. Pollock BE, Kondziolka D, Lunsford LD, et al: Repeat stereotactic radiosurgery of arteriovenous malformations: factors associated with incomplete obliteration. Neurosurgery 1996;38:318–324.
48. Gallina P, Merienne L, Meder JF, et al: Failure in radiosurgery treatment of cerebral arteriovenous malformations. Neurosurgery 1998;42:996–1004.
49. Karlsson B, Kihlström L, Lindquist C: Gamma knife surgery for previously irradiated arteriovenous malformations. Neurosurgery 1998;42:1–6.
50. Steiner L, Lindquist C, Adler JR, et al: Clinical outcome of radiosurgery for cerebral arteriovenous malformations. J Neurosurg 1992;77:1–8.

51. Kurita H, Kawamoto S, Suzuki I, et al: Control of epilepsy associated with cerebral headache in patients with arteriovenous malformations after radiosurgery. J Neuro Neurosurg Psychiatry 1998;65:648–655.
52. Kurita H, Ueki K, Shin M, et al: Headache in patients with radiosurgically treated occipital arteriovenous malformations. J Neurosurg 2000;93:224–228.
53. Riva D, Pantaleoni C, Devoti M, et al: Radiosurgery for cerebral AVMs in children and adolescents: the neurobehavioral outcome. J Neurosurg 1997;86: 207–210.
54. Karlsson B, Lindquist C, Steiner L: Effect of gamma knife surgery on the risk of rupture prior to AVM obliteration. Minim Invas Neurosurg 1996;39:21–27.
55. Pollock BE, Flickinger JC, Lunsford LD, et al: Hemorrhage risk after stereotactic radiosurgery of cerebral arteriovenous malformations. Neurosurgery 1996;38:652–661.
56. Flickinger JC, Kondziolka D, Lunsford LD, et al: A multi-institutional analysis of complication outcomes after arteriovenous malformation radiosurgery. Int J Radiat Oncol Biol Phys 1999;44:67–74.
57. Karlsson B, Lax I, Söderman M: Factors influencing the risk for complications following Gamma Knife radiosurgery of cerebral arteriovenous malformations. Radiother Oncol 1997;43:275–280.
58. Lax I, Karlsson B: Prediction of complications in gamma knife radiosurgery of arteriovenous malformation. Acta Oncol 1996;35:49–55.
59. Yamamoto M, Hara M, Ide M, et al: Radiation-related adverse effects observed on neuro-imaging several years after radiosurgery for cerebral arteriovenous malformations. Surg Neurol 1998; 49: 385–398.
60. Sakaki T, Morimoto T, Hoshida T, et al: Surgery for AVM around the sensory motor cortex. Presented at the 3rd International Symposium on Cerebral and Spinal Cord AVM. Tokyo, April 23–24, 2000 (abstract book, p 34).
61. Kihlström L, Guo WY, Karlsson B, et al: Magnetic resonance imaging of obliterated arteriovenous malformations up to 23 years after radiosurgery. J Neurosurg 1997;86:589–593.

Comment

Chapter 5

Fredric B. Meyer

The treatment of intracranial AVMs continues to be an evolving science which reflects the influence of new technologies including advanced stereotactic radiation and endovascular techniques. Unfortunately, there are no prospective clinical trials; therefore, by default, clinicians must attempt to analyze published treatment series, which introduces profound bias and error into any attempt at comparison between therapeutic modalities. Furthermore, it is apparent that the lesions that are the most optimal for stereotactic radiation are also those that are most successfully treated with surgery.

This chapter discusses the published data on stereotactic radiation for AVMs. To summarize, the reported angiographic obliteration rate is 70 to 80%, the recurrent hemorrhage risk following treatment is 3.0 to 11.5% with a mortality of 30%, and the risk of radiation-induced complications is 3.0 to 12.5%. The difficulty with relying on these statistics is that they include a broad spectrum of AVMs with different sizes, locations, and treatment plans. Also, the completeness of patient follow-up is suspect, which is important when determining the true rate of obliteration and the risk of recurrence. Therefore, these data need to be considered as estimates for comparison with other treatment interventions. For example, a small, less than 3.0 cm AVM in a noneloquent region would likely receive a higher radiation dosage with a resultant higher rate of obliteration and less risk of neurological sequelae.

By comparison, the published data by experienced neurovascular surgeons report the following results for AVMs less than 3.0 cm in size: an obliteration rate approaching 100% with a mortality rate of less than 1.0% and permanent new neurological morbidity of 0 to 3.5%. Once again, these series contain a mixture of lesions with different locations, configurations, and vascular anatomy. Of note is that approximately 45 to 50% of AVMs in the major surgical series reside in functional brain regions.[1–8]

Given the above data combined with personal experience, my recommendations for treating AVMs are as follows:

1. The best treatment regimen should be determined by a multidisciplinary team consisting of neurovascular surgeons, radiation therapists, and endovascular neuroradiologists. Required imaging for this evaluation includes a high-resolution MRI scan including coronal images to determine the anatomical location of the vascular lesion and a

detailed complete angiogram–examining not only the AVM, but also searching for intranidal and feeding pedicle artery aneurysms and possible venous outflow obstruction.

2. Convexity AVMs with a Spetzler-Martin Grade I-III should be treated with microsurgical resection. Another way of stating this is that the lesion should be resected if the surgeon estimates a perioperative risk of 10% or less. This is especially true if the patient has suffered a hemorrhage or is having significant seizures. Risk factors for hemorrhage including an intranidal or feeding pedicle aneurysm, or evidence for venous outflow stenosis or obstruction should be a decisive factor favoring surgery.
3. Preoperative embolization is a useful adjunct in decreasing intraoperative hemorrhage and the risk of postoperative hyperemia and should be utilized routinely.
4. Following surgical resection, an angiogram should be performed prior to patient discharge. If there is some intraoperative concern about the completeness of resection, then the angiogram should be performed immediately after surgery while the patient is still anesthetized.
5. Complex large AVMs will often require a team approach with multiple interventions including embolization, surgical resection, and possibly stereotactic radiation of a residual lesion if present.
6. Deep-seated AVMs in the midbrain and basal ganglia should be treated with stereotactic radiation. In patients who have suffered a hemorrhage, preradiation embolization of feeding pedicle or intranidal aneurysms should be strongly considered to decrease the risk of hemorrhage during the latency period following radiation.
7. The treatment of giant hemispheric AVMs remains a Herculean challenge in which there are currently no definitive good treatment options. Fractionated radiation, multistage embolization and surgery, surgery with hypothermia techniques, and a combination of these modalities have been attempted with only fair results.
8. Long-term radiographic and clinical follow-up is mandatory for AVMs irrespective of the treatment rendered.

References

1. Hamilton MG, Spetzler RF: The prospective application of a grading system for arteriovenous malformations. Neurosurgery 1994;34:2–7.
2. Heros RC, Korosue K, Diebold PM: Surgical excision of cerebral arteriovenous malformations: late results. Neurosurgery 1990;26:570–578.
3. Pickus HJ, Beach ML, Harbaugh RE: Microsurgical treatment of arteriovenous malformations: analysis and comparison with stereotactic radiation. J Neurosurg 1998;88:641–646.
4. Porter PJ, Shin AY, Detsky AS, et al: Surgery verses stereotactic radiosurgery for small, operable cerebral arteriovenous malformations: a clinical and cost comparison. Neurosurgery 1997;41:757–764.

5. Schaller C, Schramm J: Microsurgical results for small arteriovenous malformations accessible for radiosurgical or embolization treatment. Neurosurgery 1997;40:664–675.
6. Sisti MB, Kader A, Stein BM: Microsurgery for 67 intracranial arteriovenous malformations less than 3 cm in diameter. J Neurosurg 1993;79:653–660.
7. Sundt TM Jr, Piepgras DG, Stevens LN: Surgery for supratentorial arteriovenous malformations. Proceedings of the Congress of Neurological Surgeons. Clin Neurosurg 1991;37:49–115.
8. Tew JM Jr, Lewis AI, Reichert KW: Management strategies and surgical techniques for deep-seated supratentorial arteriovenous malformations. Neurosurgery 1995;36:1065–1072

Chapter 6

Stereotactic Radiosurgery for Dural Arteriovenous Fistulae

Michael J. Link, Bruce E. Pollock, Douglas A. Nichols, Jonathan A. Friedman, Deborah A. Gorman, Robert L. Foote, Scott L. Stafford

Introduction

Dural arteriovenous fistulae (DAVFs) are acquired vascular malformations that are distinct from parenchymal arteriovenous malformations (AVMs). The first DAVF was described in 1951.[1] Currently, DAVFs are believed to represent approximately 10 to 15% of all intracranial vascular malformations.[2] Houser et al, in the early 1970s, further defined the angiographic characteristics of DAVFs and related their development to venous sinus thrombosis.[3,4] The etiology, natural history, and treatment of these lesions have been extensively studied over the past three decades. Stereotactic radiosurgery, often accompanied by embolization, has emerged as a safe and effective treatment for DAVFs. We have treated 105 patients with DAVFs in various locations using this strategy over the past 10 years. This chapter will review patient selection, technique, results, and complications of DAVF radiosurgery.

Pathogenesis

Dural arteriovenous fistulae consist of a nidus of arteriovenous shunting within the dura mater. Usually, this occurs in proximity or continuity to a major dural venous sinus or cortical vein. Multiple hypotheses have been advanced regarding the pathogenesis of DAVFs based on

From Pollock BE (ed). *Contemporary Stereotactic Radiosurgery: Technique and Evaluation.* Armonk, NY, Futura Publishing Company, Inc. © 2002.

clinical observation, examination of resected pathological specimens, and animal experiments investigating various possible provocative factors. One of the main theories regarding the development of DAVFs relates dural sinus thrombosis and the development of venous hypertension as the hallmark events.[5,6] It is hypothesized that normal microscopic arteriovenous shunts in the dural sinus wall enlarge following sinus thrombosis in response to venous hypertension. Increased blood flow through these fistulous channels leads to further venous hypertension as the patent portion of the sinus is exposed to arterial inflow pressure. This induces further thrombosis related to turbulent flow within the sinus and high pressures, and a spiral of events that increases the size of the lesion and the arteriovenous shunting. This theory has been tested in a rodent model in which carotid to external jugular vein anastomoses, often combined with experimentally induced sinus thrombosis, resulted in venous hypertension and the development of DAVFs.[7,8] While an association between dural sinus thrombosis and DAVF development has been well established, there must be additional factors in their genesis. Not all patients with sinus thrombosis develop DAVFs, and conversely, some DAVFs are seen without evidence of sinus thrombosis and even without association with a venous sinus at all, such as those of the anterior cranial fossa.

Another theory on DAVF formation posits that angiogenic factors released from the brain or dura causes blood vessels to develop in response to local factors such as venous hypertension resulting in a DAVF. Surgical DAVF specimens have been shown to contain basic fibroblastic growth factor (bFGF), a potent angiogenic growth stimulator.[9] Lawton et al demonstrated increased angiogenesis in a rat model of venous hypertension and sinus thrombosis.[10] They suggested that venous hypertension induces angiogenic activity by decreasing cerebral perfusion, causing ischemia, and that DAVFs may be the result of this induced aberrant angiogenesis. If this is the case, antiangiogenic mediators could provide an additional treatment strategy for DAVFs.

Another possible factor in the pathogenesis of DAVFs that has received little attention in the literature is hypercoagulability.[11] It has been our clinical impression that many patients with DAVFs are hypercoagulable. This may predispose them to venous sinus thrombosis and the development of DAVFs, and also account for their spontaneous obliteration in some patients. We have sporadically screened patients for hypercoagulability, particularly those with a suggestive history, e.g., prior deep venous thrombosis, multiple miscarriages, and stroke. The screening includes prothrombin, partial thromboplastin, thrombin and bleeding times, protein S and C levels, screening for antiphospholipid and anticardiolipin antibodies, Leiden factor V mutation, homocysteine levels, and complete blood count. Although we have been unable to demonstrate a specific coagulation abnormality in these patients, we continue to feel that they are at risk for thrombotic complications.

The issue of whether DAVFs result from "enlargement" of preexisting vessels in the dura or from newly formed aberrant vessels has implications for the predicted success of radiosurgery. Animal models confirm the clinical observation that normal blood vessels are relatively radioresistant to single-fraction gamma irradiation.[12,13] On the other hand, if newly formed vessels in DAVFs are analogous to congenital AVM vessels, with thin walls and absent, discontinuous, or reduplicated elastic laminae, they would be predicted to respond to radiosurgery as do true AVMs.[14,15] To date, histologic review of resected specimens has not answered this question definitively.[4,9,16]

Natural History

Several authors have performed extensive reviews of published cases to elucidate the natural history of DAVFs.[17–19] No lesion location is immune from potential aggressive behavior (i.e., hemorrhage, seizures, progressive neurological deficit) (Table 1). Angiographic findings of retrograde cortical venous drainage, variceal or aneurysmal venous structures, and galenic venous drainage are reported to predispose DAVFs to aggressive clinical behavior.[18] However, the frequency with which these features might also be present in more benign cases remains unknown because of the bias toward discovering and reporting symptomatic or aggressive cases.

Brown et al reported 54 untreated patients with DAVFs who were followed for a mean of 6.6 years. Five patients experienced an intracranial hemorrhage for an estimated annual risk of bleeding of 1.8%.[20] Most hemorrhages occurred early, within 3 years of diagnosis. They concluded that only variceal venous drainage was a predictor of future hemorrhage. The

Table 1
Reported Frequency of Hemorrhage for Dural Arteriovenous Fistulae*

Location	*% Presenting with Hemorrhage*
Tentorial-incisura	80–90%
Anterior cranial fossa	60–80%
Sylvian-middle fossa	60–70%
Convexity-SSS	50–60%
Transverse-sigmoid	15–20%
Cavernous sinus	10–15%

SSS, superior sagittal sinus.
*Adapted from Awad IA, et al.[18]

risk of rebleeding was recently addressed by Duffau et al.[21] These investigators followed 20 patients who presented with hemorrhage from DAVFs. All of the patients had cortical venous drainage. Four patients had radiographic documented rebleeding and another three had clinical suspicion of rebleeding for a recurrent hemorrhage rate of 20 to 35%. These rebleeding episodes all occurred within 2 weeks of the original presenting hemorrhage and were associated with worsened neurological deficits.

Presentation

Lesions of the transverse/sigmoid sinus region, including the petrosal sinuses, jugular bulb, and marginal sinus usually present with pulsatile tinnitus. By the time the patient is referred for neurosurgical consultation, a bruit is often audible over the mastoid or temporal regions. The majority of patients report tinnitus that starts rather insidiously and becomes progressively louder over the ensuing months or years prior to presentation. Provided that there is no cortical venous drainage, these are usually benign lesions. However, the tinnitus may be so distracting to the patient that it prevents sleep. For this reason, curative or at least palliative treatment is indicated.

Carotid cavernous sinus DAVFs may also present with intractable tinnitus. More often, however, patients have prominent eye findings including proptosis, chemosis, extraocular motion palsies, and progressive visual loss. This usually occurs when the normal drainage from the cavernous sinus is thrombosed and the ophthalmic venous system is subjected to arterial pressure. The intraocular pressure may be acutely elevated with significant risk to vision. In these cases, urgent treatment is indicated. As before, if there is prominent cortical venous drainage, hemorrhage is also a risk.

DAVFs not associated with a major venous sinus, such as those of the anterior cranial fossa or the tentorial incisura, are felt by most authors to remain asymptomatic until they present with hemorrhage. Seizures or progressive neurological deficits without hemorrhage, related to venous hypertension and ischemia, are also possible. Because the only potential venous drainage for these lesions is into leptomeningeal veins, they are always considered for treatment.

Treatment Options

Treatment for DAVFs has evolved over the past three decades. For minimally symptomatic or asymptomatic lesions, observation alone has often been recommended, principally because there are many documented cases of spontaneous regression of DAVFs.[22–32] Intermittent manual vascular compression of the ipsilateral carotid or occipital arteries has also been effective in producing thrombosis of the arteriovenous shunts in select patients.[33,34] Surgical resection of the fistulous dura, often including a portion of the sinus, became a prominent method of treatment through the 1970s and 1980s.[18,19,35–38] As the pathophysiology of DAVFs has become better elucidated, some authors have reported success with surgical disconnection of the arterialized cortical veins, preserving a patent sinus.[39–43]

Endovascular treatment has emerged as the primary treatment for the majority of patients with DAVFs, particularly for lesions involving the cavernous sinus which are difficult to cure with acceptable morbidity by direct surgical approaches.[26,30,33,34,44–63] However, recanalization of DAVFs occurs particularly with long-term follow-up.[4,26,30,34,44,49,50,53,62–68] More recently, transvenous embolization has been advocated as the preferred endovascular treatment route, reporting greater success with fewer complications compared to transarterial embolization.[67–74]

Radiosurgery, using a variety of techniques, has also come to light as a viable treatment option for DAVFs.[75–87] We reported our initial experience with 29 patients in 1996.[88] Since that time, radiosurgery has become the main treatment modality for DAVFs at our institution (Table 2).

Treatment Rationale

Radiosurgery was expected to cause obliteration of the DAVFs between 1 and 3 years after treatment analogous to the AVM experience. Transarterial embolization, usually performed within 48 hours following

Table 2
Number of Cases of Dural Arteriovenous Fistulae Treated with Radiosurgery at the Mayo Clinic 1990–October 2000*

Years	*No. of DAVF Radiosurgical Procedures*	*No. of DAVF Microsurgical Procedures*
1990–1993	23	26
1994–1996	33	21
1997–1999	45	13
2000†	11	1

DAVF, dural arteriovenous fistula.

*One hundred five patients treated; five patients treated with two sessions and one patient treated with three sessions. Number of cases treated primarily with microsurgical resection during the same time period.

†January–October 2000.

radiosurgery, provided early palliative relief of intractable tinnitus, orbital venous congestion, diplopia, etc. In addition, it substantially reduced or eliminated the cortical venous drainage, reducing the risk of hemorrhage during the radiosurgery latency period. Even if recanalization of the embolized fistula were to occur, the fistula would be undergoing simultaneous radiosurgery-induced obliteration. Embolization is performed after radiosurgery to avoid the pitfall of having embolization temporarily obscure portions of the nidus that would not be irradiated during the radiosurgical procedure. Thus, the combination of radiosurgery and transarterial embolization, whenever possible, provides both rapid symptom relief and long-term cure of DAVFs.

Patient Characteristics and Radiosurgery Technique

Patients

Between October 1990 and October 2000 we managed 105 DAVF patients with radiosurgery using the Gamma Knife® (Elekta Instruments, Norcross, GA) combined with particulate embolization of accessible external carotid artery (ECA)-feeding vessels in selected cases. Five patients were treated with two sessions of radiosurgery and one patient was treated with three sessions. The patients included 75 women and 30 men. The mean age at the time of treatment was 58.5 years (range, 20–80 years). All but a few patients, whose DAVFs were incidentally discovered during work-up for unrelated neurological complaints, had symptoms and/or signs referable to their fistula at the time of diagnosis (Table 3).

Table 3
Clinical Presenting Signs and Symptoms of 105 Patients with Dural Arteriovenous Fistulae Treated with Gamma Knife Radiosurgery*

Signs/Symptoms	*No. of Patients*
Intractable tinnitus/bruit or vascular headache	66
Chemosis, ophthalmoplegia or visual loss	41
Hemorrhage	11
Altered mental status	4
Seizures	2
Other neurological deficit	4

*Some patients experienced more than one category of signs/symptoms.

Two patients underwent surgical ligation of ECA-feeding vessels prior to referral for radiosurgery. Another two patients had undergone successful surgical obliteration of DAVFs at other locations prior to radiosurgery. In these cases, the microsurgically treated lesions had significant cortical venous drainage. Six patients had undergone noncurative transarterial embolization, and one patient also had transvenous embolization, of their DAVFs before being referred for radiosurgery. Treatment prior to radiosurgery did not completely obliterate the fistula in any of the cases.

Characteristics of DAVFs

All patients underwent thorough neurological, and for the patients with cavernous sinus DAVFs, ophthalmological evaluation, prior to treatment to provide baseline data for comparison during follow-up. All DAVFs were defined using conventional transfemoral cerebral angiography. This often included bilateral selective internal carotid artery (ICA), ECA, and vertebral artery (VA) injections to completely define the areas of arteriovenous shunting and venous drainage. Super selective injection of ECA branches was occasionally performed to delineate very complex lesions, and to better assess the feasibility of postradiosurgical embolization. The locations of the DAVFs in this series are summarized in Table 4. Thirty patients had evidence of cortical venous drainage on the initial diagnostic angiogram.

Table 4
Location of Dural Arteriovenous Fistulae in 105 Patients Treated with Gamma Knife Radiosurgery

Location	*No. of Patients*
Transverse/sigmoid sinus*	39
Cavernous sinus	33
Petrosal sinus	10
Jugular/condylar	8
Convexity dura	5
Torula-SSS	5
Tentorial notch	2
Vein of Galen	2
Multiple locations	1

SSS, superior sagittal sinus.

*Includes dural arteriovenous fistulae that also had a component involving the petrosal sinuses, torcula, straight sinus, SSS, and/or jugular bulb.

Radiosurgical Treatment Planning

All patients were treated using local anesthesia and oral benzodiazepine sedation for head frame placement. Proper head frame placement is critical when treating DAVFs at the periphery of the head, such as those of the transverse-sigmoid region or jugular bulb. In order to reach very inferior targets and avoid collisions of the head frame with the collimator helmet when using the Model U, it was sometimes necessary to place the anterior pins of the head frame in the maxillary prominences. Also, many patients had to be treated in the prone position when using the Model U. We have not found this necessary with the Model B, but correct head frame placement remains critically important.

High-resolution biplane, stereotactic cerebral angiography that included selective ECA, ICA, and/or VA injections, when appropriate, was used for targeting. For most cases, stereotactic computed tomography (CT) or magnetic resonance imaging (MRI) was also used. This is particularly helpful in identifying adjacent critical structures such as the optic nerves for cavernous sinus DAVFs, and the brainstem and cerebellum for transverse/sigmoid DAVFs. With current dose-planning software, the dose to these structures can be easily calculated, and the dose plan adjusted accordingly.

Based on the acquired stereotactic imaging, dose plans were constructed using the dose-planning systems available during the past 10 years (KULA system, 1990–1992; Gamma Plan System, 1993–present) to cover the entire fistulous site within the 50% isodose line. There are important distinctions between dose planning for parenchymal AVMs and DAVFs. For parenchymal AVMs, the nidus usually receives 50 to 100% of the prescribed dose due to the inhomogeneity of the radiation delivered, with the expectation that the shunting vessels within the nidus of an AVM receive the highest dose or close to it, for maximal benefit. For DAVFs, because they are often located in the wall of a venous sinus, the highest dose is delivered to the flowing blood elements within the lumen of the sinus, and the targeted fistulous vessels may only receive the margin dose. However, because most DAVFs are surrounded by non-neurological tissue (bone, cerebrospinal fluid, scalp), even extensive fistulae with large-volume dose plans can be safely treated (Fig. 1). The median radiation dose to the margin in the 105 patients treated was 19 Gy (range, 15–25 Gy). The median maximum dose was 38 Gy (range, 22–50 Gy). The mean prescription isodose volume was 6.4 cm^3 (range, 0.35–30.8 cm^3) using one to eleven isocenters (median, 5).

Embolization

Transarterial particulate embolization was undertaken in addition to radiosurgery in 68 patients, usually within 48 hours after the radiosurgi-

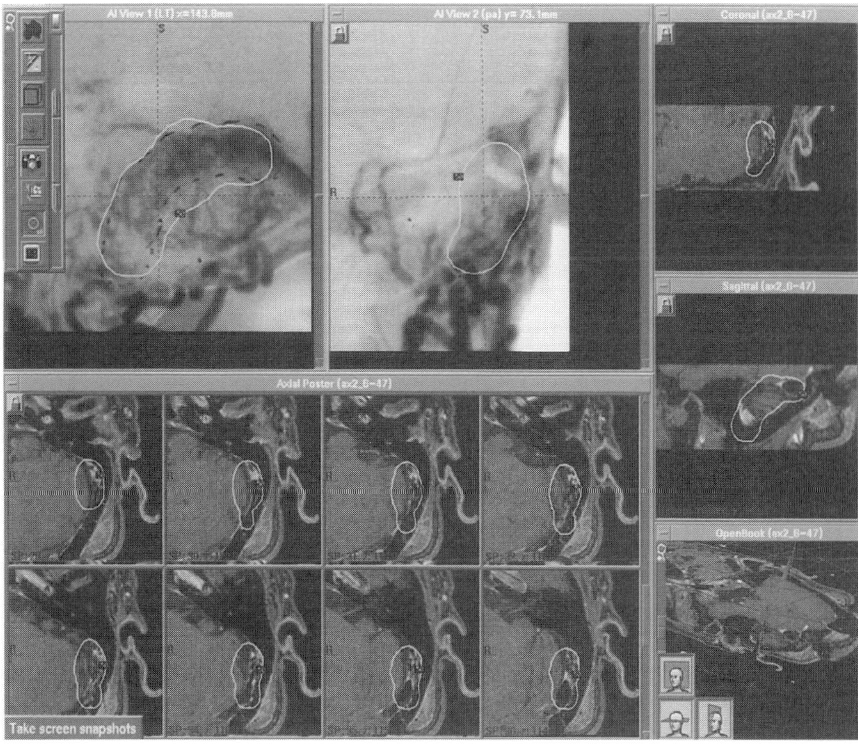

Figure 1. Typical radiosurgical dose plan for a transverse-sigmoid dural arteriovenous fistula (DAVF) without cortical venous drainage. The stereotactic lateral and AP digital subtraction angiograms are scanned directly into GammaPlan (Elekta Instruments, Norcross, GA) and the dose plan can be directly correlated to the stereotactic MRI scan in axial, coronal, and sagittal imaging planes.

cal procedure. The goal of embolization was to reduce cortical venous drainage, intractable tinnitus, or ocular/visual symptoms. Five patients underwent embolization procedures elsewhere prior to being referred for radiosurgery; four via a transarterial route and one via a transarterial and transvenous approach. One patient with a complicated bilateral cavernous carotid DAVF was embolized at our institution prior to undergoing radiosurgery. She had such extensive cortical venous drainage that it significantly impeded angiographic visualization of the fistula site before embolization. Embolization was successful in substantially reducing (n=26) or eliminating (n=4) cortical venous drainage in all cases. All patients with intractable tinnitus noted immediate and substantial relief after embolization. Polyvinyl alcohol particles were the primary embolization materials used; in conjunction with silk suture, gelfoam, and fibered microcoils in select cases.

Follow-Up

Most patients were observed in the hospital 24 hours after treatment. Recently, we have begun to perform both radiosurgery and embolization in the outpatient setting without complication. Patients were scheduled to return 1-year post treatment for follow-up neurological and/or ophthalmological evaluation. If new neurological symptoms developed, CT and/or MRI scanning was performed to investigate for hemorrhage or adverse radiation effects. If presenting symptoms of tinnitus or ocular/visual difficulties recurred, angiography was performed. Four patients had recurrence of a portion of the fistula that was subsequently re-embolized with resolution of their symptoms.

Formal cerebral angiography was planned for 1 to 3 years after treatment to document obliteration of the DAVFs. While some MRI techniques are showing promise with regard to delineating DAVFs,[89] we feel digital subtraction angiography is necessary to definitively assess the results of treatment. We considered additional treatment if complete angiographic obliteration of DAVFs did not occur by 3 years after the initial radiosurgical procedure.

Results

The clinical and angiographic results of this series regarding the first 29 and 67 patients have been reported in 1996 and 1998, respectively.[88,90] For the entire series of 105 patients, there have been no adverse radiation-related complications. Symptomatic long-term improvement included diminished or absent bruit, relief of intractable vascular headaches, disappearance of chemosis, proptosis, and/or resolution of extraocular motion deficits. Fifty of 105 patients have undergone follow-up angiography a median of 14 months following treatment (mean, 20 months; range, 11–62 months). Thirty-four of 50 (68%) patients had documented total obliteration of their DAVFs. Seven additional patients (14%) had near-total obliteration, with only a very focal low-flow fistula remaining, and no cortical venous drainage. Nine patients (18%) have obtained only subtotal obliteration and have been encouraged to return for further follow-up and possible treatment. The results for patients with cavernous sinus DAVFs and transverse-sigmoid DAVFs, the two most common types, are reviewed in detail.[83,91]

Cavernous Sinus DAVFs

The results of treatment for the first 20 patients with cavernous sinus DAVFs were reviewed from a prospectively established database.[83] The patients included 17 women and 3 men. The median patient age was

67 years old (range, 34–80 years old). All patients had symptoms referable to their fistula at the time of presentation. There was no history of intracranial hemorrhage. Four patients had cortical venous drainage on pretreatment diagnostic angiography. The median prescription isodose volume was 2.8 cm^3 (range, 0.7–7.5 cm^3). The median marginal radiation dose was 20 Gy (range, 18–20 Gy). The median maximal radiation dose was 40 Gy (range, 22.2–40 Gy). Twelve patients underwent particulate embolization following radiosurgery.

Clinical follow-up data were available for all patients for a median of 36 months after radiosurgery (range, 4–59 months). Overall, 19 patients (95%) experienced some symptom improvement. Chemosis and/or proptosis improved significantly ($n = 2$) or resolved completely ($n = 15$) for 17 of 18 affected individuals (94%). Most notably, seven of eight patients (88%) with decreased visual fields or visual acuity regained normal vision. One patient experienced worsened vision secondary to choroidal detachment and closed-angle glaucoma. Diplopia completely resolved ($n = 8$) or improved ($n = 2$) in 10 of 13 patients (77%) with this symptom prior to treatment. One patient with persistent diplopia related to sixth nerve palsy underwent medial rectus muscle resection 34 months after radiosurgery. No difference in symptom improvement was noted between patients treated using radiosurgery alone (100%) and patients treated using radiosurgery and transarterial embolization (92%, $p = 1.0$). However, the median time to symptom improvement was shorter for the patients who underwent both radiosurgery and embolization, compared with the patients who underwent only radiosurgery (2 weeks vs. 6 months, $p<0.001$).

Two patients underwent repeat transarterial particulate embolization procedures at our institution, 7 and 12 months, respectively, after the initial procedures, because of recurrent symptoms. Both patients again noted resolution of their symptoms but had residual arteriovenous shunting seen on angiography at the conclusion of the repeat embolization procedures. Subsequent follow-up angiograms revealed complete obliteration of their fistulae and they had no further symptoms. One other patient experienced increasing intraocular pressure and worsening of her vision 4 months after radiosurgery and embolization. Transvenous coil occlusion of the cavernous sinus was performed at another institution with rapid improvement in her chemosis and intraocular pressure. Her visual acuity has returned to normal, but diplopia persists.

Thirteen of 15 patients (87%) for whom follow-up angiography could be obtained experienced complete obliteration of their DAVFs. Follow-up angiograms were acquired a median of 12 months (range, 4–33 months) after treatment. One patient underwent repeat angiography and transvenous embolization elsewhere, 4 months after treatment as detailed above, with complete angiographic obliteration. One patient had marked improvement of her chemosis, proptosis, and visual loss 13 months after radiosurgery. Follow-up angiography at that time revealed 95% obliteration of her fistula with only a small component from the intracavernous ICA remaining. She remains asymptomatic 33 months after radiosurgery and refuses to undergo further angiography. Five additional patients remain asymptomatic and have refused follow-up angiography.

Transverse-Sigmoid DAVFs

The clinical and angiographic results of the first 25 patients with pure transverse-sigmoid DAVFs (excluding patients who also had a component involving the petrosal sinuses, jugular bulb, straight sinus, or torcula) were also reviewed.[91] The patients included 18 women and 7 men. The median age at the time of treatment was 57 years old (range, 33–79 years old). Twenty-two patients presented with pulsatile tinnitus, two patients had a prior history of intracranial hemorrhage, and one transverse-sigmoid DAVF was discovered incidentally. Four patients in this subgroup also had evidence of cortical venous drainage pretreatment, two of which had a history of hemorrhage. All four of these patients were felt to be high risk for open surgery due to advanced age and medical comorbidity. The median prescription isodose volume was 9.6 cm^3 (range, 2.7–29.6 cm^3) reflecting how anatomically extensive these fistulae can be in comparison with the more localized cavernous sinus DAVFs. The median margin dose was 18 Gy (range, 16–20 Gy). The median maximum radiation dose was 36 Gy (range, 32–40 Gy). Seventeen patients underwent transarterial embolization following radiosurgery during one ($n = 13$) or more ($n = 4$) sessions.

The mean clinical follow-up after radiosurgery was 50 months (range, 33–79 months). Symptoms completely resolved in 20 patients (87%) and were significantly improved in two (9%). One patient was clinically unchanged, but declined further treatment. No clinical follow-up could be obtained for two patients. Two patients who initially had good resolution of their symptoms after radiosurgery and embolization had recurrence of their symptoms at 10 and 12 months, respectively. Follow-up angiography in one patient showed greater than 50% reduction in the size of the fistula. This patient ultimately underwent repeat radiosurgery and embolization 38 months after the initial procedure. In the other patient, a greater than 50% reduction in the size of the fistula was also seen on follow-up angiography. However, a new area of fistulization had developed adjacent to the previously treated DAVF. This patient was also retreated with stereotactic radiosurgery and transarterial embolization 21 months after the initial procedure. No patient suffered an intracranial hemorrhage or radiation-related complication during the follow-up period.

Seventeen patients had angiographic follow-up at a mean of 21 months after radiosurgery (range, 11–38 months). Total angiographic obliteration of the DAVF was seen in seven patients (41%). Four patients

(24%) had greater than 95% obliteration. The remaining six patients (35%) for which follow-up angiography could be obtained had greater than 50% reduction in the size of the fistulae.

Complications

In the series of 105 patients, complications from treatment were rare. Six patients developed new neurological symptoms during diagnostic angiography before treatment or during follow-up. Three patients developed confusion without focal neurological deficit that resolved within 24 hours. One patient developed left hemiparesis and was discovered to have an embolus in the right middle cerebral artery. Immediate intra-arterial thrombolysis was performed with resolution of the neurological deficit. Another patient developed dysarthria and hemiparesis that resolved completely over several months. During transarterial embolization procedures for transverse-sigmoid or petrosal DAVFs, three patients developed transient facial weakness. This was undoubtedly due to occlusion of vasa nervosa to the facial nerve from embolized ECA branches. Occasional patients also reported facial or head pain ipsilateral to embolized ECA branches that resolved within days to weeks. One patient with a cavernous sinus DAVF developed a small venous infarct during postradiosurgical embolization, resulting in transient aphasia, which improved in the months after the procedure. Another patient developed transient vertigo with permanent unilateral hearing loss 1 year after radiosurgery and embolization of an ipsilateral transverse sinus DAVF. Review of the radiosurgical dose plan revealed that the vestibulocochlear system was well outside the radiosurgical treatment field. The symptoms may have been secondary to propagation of venous thrombus to the cochlear venous system as the DAVF became obliterated.[27]

One patient experienced a fatal hemorrhage, 17 months after radiosurgery for a superior sagittal sinus (SSS) DAVF. This 44-year-old man initially presented in 1992 with seizures, and was discovered to have a high-flow Spetzler-Martin Grade III AVM in the right occipital lobe. He was treated with Gamma Knife radiosurgery in 1993. A dose plan consisting of 11 isocenters of radiation was used to cover a volume of 36.4 cm^3. The dose to the margin was 16 Gy and the maximum dose was 32 Gy. Follow-up angiography in 1997 revealed complete obliteration of the parenchymal AVM. However, a DAVF, previously angiographically obscured by the AVM, became apparent, fed by branches of the ECA and draining via a single right occipital cortical vein to the SSS. The DAVF was treated in 1997, also with 11 isocenters of radiation to cover a volume of 8.8 cm^3. The dose to the margin was 16 Gy and the maximum dose was 32 Gy. Seventeen months after treatment, he was admitted to his local hospital after collapsing at work. A non-contrast CT scan showed diffuse subarachnoid blood without intraparenchymal hemorrhage. He died 3 days later. While autopsy could not confirm it, the hemorrhage was most likely secondary to the DAVF. There have been no other clinical or radiographic hemorrhages in the 105 patients treated to date, including those patients who initially presented with hemorrhage, and/or had cortical venous drainage.

Illustrative Cases

Case 1

M.J.P. is a 54-year-old man who presented in 1992 with a 3- to 4-year history of progressive left greater than right pulsatile tinnitus. On examination he had mild left eye proptosis and an audible bruit over the left temporal region. An angiogram revealed a DAVF involving the left cavernous sinus with no cortical venous drainage (Figs. 2A–2D). On May 1, 1992 he underwent Gamma Knife radiosurgery using five isocenters of radiation. The fistula was covered by the 50% isodose line and received 18 Gy. The maximum dose was 36 Gy. His symptoms gradually resolved over the ensuing year, and follow-up angiography 16 months later confirmed complete obliteration of the DAVF (Figs. 2E and 2F).

Case 2

B.A. is a 47-year-old woman who presented in 1996 with a 1-year history of progressive pulsatile tinnitus involving the right ear. Her neurological examination was normal. A pulsatile bruit, synchronous with her pulse, was audible over her right mastoid region and temporal bone. A transfemoral cerebral angiogram revealed a right transverse-sigmoid DAVF fed by branches of the right ICA and ECA (Figs. 3A and 3B). It drained antegrade into the transverse-sigmoid sinus. There was no evidence of cortical venous drainage or sinus thrombosis. She was treated with five isocenters of radiation to cover a volume of 13.3 cm^3. The dose to the margin was 18 Gy and the maximum dose was 36 Gy. The following day she underwent transarterial embolization of the accessible ECA feeding vessels. Her tinnitus was significantly reduced following embolization, but angiography at the conclusion of this procedure did reveal some persistent arteriovenous shunting. Her tinnitus completely resolved by 1-year post treatment and follow-up angiography 14 months after radiosurgery and embolization revealed complete obliteration of the DAVF (Figs. 3C–3F).

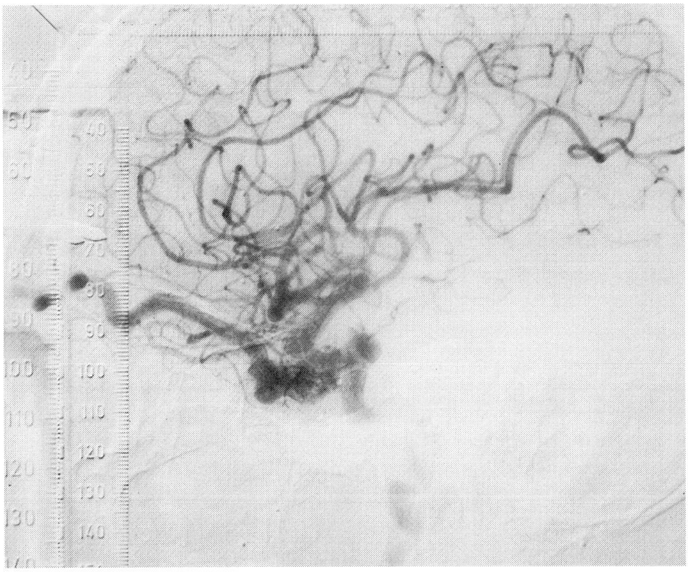

A

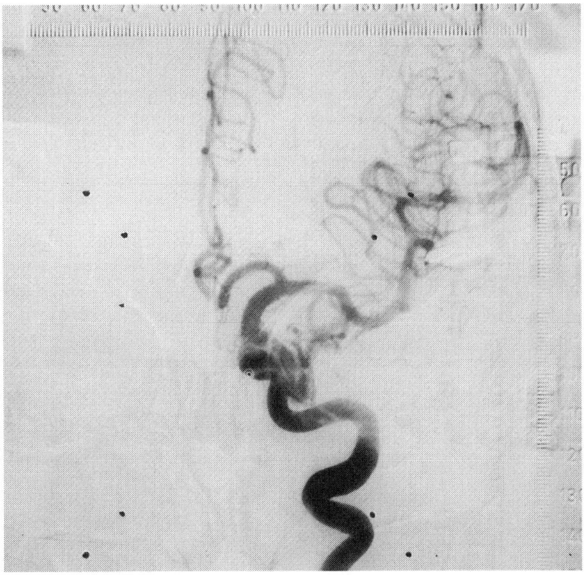

B

Figures 2A–2D. Lateral (**A**) and AP (**B**) selective left internal carotid artery and lateral (**C**) and anterior-posterior (**D**) selective left external carotid artery injections reveal a left cavernous DAVF with venous drainage via the left superior ophthalmic vein. *(Continued.)*

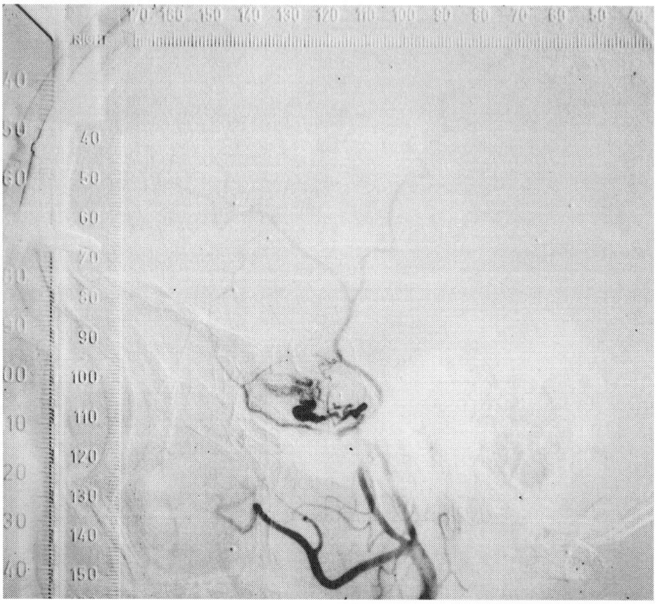

C

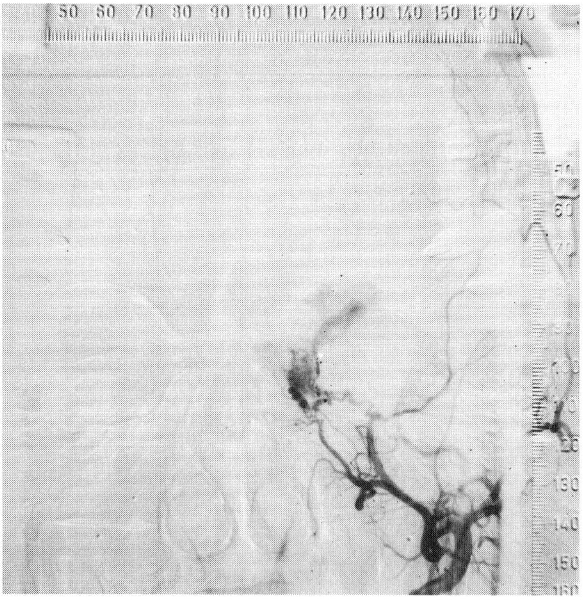

D

Figure 2.

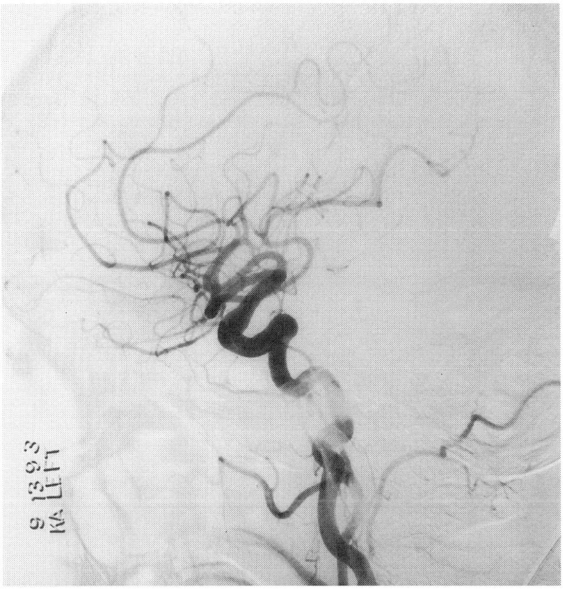

E

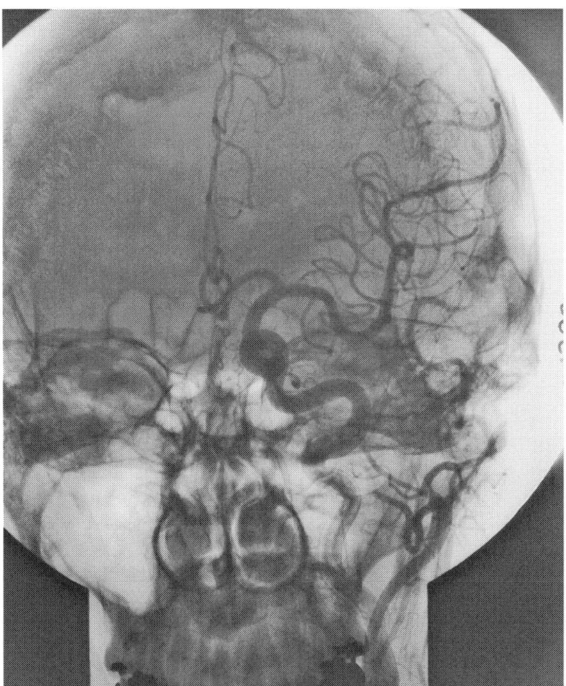

F

Figures 2E and 2F. Lateral (**E**) and (AP) (**F**) common carotid artery injections 16 months later reveal complete obliteration of the DAVF.

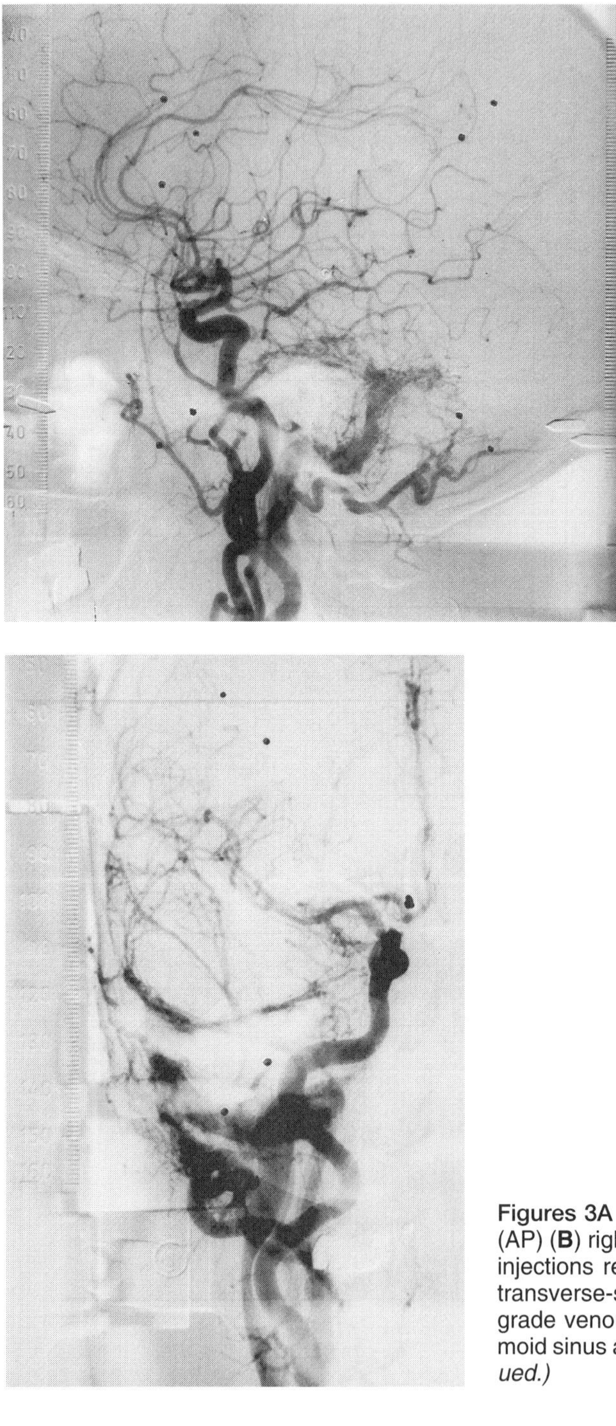

A

B

Figures 3A and 3B. Lateral (**A**) and (AP) (**B**) right common carotid artery injections reveal a DAVF of the left transverse-sigmoid sinus with antegrade venous drainage into the sigmoid sinus and jugular vein. *(Continued.)*

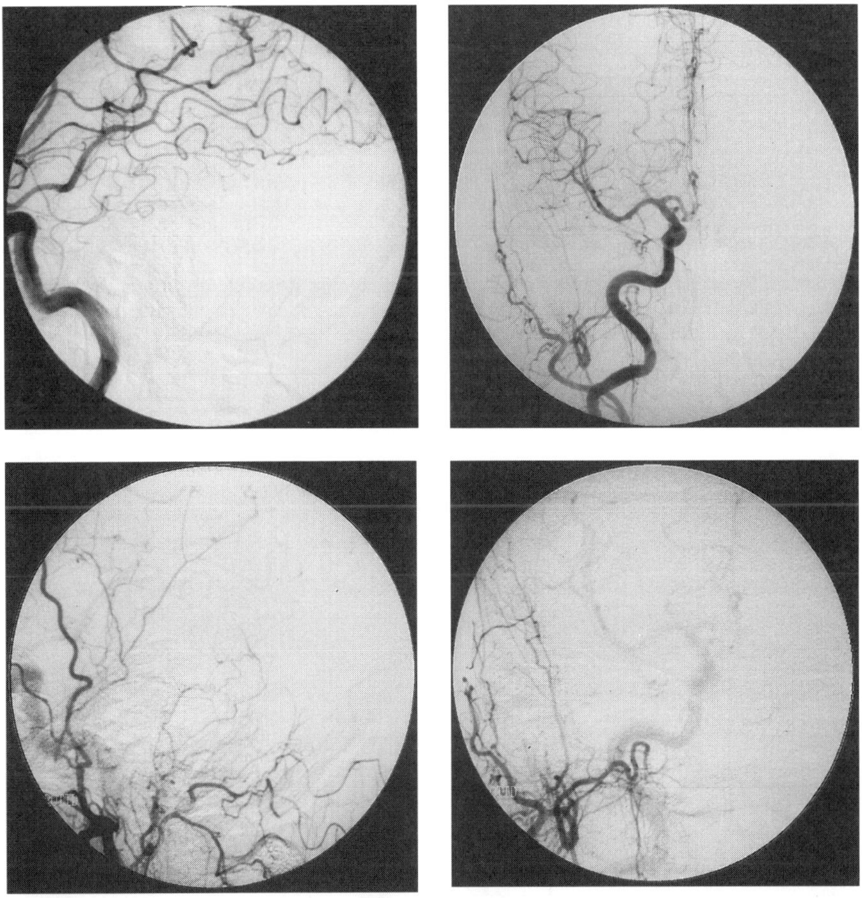

C D E F

Figures 3C–3F. Lateral (**C**) and (AP) (**D**) selective right internal carotid artery and lateral (**E**) and anterior-posterior (**F**) selective right external carotid artery injections 14 months after treatment reveal complete obliteration of the DAVF.

Case 3

G.M. is a 58-year-old woman who presented in 1999 with a 3-month history of right greater than left pulsatile tinnitus and headache. Her neurological examination was normal except for absence of venous pulsations on funduscopy. A transfemoral cerebral angiogram revealed a DAVF involving the posterior SSS, torcula, straight sinus, right transverse, and sigmoid sinuses (Fig. 4A–4D). The left transverse-sigmoid system appeared occluded. There was no cortical venous drainage. She was treated with two sessions of radiosurgery to cover the entire fistulous site. During the first session, 11 isocenters of radiation were used to cover a volume of 15.2 cm^3. The dose to the prescription isodose line was 16 Gy with a maximum dose of 32 Gy. This corresponded to the straight sinus-right transverse-sigmoid component. One week later, three isocenters of radiation were used to cover a volume of 1.4 cm^3. The margin dose was 20 Gy with a maximum dose of 40 Gy. This corresponded to the SSS component. She subsequently underwent two-staged particulate embolization of the DAVF, separated by 48 hours. There were no complications following the treatment. Her tinnitus was improved and her headaches were unchanged. One month later, her tinnitus completely resolved and her headaches also did not recur. Follow-up angiography 9-months post treatment showed complete obliteration of the DAVF (Figs. 4E and 4F).

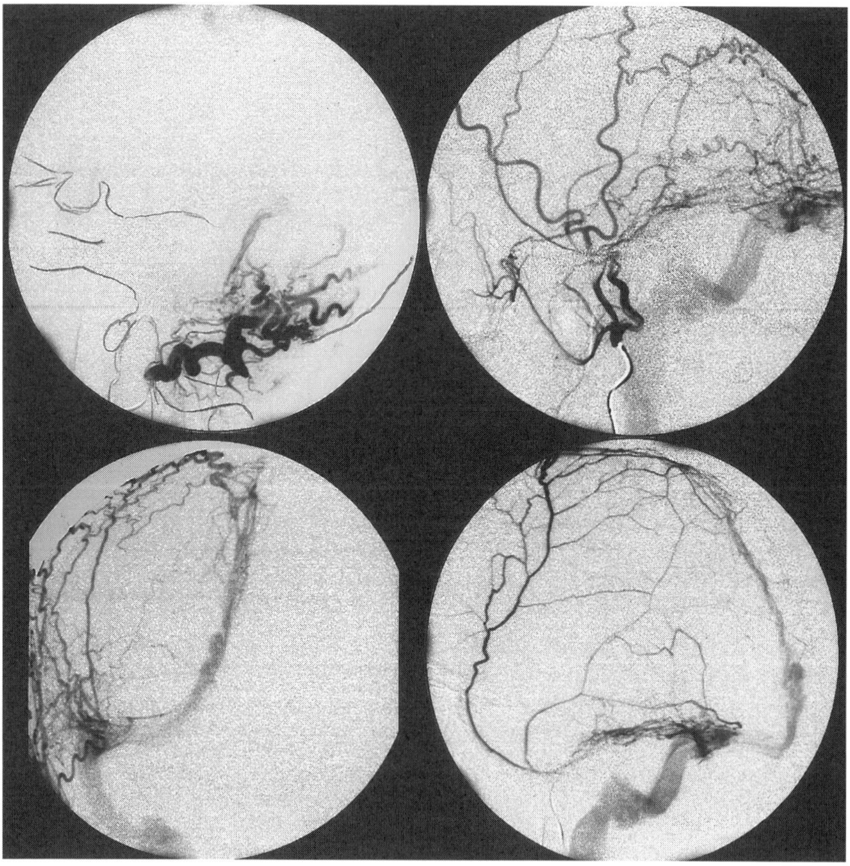

Figure 4A. Lateral selective right occipital artery (upper left), lateral selective right superficial temporal artery (upper right), anterior-posterior selective right superficial temporal artery (lower left), and selective right middle meningeal artery (lower right) injections reveal a complicated DAVF involving the superior sagittal sinus, torcula, distal straight sinus, and right transverse-sigmoid sinuses. The left transverse-sigmoid sinus was occluded. Venous drainage was antegrade into the right sigmoid sinus-jugular vein. *(Continued.)*

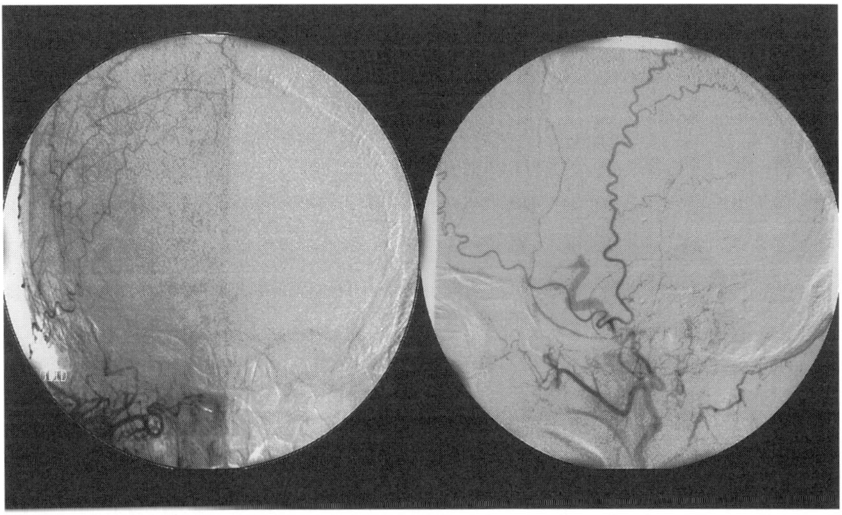

Figure 4B. Anterior-posterior (left) and lateral (right) selective right external carotid artery injections 9-months post treatment reveal complete obliteration of the DAVF.

The extensive nature of this fistula precluded single session treatment. To encompass the entire DAVF, the dose plan was too large for a single radiation treatment matrix using the available dose-planning software at the time. In addition, for such circuitous lesions at the periphery of the skull, a single head frame placement was not possible to avoid collisions of the head frame with the collimator helmet when trying to reach all shots. Current gamma plan software that includes the capability of multiple matrices has solved the former limitation.

Discussion

The treatment of DAVFs has evolved significantly over the past 30 years as the information regarding the etiology, pathophysiology, and natural history of these lesions has progressed. Patients with DAVFs that have bled or are associated with significant symptoms warrant treatment. Also, those with angiographic features suggestive of an aggressive clinical course should be considered for treatment, independent of symptom severity.

Our management strategy involving radiosurgery and particulate embolization has proven to be safe and effective. The rationale for this approach is that radiosurgery should cause obliteration of most DAVFs within 1 to 3 years. Embolization after radiosurgery keeps the DAVF angiographically visible for radiosurgical targeting, palliates the patient's symptoms, and protects the patient to some extent from early hemorrhage. Even if the embolized portion of the DAVF were to recanalize, the entire lesion is simultaneously undergoing radiosurgery-induced occlusion. Overall, we estimate that the angiographic obliteration rate for DAVFs at all locations is 68%, with another 14% achieving near-total (>95%) obliteration. For patients with subtotal obliteration, continued follow-up is warranted. Retreatment is considered for patients with recurrent intractable symptoms or persistent cortical venous drainage.

Patients with cavernous sinus DAVFs have had the most gratifying results from this treatment paradigm with an 87% complete angiographic obliteration rate. The reason that these lesions respond so favorably in comparison to other DAVFs is uncertain, but may relate to the larger size, longer segment of involved sinus, more complex geometry, multiplicity and variety of feeding vessels, or flow characteristics of noncavernous DAVFs. Barcia-Salorio et al also reported good results when treating low-flow carotid-cavernous fistulae.[75] They treated 22 spontaneous, cavernous sinus DAVFs with a cobalt source, with 5- to 10-mm collimators. A total dose of 30 to 40 Gy was delivered in all cases. Twenty of 22 fistulae (90.9%) completely closed in a mean period of 7.5 months (range, 2–20 months) after radiosurgery.[75] Guo et al likewise treated 18 patients with cavernous sinus DAVFs with Gamma Knife radiosurgery.[87] The mean prescription dose was 28 Gy (range, 22–38 Gy) to the 50 to 90% isodose lines. The DAVFs were obliterated in 12 of 15 patients (80%) in which follow-up angiography was available.[87]

Other centers have also reported success with radiosurgery for DAVFs. Chandler and Friedman successfully treated one case of an anterior cranial fossa DAVF using linear accelerator radiosurgery.[76] Lewis et al[80] reported seven patients with tentorial DAVFs treated with combination transarterial embolization and linear accelerator radiosurgery. After a mean follow-up period of 24 months, three fistulae were obliterated; another fistula was obliterated after a third embolization procedure (overall obliteration rate, 57%). One patient suffered a transient radiation injury to the brainstem. Shin et al treated two patients with DAVFs draining into the vein of Galen with Gamma Knife radiosurgery. The margin dose used was 20 and 25 Gy, respectively, to the 50% isodose line. Complete obliteration was confirmed at approximately 2 years after radiosurgery in both patients.[86]

Endovascular therapy alone has also been touted as a safe and effective treatment for DAVFs. Purely transarterial embolization is rarely curative and seldom sufficiently decreases shunting to induce spontaneous thrombosis of the lesion.[69] Transvenous embolization offers more dependable results, as long as the diseased segment of the sinus is completely and permanently occluded with the embolic agent, and if the normal venous drainage is rerouted through another pathway. Roy and Raymond reported anatomical cure in 21 of 24 patients (87.5%) with DAVFs in various locations utilizing primarily transvenous embolization.[70] Clinical cure was obtained in 23 patients (96%). Five transient and one permanent sixth nerve palsy occurred in 12 patients with cavernous sinus DAVFs, related to mass effect of the coils in the cavernous sinus. Halbach et al reported clinical cures in 81% and 55% of patients with cavernous sinus and transverse-sigmoid DAVFs, respectively.[92] Permanent complications occurred in 4% of patients with cavernous lesions and 5% of patients with transverse-sigmoid fistulae. Urtasun et al also reported a permanent complication rate of 5% for transverse-sigmoid DAVFs but achieved an 80% anatomical cure.[67] Our results are very comparable. In addition, radiosurgery has the distinct advantages of not requiring sacrifice of a portion of the sinus, and there is no mass effect generated as when coils are deposited in the cavernous sinus. We have not encountered any radiation related cranial neuropathies in the 33 patients treated with cavernous sinus DAVFs in our series.

For patients who present with hemorrhage or progressive neurological deficit and cortical venous drainage on angiography, surgical obliteration of the DAVF is considered, often accompanied by preoperative embolization. For cavernous sinus DAVFs this is a formidable undertaking, but has been reported with acceptable results.[93] Early experience with surgical treatment of transverse-sigmoid DAVFs at our institution yielded good outcomes in 85% of patients and a mortality rate of 7%.[38] For patients with significant medical comorbidity, or for patients unwilling to accept the risk of an open operation, Gamma Knife radiosurgery has been an excellent alternative.

Overall, the complication rate from stereotactic radiosurgery and transarterial particulate embolization is 4% transient and 2% permanent complications. One patient with a mixed AVM-DAVF hemorrhaged and died after his AVM was obliterated and his DAVF had been treated 17 months prior, for a 1% mortality rate. Almost all complications were secondary to thromboembolic events at the time of diagnostic or therapeutic angiography. This may relate to an underlying hypercoagulable state in these patients. Our current treatment paradigm requires patients undergo a minimum of three, and often four angiograms. One angiogram is done to diagnose and characterize the DAVF. Another is necessary for radiosurgical targeting on the day of radiosurgical treatment. A third angiogram is performed at the time of transarterial embolization, usually within 48 hours of radiosurgery. A final angiogram is necessary 1 to 3 years after treatment to document obliteration of the fistula. Currently, we do not feel that MRI or magnetic resonance angiography (MRA) is sufficient for either diagnosis or treatment. However, we are currently reviewing a bolus gadolinium technique of MRA for use in lieu of digital subtraction stereotactic angiography, on the day of radiosurgical treatment, to attempt to further reduce the risk to patients.[94]

We have obtained an angiographic follow-up rate of only 48% for 105 patients treated over the past 10 years. In our experience, many patients, the majority of whom are elderly, are reluctant to undergo follow-up angiography once their symptoms have resolved. Even patients with associated cortical venous drainage, who are strongly counseled regarding the possible future risk of hemorrhage, are satisfied with palliation of their symptoms and may not wish to return for radiographic proof of cure.

DAVFs are dynamic lesions and may change their pattern of venous drainage from benign sinus drainage to retrograde cortical venous drainage, as further thrombosis within the fistula occurs. Usually, this is associated with worsened or new symptoms. Therefore, careful clinical follow-up is very important. We have been able to maintain clinical follow-up for 95% of treated patients. We have not encountered either recanalization of an obliterated DAVF or recurrent symptoms following near-total obliteration. Currently, we feel that radiosurgery is a durable treatment for DAVFs.

Acknowledgments: The authors wish to express their gratitude to Robert J. Coffey, MD, for his contribution to the Mayo Clinic Radiosurgery program, 1990–1997, and Lynn Root, RN, for her assistance with collection of data.

References

1. Fincher EF: Arteriovenous fistula between the middle meningeal artery and the greater petrosal sinus: case report. Ann Surg 1951;133:886–888.
2. Newton TH, Cronqvist S: Involvement of dural arteries in intracranial arteriovenous malformations. Radiology 1969;93:1071–1078.
3. Houser OW, Baker HL Jr, Rhoton AL Jr, Okazaki H: Intracranial dural arteriovenous malformations. Radiology 1972;105:55–64.
4. Houser OW, Campbell JK, Campbell RJ, Sundt TM Jr: Arteriovenous malformation affecting the transverse dural venous sinus: an acquired lesion. Mayo Clin Proc 1979;54:651–661.
5. Chaudhary MY, Sachdev VP, Cho SH, et al: Dural arteriovenous malformation of the major venous sinuses: an acquired lesion. Am J Neuroradiol 1982;3:13–19.
6. Kutluk K, Schumacher M, Mironov A: The role of sinus thrombosis in occipital dural arteriovenous malformations-development and spontaneous closure. Neurochirurgica 1991;34:144–147.
7. Terada T, Higashida RT, Halbach VV, et al: Development of acquired arteriovenous fistulas in rats due to venous hypertension. J Neurosurg 1994;80: 884–889.
8. Herman JM, Spetzler RF, Bederson JB, et al: Genesis of a dural arteriovenous malformation in a rat model. J Neurosurg 1995;83:539–545.
9. Terada T, Tsuura M, Komai N, et al: The role of angiogenic factor bFGF in the development of dural AVFs. Acta Neurochir 1996;138:877–883.
10. Lawton MT, Jacobowitz R, Spetzler RF: Redefined role of angiogenesis in the pathogenesis of dural arteriovenous malformations. J Neurosurg 1997;87: 267–274.
11. Kraus JA, Stuper BK, Berlit P: Association of resistance to activated protein C and dural arteriovenous fistulas. J Neurol 1998;245:731–733.
12. Kamiryo T, Lopes MB, Berr SS, et al: Occlusion of the anterior cerebral artery after Gamma Knife irradiation in a rat. Acta Neurochir 1996;138:983–991.
13. Nilsson A, Wennerstrand J, Leksell D, Backlund EO: Stereotactic gamma irradiation of basilar artery in cat: preliminary experiences. Acta Radiol Oncol Radiat Phys Biol 1978;17:150–160.

14. Schneider BF, Eberhard DA, Steiner LE: Histopathology of arteriovenous malformations after gamma knife radiosurgery. J Neurosurg 1997;87:352–357.
15. Szeifert GT, Kemeny AA, Timperley WR, Foster DM: The potential role of myofibroblasts in the obliteration of arteriovenous malformations after radiosurgery. Neurosurgery 1997;40:61–66.
16. Nishijima M, Takaku A, Endo S, et al: Etiological evaluation of dural arteriovenous malformations of the lateral and sigmoid sinuses based on histopathological examinations. J Neurosurg 1992;76:600–606.
17. Lasjaunias P, Chiu M, Ter Brugge K, et al: Neurological manifestations of intracranial dural arteriovenous malformations. J Neurosurg 1986;64:724–730.
18. Awad IA, Little JR, Akarawi WP, Ahl J: Intracranial dural arteriovenous malformations: factors predisposing to an aggressive neurological course. J Neurosurg 1990;72:839–850.
19. Malik GM, Pearce JE, Ausman JI, Mehta B: Dural arteriovenous malformations and intracranial hemorrhage. Neurosurgery 1984;15:332–339.
20. Brown RD Jr, Wiebers DO, Nichols DA: Intracranial dural arteriovenous fistulae: angiographic predictors of intracranial hemorrhage and clinical outcome in nonsurgical patients. J Neurosurg 1994;81:531–538.
21. Duffau H, Lopes M, Janosevic V, et al: Early rebleeding from intracranial dural arteriovenous fistulas: report of 20 cases and review of the literature. J Neurosurg 1999;90:78–84.
22. Aminoff MJ, Kendall BE: Asymptomatic dural vascular anomalies. Br J Radiol 1973;46:662–667.
23. Bitoh S, Sakaki S: Spontaneous cure of dural arteriovenous malformation in the posterior fossa. Surg Neurol 1979;12:111–114.
24. Eisenman JI, Alekoumbides A, Pribram H: Spontaneous thrombosis of vascular malformations of the brain. Acta Radiol (Diagn) 1972;13:77–85.
25. Kataoka K, Taneda M: Angiographic disappearance of multiple dural arteriovenous malformations: case report. J Neurosurg 1984;60:1275–1278.
26. Kupersmith MJ, Berenstein A, Choi IS, et al: Management of nontraumatic vascular shunts involving the cavernous sinus. Ophthalmology 1988;95:121–130.
27. Landman JA, Braun IF: Spontaneous closure of a dural arteriovenous fistula associated with acute hearing loss. Am J Neuroradiol 1985;6:448–449.
28. Magidson MA, Weinberg PE: Spontaneous closure of a dural arteriovenous malformation. Surg Neurol 1976;6:107–110.
29. Olutola PS, Eliam M, Molot M, Talalla A: Spontaneous regression of a dural arteriovenous malformation. Neurosurgery 1983;12:687–690.
30. Vinuela F, Fox AJ, Debrun GM, et al: Spontaneous carotid-cavernous fistulas: clinical, radiological, and therapeutic considerations. Experience with 20 cases. J Neurosurg 1984;60:976–984.
31. Voigt K, Sauer M, Dichgans J: Spontaneous occlusion of a bilateral caroticocavernous fistula studied by serial angiography. Neuroradiology 1971;2:207–211.
32. Hansen JH, Sogaard I: Spontaneous regression of an extra- and intracranial arteriovenous malformation: case report. J Neurosurg 1976;45:338–341.
33. Halbach VV, Higashida RT, Hieshima GB, et al: Dural fistulas involving the cavernous sinus: results of treatment in 30 patients. Radiology 1987;163:437–442.
34. Halbach VV, Higashida RT, Hieshima GB, et al: Dural fistulas involving the transverse and sigmoid sinuses: results of treatment in 28 patients. Radiology 1987;163:443–447.
35. Barnwell SL, Halbach VV, Higashida RT, et al: Complex dural arteriovenous fistulas: results of combined endovascular and neurosurgical treatment in 16 patients. J Neurosurg 1989;71:352–358.

36. Grisoli F, Vincentelli F, Fuchs S, et al: Surgical treatment of tentorial arteriovenous malformations draining into the subarachnoid space: report of four cases. J Neurosurg 1984;60:1059–1066.
37. Hugosson R, Bergstrom K: Surgical treatment of dural arteriovenous malformation in the region of the sigmoid sinus. J Neurol Neurosurg Psychiatry 1974;37:97–101.
38. Sundt TM Jr, Piepgras DG: The surgical approach to arteriovenous malformations of the lateral and sigmoid dural sinuses. J Neurosurg 1983;59:32–39.
39. Thompson BG, Doppman JL, Oldfield EH: Treatment of cranial dural arteriovenous fistulae by interruption of leptomeningeal venous drainage. J Neurosurg 1994;80:617–623.
40. Hoh BL, Choudhri TF, Connolly ES Jr, Solomon RA: Surgical management of high-grade intracranial dural arteriovenous fistulas: leptomeningeal venous disruption without nidus excision. Neurosurgery 1998;42:796–805.
41. Lucas CP, DeOliveira E, Tedeschi H, et al: Sinus skeletonization: a treatment for dural arteriovenous malformations of the tentorial apex. Report of two cases. J Neurosurg 1996;84:514–517.
42. Collice M, D'Aliberti G, Talamonti G, et al: Surgical interruption of leptomeningeal drainage as treatment for intracranial dural arteriovenous fistulas without dural sinus drainage. J Neurosurg 1996;84:810–817.
43. Collice M, D'Aliberti G, Arena O, et al: Surgical treatment of intracranial dural arteriovenous fistulae: role of venous drainage. Neurosurgery 2000;47: 56–67.
44. Barnwell SL, Halbach VV, Dowd CF, et al: Dural arteriovenous fistulas involving the inferior petrosal sinus: angiographic findings in six patients. Am J Neuroradiol 1990;11:511–516.
45. Black P, Uematsu S, Perovic M, Walker AE: Carotid-cavernous fistula: a controlled embolus technique for occlusion of fistula with preservation of carotid blood flow: technical note. J Neurosurg 1973;38:113–118.
46. Costin JA, Weinstein MA, Berlin AJ, et al: Dural arterio-venous malformations involving the cavernous sinus: a case report. Br J Ophthalmol 1978; 62:478–482.
47. Courtheoux P, Labbe D, Hamel C, et al: Treatment of bilateral spontaneous dural carotid-cavernous fistulas by coils and sclerotherapy: case report. J Neurosurg 1987;66:468–470.
48. Fardoun R, Adam Y, Mercier P, Guy G: Tentorial arteriovenous malformation presenting as an intracerebral hematoma: case report. J Neurosurg 1981;55: 976–978.
49. Fermand M, Reizine D, Melki JP, et al: Long term follow-up of 43 pure dural arteriovenous fistulae (AVF) of the lateral sinus. Neuroradiology 1987;29: 348–353.
50. Gobin YP, Rogopoulos A, Aymard A, et al: Endovascular treatment of intracranial dural arteriovenous fistulas with spinal perimedullary venous drainage. J Neurosurg 1992;77:718–723.
51. Grossman RI, Sergott RC, Goldberg HI, et al: Dural malformations with ophthalmic manifestations: results of particulate embolization in seven patients. Am J Neuroradiol 1985;6:809–813.
52. Halbach VV, Higashida RT, Hieshima GB, et al: Treatment of dural fistulas involving the deep cerebral venous system. Am J Neuroradiol 1989;10:393–399.
53. Hardy RW Jr, Costin JA, Weinstein M, et al: External carotid cavernous fistula treated by transfemoral embolization. Surg Neurol 1978;9:255–256.
54. Ishimori S, Hattori M, Shibata Y, et al: Treatment of carotid-cavernous fistula by gelfoam embolization. J Neurosurg 1967;27:315–319.

55. Kendall B: Percutaneous embolic occlusion of dural arteriovenous malformation. Br J Radiol 1973;46:520–523.
56. Mahalley MS Jr, Boone SC: External carotid-cavernous fistula treated by arterial embolization: case report. J Neurosurg 1974;40:110–114.
57. Manaka S, Izawa M, Nawata H: Dural arteriovenous malformation treated by artificial embolization with liquid silicone. Surg Neurol 1977;7:63–65.
58. Mullan S: Treatment of carotid-cavernous fistulas by cavernous sinus occlusion. J Neurosurg 1979;50:131–144.
59. Peeters FLM, Kroger R: Dural and direct cavernous sinus fistulas. Am J Roentgenol 1979;132:599–606.
60. Pugatch RD, Wolpert SM: Transfemoral embolization of an external carotid-cavernous fistula: case report. J Neurosurg 1975;42:94–97.
61. Sano H, Jain VK, Kato Y, et al: The treatment of dural AVM by embolization with Aron Alpha (ethyl-2-cyanoacrylate). Acta Neurochir 1987;88:10–19.
62. Vinuela F, Fox AJ, Pelz DM, Drake CG: Unusual clinical manifestations of dural arteriovenous malformations. J Neurosurg 1986;64:554–558.
63. Vinuela FV, Debrun GM, Fox AJ, Kan S: Detachable calibrated-leak balloon for superselective angiography and embolization of dural arteriovenous malformations. J Neurosurg 1983;58:817–823.
64. Mendelowitsch A, Gratzl O, Radu EW: Current therapeutic methods of dural arteriovenous malformation: are there any alternatives? Two case reports of infratentorial AVMs. Neurosurg Rev 1989;12:141–145.
65. Cognard C, Gobin YP, Pierot L, et al: Cerebral dural arteriovenous fistulas: clinical and angiographic correlation with a revised classification of venous drainage. Radiology 1995;194:671–680.
66. Hirabuki N, Mitomo M, Miura T, et al: External carotid artery embolization of dural arteriovenous malformations involving the cavernous sinus: outcome and role of venous thrombosis. Acta Radiol 1990;31:197–201.
67. Urtasun F, Biondi A, Casasco A, et al: Cerebral dural arteriovenous fistulas: percutaneous transvenous embolization. Radiology 1996;199:209–217.
68. Teng MM, Guo WY, Huang CI, et al: Occlusion of arteriovenous malformations of the cavernous sinus via the superior ophthalmic vein. Am J Neuroradiol 1988;9:539–546.
69. Malek AM, Halbach VV, Higashida RT, et al: Treatment of dural arteriovenous malformations and fistulas. Neurosurg Clin N Am 2000;11:147–166.
70. Roy D, Raymond J: The role of transvenous embolization in the treatment of intracranial dural arteriovenous fistulas. Neurosurgery 1997;40:1133–1144.
71. Halbach VV, Higashida RT, Hieshima GB, et al: Transvenous embolization of dural fistulas involving the cavernous sinus. Am J Neuroradiol 1989;10:377–383.
72. Halbach VV, Higashida RT, Hieshima GB, et al: Transvenous embolization of dural fistulas involving the transverse and sigmoid sinuses. Am J Neuroradiol 1989;10:385–392.
73. Nakamura M, Tamaki N, Kawaguchi T, Fujita S: Selective transvenous embolization of dural carotid-cavernous sinus fistulas with preservation of sylvian venous outflow: report of three cases. J Neurosurg 1998;89:825–829.
74. Dawson RC 3rd, Joseph GJ, Owens DS, Barrow DL: Transvenous embolization as the primary therapy for arteriovenous fistulas of the lateral and sigmoid sinuses. Am J Neuroradiol 1998;19:571–576.
75. Barcia-Salorio JL, Soler F, Barcia JA, Hernandez G: Stereotactic radiosurgery for the treatment of low-flow carotid-cavernous fistulae: results in a series of 25 cases. Stereotact Funct Neurosurg 1994;63:266–270.
76. Chandler HC Jr, Friedman WA: Successful radiosurgical treatment of a dural arteriovenous malformation: case report. Neurosurgery 1993;33:139–142.

77. Fabrikant JI, Lyman JT, Hosobuchi Y: Stereotactic heavy-ion Bragg peak radiosurgery for intra-cranial vascular disorders: method for treatment of deep arteriovenous malformations. Br J Radiol 1984;57:479–490.
78. Hosobuchi Y, Fabrikant J, Lyman JT: Stereotactic heavy-particle irradiation of intracranial arteriovenous malformations. Appl Neurophysiol 1987;50: 248–252.
79. Kobayashi H, Hayashi M, Noguchi Y, et al: Dural arteriovenous malformations in the anterior cranial fossa. Surg Neurol 1988;30:396–401.
80. Lewis AI, Tomsick TA, Tew JM Jr: Management of tentorial arteriovenous malformations: transarterial embolization combined with stereotactic radiation or surgery. J Neurosurg 1994;81:851–859.
81. Lunsford LD, Kondziolka D, Flickinger JC, et al: Stereotactic radiosurgery for arteriovenous malformations of the brain. J Neurosurg 1991;75:512–524.
82. Steiner L, Lindquist C, Adler JR, et al: Outcome of radiosurgery for cerebral arteriovenous malformations. J Neurosurg 1992;77:771–778.
83. Pollock BE, Nichols DA, Garrity JA, et al: Stereotactic radiosurgery and particulate embolization for cavernous sinus dural arteriovenous fistulae. Neurosurgery 1999;45:459–467.
84. Ratliff J, Voorhies RM: Arteriovenous fistula with associated aneurysms coexisting with dural arteriovenous malformation of the anterior inferior falx: case report and review of the literature. J Neurosurg 1999;91:303–307.
85. Bavinzski G, Richling B, Killer M, et al: Evolution of different therapeutic strategies in the treatment of cranial dural arteriovenous fistulas: report of 30 cases. Acta Neurochir 1996;138:132–138.
86. Shin M, Kurita H, Tago M, Kirino T: Stereotactic radiosurgery for tentorial dural arteriovenous fistulae draining into the vein of Galen: report of two cases. Neurosurgery 2000;46:730–734.
87. Guo W, Pan DHC, Wu H, et al: Radiosurgery as a treatment alternative for dural arteriovenous fistulas of the cavernous sinus. Am J Neuroradiol 1998; 19:1081–1087.
88. Link MJ, Coffey RJ, Nichols DA, Gorman DA: The role of radiosurgery and particulate embolization in the treatment of dural arteriovenous fistulas. J Neurosurg 1996;84:804–809.
89. Wetzel SG, Bilecen D, Lyrer P, et al: Cerebral dural arteriovenous fistulas: detection by dynamic MR projection angiography. Am J Roentgenol 2000;174: 1293–1295.
90. Coffey RJ, Link MJ, Nichols DA, et al: Gamma knife radiosurgery and particulate embolization of dural arteriovenous fistulas, with a special emphasis on the cavernous sinus. In Lunsford LD, Kondziolka D, Flickinger JC (eds): Gamma Knife Brain Surgery. Basel, Karger, 1998, pp 60–77.
91. Friedman JA, Pollock BE, Nichols DA, et al: Results of combined stereotactic radiosurgery and transarterial embolization for dural arteriovenous fistulas of the transverse and sigmoid sinuses. J Neurosurg 2001;94:886–891.
92. Halbach VV, Higashida RT, Hieshima GB, Christopher FD: Endovascular therapy of dural fistulas. In Vinuela F, Halbach VV, Dion JE (eds): Interventional Neuroradiology: Endovascular Therapy of the Central Nervous System. New York, Raven, 1992, pp 29–50.
93. Tu YK, Liu HM, Hu SC: Direct surgery of carotid cavernous fistulae and dural arteriovenous malformations of the cavernous sinus. Neurosurgery 1997; 41:798–806.
94. Wang Y, Johnston DL, Breen JF, et al: Dynamic MR digital subtraction angiography using contrast enhancement, fast data acquisition, and complex subtraction. Mag Res Med 1996;36:551–556.

Comment
Chapter 6

Daniel L. Barrow

The authors have reported their extensive series of patients with various dural arteriovenous malformations (DAVMs) treated by radiosurgery, most combined with transarterial embolization. They state that radiosurgery has become the primary treatment modality for DAVMs at the Mayo Clinic. Their protocol involves radiosurgical treatment followed by transarterial embolization 48 hours after the radiosurgery for early palliative treatment of symptoms.

Although the authors report good results in their short-term follow-up, I find this therapeutic approach to be somewhat illogical. The overwhelming majority of the 105 patients reported in this series had DAVMs in locations readily treatable by endovascular techniques alone. The therapeutic regimen advocated by the authors exposes the patient to two procedures, which markedly increase risks as well as costs, and is associated with the need for multiple follow-up angiograms. The risks of the multiple interventions is evident in the results where six patients experienced new neurological deficits during diagnostic angiography alone, five experienced complications of embolization, and one patient suffered a fatal hemorrhage while awaiting the potential benefits of the radiosurgery.

Although our knowledge of the natural history of DAVMs is incomplete, it is well recognized that those associated with retrograde leptomeningeal venous drainage (Borden Grades II and III[1]) are associated with a very aggressive natural history compared to their counterparts with venous drainage purely into a dural sinus. The best information regarding the natural history comes from the publication by Davies et al from the University of Toronto.[2] In this study, a cohort of 46 patients with Borden Grade II and III DAVMs was seen at a single institution. All were offered treatment but 14 selected conservative therapy. During the follow-up period (249 lesion months) for the conservatively treated group, four (29%) patients died. Excluding presentation, these patients were observed to have interval rates of intracranial hemorrhage, nonhemorrhagic neurological deficit, and mortality of 19.2%, 10.9%, and 19.3% per lesion year, respectively. This study also demonstrated that persistence of retrograde leptomeningeal venous drainage after inadequate treatment results in adverse outcomes.

Thirty of the patients in this series had DAVMs associated with retrograde leptomeningeal venous drainage. In the limited follow-up, only four of these lesions were eliminated and 26 were reported to have "substantially reduced" cortical venous drainage. Once again, most DAVMs with retrograde leptomeningeal venous drainage are amenable to immediate cure by either transvenous embolization or surgical interruption of the venous drainage. The use of stereotactic radiosurgery with its long interval to therapeutic benefit seems to expose the patient to unnecessary risks.

Although the results in this series appear to be acceptable, the reported results are somewhat misleading. As with much of the literature dealing with radiosurgery, the obliteration rate is reported as a percentage of only those patients that have undergone follow-up angiography, which is less than 50% in the current series. Of the 105 patients, only 50 have undergone follow-up angiography. The authors report that 34 of 50 (68%) had total obliteration of their DAVMs. In fact, only 32% of patients (34 of 105) have been *documented* to have total obliteration of their malformation.

In addition to the need for multiple treatment modalities, the long interval to cure, and the paucity of follow-up angiography, this therapeutic approach also raises concern about the possibility of partial treatment of DAVMs. It is well recognized that partial treatment by any modality including surgery or embolization can result in alteration of venous drainage. If that alteration of venous drainage includes the development of retrograde leptomeningeal venous drainage, a benign DAVM may be converted into one with a much more aggressive natural history.

Advances in interventional neuroradiology have provided an opportunity for the overwhelming majority of DAVMs to be treated by endovascular techniques, most commonly transvenous embolization. For those that are not amenable to endovascular techniques, surgical interruption of the venous drainage provides safe and prompt elimination of the lesion. If that lesion is associated with retrograde leptomeningeal venous drainage, one can provide an immediate elimination of the grave risks associated with the malformation.

References

1. Borden JA, Wu KW, Schucart WA: A proposed classification for spinal and cranial dural arteriovenous fistulous malformations and implications for treatment. J Neurosurg 1995;82:166–179.
2. Davies MA, Ter Brugge K, Willinsky R, Wallace MC: The natural history and management of intracranial dural arteriovenous fistulae. Part 2: Aggressive lesions. Intervent Neuroradiol 1997;3:303–321.

Chapter 7

Stereotactic Radiosurgery for Cavernous Malformation

Steven D. Chang, Richard P. Levy, David P. Martin, Gary K. Steinberg, John R. Adler, Jr.

Introduction

Cavernous malformations (CMs) represent a subset of angiographically occult vascular malformations (AOVMs),[1–6] and are a well-recognized cause of neurological morbidity and mortality.[7,8] The true incidence of CMs is not known, but studies suggest that they account for 8 to 15% of intracranial and spinal vascular malformations[4] and 31% of AOVMs.[5] Increased utilization and improvements in magnetic resonance imaging (MRI) have led to the clinical recognition of these lesions with increasing frequency,[9,10] and to a better understanding of their natural history.[6,11]

Historically, treatment of superficial or subcortical CMs consisted of surgical resection. Improvements in surgical techniques,[8,12] and the use of stereotactic navigation instruments and electrophysiological monitoring,[8,12,13] have made possible resection of some CMs in previously "unresectable" locations such as the brainstem, thalamus, and basal ganglia.[8,12] Despite these advances, some CMs are located in regions that pose an unacceptable surgical risk. For these patients and for those with medical contraindications to surgery, stereotactic radiosurgery has been advocated as an alternative treatment.[7,14–18] This chapter will review the indications, results, and potential complications that follow the treatment of CMs with stereotactic radiosurgery.

This work was supported in part by funding from Bernard and Ronni Lacroute (GKS), the William Randolph Hearst Foundation (GKS), John and Dodie Rosekrans (GKS), and from the Lorraine Ulshaefer Memorial Fund (JRA).

From Pollock BE (ed). *Contemporary Stereotactic Radiosurgery: Technique and Evaluation.* Armonk, NY, Futura Publishing Company, Inc. © 2002.

Rationale for Radiosurgery: Which Patients Should Be Treated?

Radiosurgery is effective in obliterating true arteriovenous malformations (AVMs),[14,19–34] but much less is known about the effects of this treatment on CMs. Several previous studies on AOVMs have suggested a reduction in hemorrhage risk after stereotactic radiosurgery,[7,14–18,27,35–37] but follow-up was relatively short (2–4 years) in all but one series. As a consequence, the true long-term outcome of CMs following radiosurgery is unclear. Furthermore, histopathological studies have shown that CMs resected several years after radiosurgery or fractionated radiotherapy showed incomplete evidence of thrombosis and obliteration.[38] Short follow-up periods, coupled with questions regarding the radiobiological effect of radiosurgery, have prevented the development of commonly accepted treatment guidelines for CM radiosurgery.

Though controversy remains, most radiosurgical centers will consider a patient with a CM for treatment with radiosurgery if the following criteria are met: (1) a lesion on MRI with radiographic characteristics of a CM (heterogenous signal indicating a region of chronic hemorrhage, without edema or other evidence of systemic or focal neoplasia)[7,39,40]; (2) an unresectable location (i.e., a deep CM in eloquent tissue that does not present to a pial surface; and (3) two or more clinical and/or radiographic hemorrhages resulting in neurological deficits. Patients who have had either no prior hemorrhage or a solitary clinical hemorrhage are not routinely considered candidates for radiosurgery. For many neurosurgeons, once an unresectable CM has declared its "aggressive" nature with multiple hemorrhages, radiosurgery represents a reasonable option; CMs associated with hemorrhage tend to hemorrhage repeatedly, resulting in considerable cumulative morbidity.[39,41] The clinical condition of patients in one series,[7] all of whom presented with hemorrhage, often multiple, is consistent with this observation as only 44% of patients in this series were in excellent clinical grade at the time of radiosurgery.

Results of Published Series

Stanford Series

Review of the medical literature reveals several series of patients with CMs treated with stereotactic radiosurgery. Over a 15-year period at Stanford University, 59 patients with AOVMs (most with the characteristic radiographic appearance of a CM) were treated with stereotactic radiosurgery. Only patients with symptomatic, deep-seated AOVMs and a history of intracranial hemorrhage were considered candidates for radiosurgery. These patients had a mean age of 35.7 years (range, 13–71

Table 1
Clinical Results of Cavernous Malformation Radiosurgery in the Stanford Series

	Excellent	*Good*	*Poor*	*Dead*
Before radiosurgery	26	27	6	0
After radiosurgery	26	25	3	5*

*Three from causes unrelated to cavernous malformation or radiosurgery treatment of cavernous malformation.

years). Patients were graded clinically according to the scale of Drake and colleagues[22,42,43] (Table 1), and by Karnofsky Performance Score (KPS) (mean, 76; range, 40–90). Forty-seven patients (80%) were treated with helium ion Bragg-peak radiosurgery (Fig. 1), a method described in detail in previous reports.[14,24,27,28] The marginal doses for these patients ranged from 7.0 to 40 GyE (GyE = gray equivalent = physical dose × relative biological effectiveness [RBE]; RBE = 1.3 for Helium ion Bragg peak[44]), but the great majority of cases received marginal doses of 13.5 to 20 GyE. Twelve patients (20%) were treated as outpatients with linear accelerator (LINAC)-based stereotactic radiosurgery using a technique modeled after that of Winston and Lutz.[45,46] Marginal doses, ranging from 12 to 20 Gy, were prescribed to the 80% isodose contour.

Twenty symptomatic hemorrhages (neurological worsening corresponding to MRI signal changes indicating rebleed) occurred in 18 patients (31%) following radiosurgery. The mean time interval between radiosurgery and intracerebral bleed was 18.8 months (range, 1–68 months). Sixteen hemorrhages occurred within 3 years after radiosurgery (9.1% annual hemorrhage rate; 16 bleeds in 175 patient-years); four hemorrhages occurred more than 3 years after treatment (1.5% annual hemorrhage rate; 4 bleeds in 261 patient-years) (chi-square; $p<0.001$). Statistical analysis comparing hemorrhage rates in the first 2 years post radiosurgery with bleeds beyond 2 years revealed an initial annual rebleed rate of 11.9% (14 bleeds in 118 patient-years) during the first 24 months compared to a 1.9% annual rehemorrhage rate (6 bleeds in 318 patient-years) thereafter (chi-square; $p<0.001$). Forty-one patients (69%) had no hemorrhages following radiosurgery. No patient treated with marginal doses greater than or equal to 27 GyE subsequently hemorrhaged (Fig. 2).

Headaches resolved in 4 of 11 patients and improved in an additional two cases. Seizures resolved in two of the four patients presenting with this symptom. The mean Karnofsky score 3 years following radiosurgery was 69 (range, 0–100), which was not significantly different from the pre-

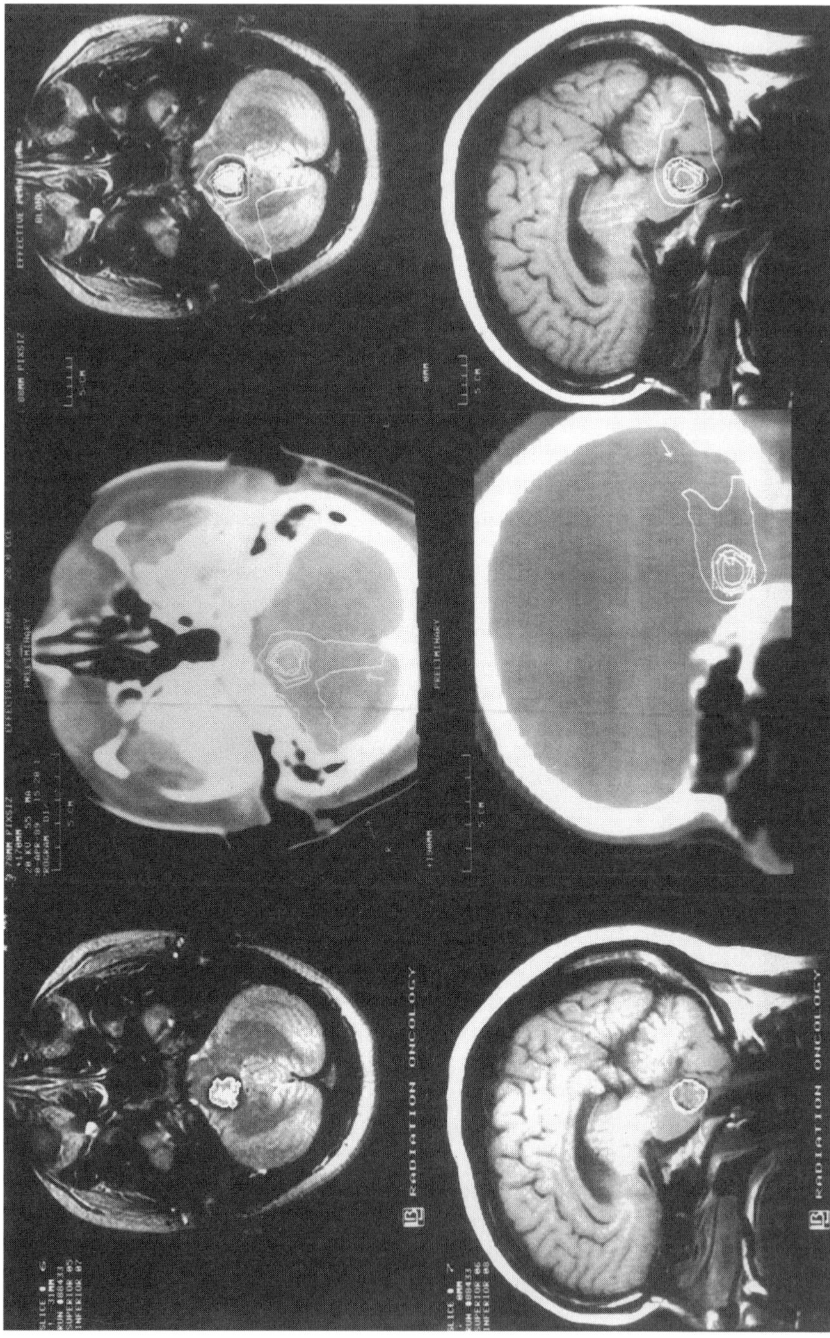

Figure 1. Stereotactic heavy-charged-particle Bragg-peak radiosurgery treatment planning for an AOVM of the pons in a 30-year-old woman.[14] Left upper and lower images show representative stereotactic MRI scans in the axial and sagittal projections used to define the target volume for stereotactic radiosurgery (ring of white dots). The target contour data are transferred to corresponding images on the stereotactic CT scans, using a VAX 11/780 computer system (middle upper and lower images). CT data are then used to identify and compensate for inhomogeneities in the tissues to be traversed by the charged particle beams and to calculate three-dimensional dose distribution contours. The dose contour information is then transferred back to the original MRI scans (right upper and lower images), in order to permit the demonstration (and modifications, where required) of isodose contour distributions in the brain in all desired anatomical planes. Isodose contours in the axial and sagittal planes are calculated for 10%, 50%, 70%, and 90% of the maximum dose. Reprinted with permission from Chang SD, et al.[7]

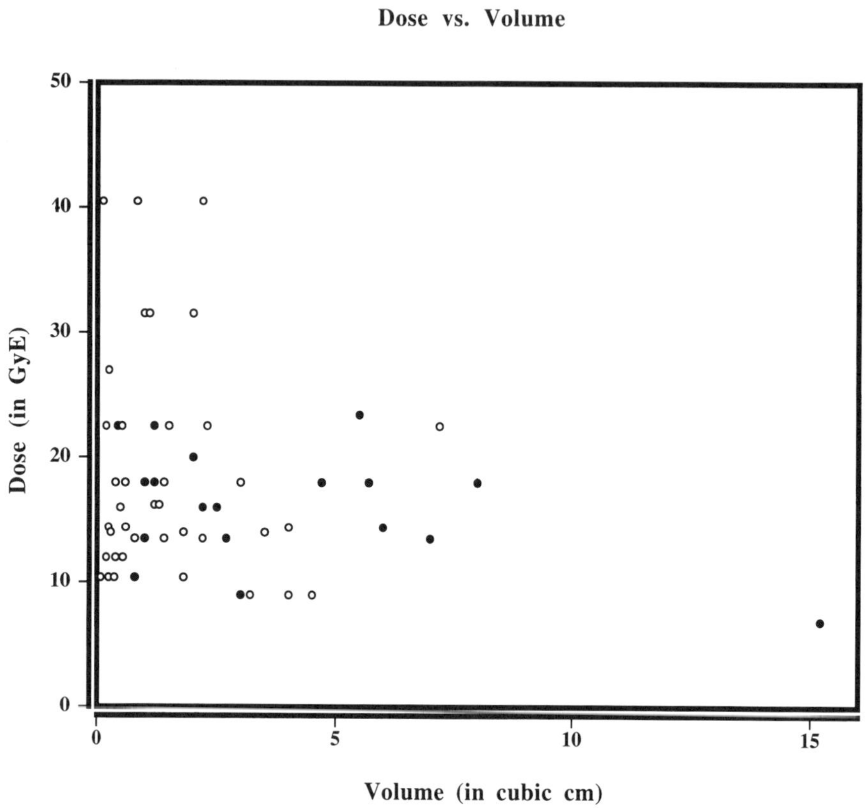

Figure 2. Scatterplot showing marginal dose in GyE vs. volume in cm^3. Patients who rehemorrhaged are denoted by dark circles. No patient treated with a marginal dose greater than or equal to 27 GyE suffered a rehemorrhage. Reprinted with permission from Chang SD, et al.[7]

treatment score. Clinical results after treatment (Table 1) were excellent (26), good (25), poor (3), and deceased (5). Three of the five patients who died during the follow-up period expired from causes unrelated to their AOVMs or radiosurgery (2 from pneumonia, 1 from renal failure). Two patients, who were in poor condition after previously receiving radiotherapy for presumed brainstem glioma, died of rebleeding 9 and 14 months after treatment. Both patients had been treated with marginal doses of 9 GyE or less.

Other Series

The University of Pittsburgh investigators analyzed their series of 47 CM patients (44 with two or more hemorrhages) treated with Gamma

Knife radiosurgery with a mean follow-up period of 3.6 years.[35] Following the first CM hemorrhage (often the event leading to diagnosis), there was a 32% annual rehemorrhage rate prior to radiosurgery, as compared to a 8.8% rehemorrhage rate the first 2 years after radiosurgery and a 1.1% rehemorrhage rate more than 2 years after radiosurgery ($p<0.0001$). These authors reported a 26% total complication rate (which corresponded to imaging changes) and a 4% new permanent deficit rate. The Harvard University group reviewed their series of 95 patients with 98 CMs treated with proton beam radiosurgery with a mean follow-up period of 5.4 years.[47] Their analysis revealed a decrease in the annual hemorrhage rate from 17.3% per lesion per year before radiosurgery to a 4.5% per lesion per year hemorrhage rate after a 2-year latency period. There was a 16% incidence of permanent neurological deficit, and a 3% mortality rate during follow-up, ascribed to a combination of radiation-related injury and clinical progression (hemorrhage) of the CMs. Both reports concluded that radiosurgery, despite some risks, may be an effective strategy in the treatment of unresectable CMs.

Conceptual Difficulties with Cavernous Malformations Radiosurgery

Pathology Cannot Be Confirmed

Cavernous malformations are a distinct subset of AOVMs. MRI features such as a hemosiderin ring and the absence of edema or mass effect have been shown to favor the diagnosis of CMs.[48] However, these features are by no means unique to this type of lesion. Although it is possible to confirm the diagnosis of a brain tumor with a stereotactic brain biopsy prior to radiosurgery, the treatment of a vascular malformation based on radiographic appearance alone allows for the potential inclusion of non-CM lesions, thus potentially biasing the results.

Radiosurgery Target Delineation

Delineation of the appropriate radiosurgical target volume in the treatment of CMs is difficult. Accurate localization of abnormal vasculature is fairly straightforward with most angiographically demonstrable AVMs, but this is not the case with CMs. Currently available neuroradiologic methods do not demonstrate the exact location of the CM itself, but rather image the characteristic magnetic resonance signal of hemorrhage within adjacent brain parenchyma.[40,49] Moreover, CMs may hemorrhage eccentrically and frequently are found during surgery only by careful exploration of the wall of the hematoma cavity.[41] Accordingly, a CM target must necessarily include the entire volume of abnormality defined by high-resolution MRI. This strategy results in treatment of both the CM and adjacent hematoma, which unfortunately increases the volume of normal brain treated with high dose.

Radiobiology of Cavernous Malformation and Optimal Radiosurgery Dose Is Unknown

The optimal radiosurgery dose for treating CMs is unknown. Among the seven patients in the Stanford series treated with marginal doses greater than or equal to 27 GyE (range, 27–40.5 GyE), no hemorrhages were documented over a mean follow-up period of 10.2 years.[7] However, two of these seven patients developed symptomatic radiation edema, and based on this experience, subsequent radiosurgery patients were treated with lower doses. Furthermore, in this same series, there was no significant difference between the volume of treated lesion ($p=0.22$) and dose ($p=0.51$) for the five patients with long-term complications (4 with symptomatic edema; 1 with radionecrosis) and the rest of the patient series.[7] However, based on the observation of higher complication rates with higher doses when treating true AVMs,[14,19,24,25,31] patients are typically treated using marginal doses of approximately 18 GyE.

Lack of Optimal Radiographic Study to Evaluate Follow-Up

No adequate radiographic study exists for follow-up of CM obliteration after radiosurgery. Most patients demonstrate little change on follow-up MRI, other than what could be explained by partial resolution or evolution of preexisting hemorrhage. In the Stanford series, no CM underwent radiologic changes that could be interpreted as demonstrating luminal obliteration[7] comparable to that seen with angiographically high-flow AVMs after radiosurgery.[28] Five patients developed findings of enhanced signal on T2-weighted MRI scans, but only four patients had concomitant clinical worsening. Follow-up computed tomography (CT) scanning is of limited value, other than for diagnosing acute recurrent hemorrhage when clinically suspected.

Rate of Hemorrhage Response

It is well established that true AVMs obliterate progressively over a period of 2 to 3 years after stereotactic radiosurgery.[14,19,24–26,29–34] As a result, a similar response and time course has been investigated among AOVMs treated with stereotactic radiosurgery. In the absence of an established neuroimaging procedure for evaluation of CMs,[14,28,35,37] the response must be assessed indirectly by hemorrhage frequency. Accordingly, rehemorrhage rates in several series were evaluated before and after both 2- and 3-year cutoff points.[7,35,47] Over a mean follow-up time of 7.5 years in the Stanford series, there was a significant difference between rehemorrhage rate in the first 3 years following radiosurgery (9.1% annual rate), and during the years thereafter (1.5% annual rate).[7] Of the four patients with rehemorrhage more than 3 years post treatment, three bled within the 4th year and subsequently underwent surgical resection of their CM. Only one patient hemorrhaged more than 4 years after radiosurgery (1 hemorrhage in 199.5 patient-years; 0.5% hemorrhage rate). This occurred in a patient who had also bled within 3 years of radiosurgery, and in whom pathology revealed a true AVM. The statistically significant reduction in hemorrhage rate more than 3 years after radiosurgery is consistent with the better understood time course of radiosurgical effects on angiographically visible AVMs. Considering that most CMs are relatively small, and that small true AVMs usually obliterate within 2 years post radiosurgery treatment, analysis was performed comparing the rebleed rate before and after 24 months post treatment. Similar to the analysis with a 3-year latency period, this comparison revealed a statistically significant decrease in the rebleed rate after 2 years.

A primary unresolved issue regarding CM treatment with radiosurgery is whether or not the observed time-dependent hemorrhage rate reflects a true improvement vis-à-vis the natural history of this lesion. Unfortunately, few studies of the natural hemorrhage risk of patients with CMs exist. Recent analysis of the natural history of CMs reveal an annual bleed rate of approximately 2.6%.[35] These same studies also note an increased rate of hemorrhage (4.5% per year) after a patient had sustained an initial hemorrhage.[6,35] Higher hemorrhage rates (8.8% per year) have been reported during the first 2 years following radiosurgery for CMs, followed by a reduction in hemorrhage rate to 1.1% per year. This latter value closely parallels the annual 0.25 to 1.1% bleed rate reported with CMs that have not previously hemorrhaged.[50–52] The results in the Stanford series are similar to that of an earlier study reported by the University of Pittsburgh in which an initial 9.4% per year bleed rate during the first 3 years after radiosurgery (12.3% per year for the first 2 years) was observed to decrease to 0.5% per year over subsequent years.[35]

Two alternative scenarios potentially explain these findings. In the first case, the natural rehemorrhage rate for symptomatic CMs increases to 4.5% or more annually after the first bleed and remains constant for subsequent years.[6,35] Here, results showing that radiosurgery reduces the rehemorrhage rate to less than 2% per year would indicate a significant protective effect. Alternatively, if untreated CMs have a period of transiently increased or accelerated hemorrhage rate (e.g., cluster hemorrhages) for several years after initial hemorrhage, followed by a return to a more quiescent state, then the reported results may only parallel the natural history of these lesions, without a significant benefit from radiosurgery. The natu-

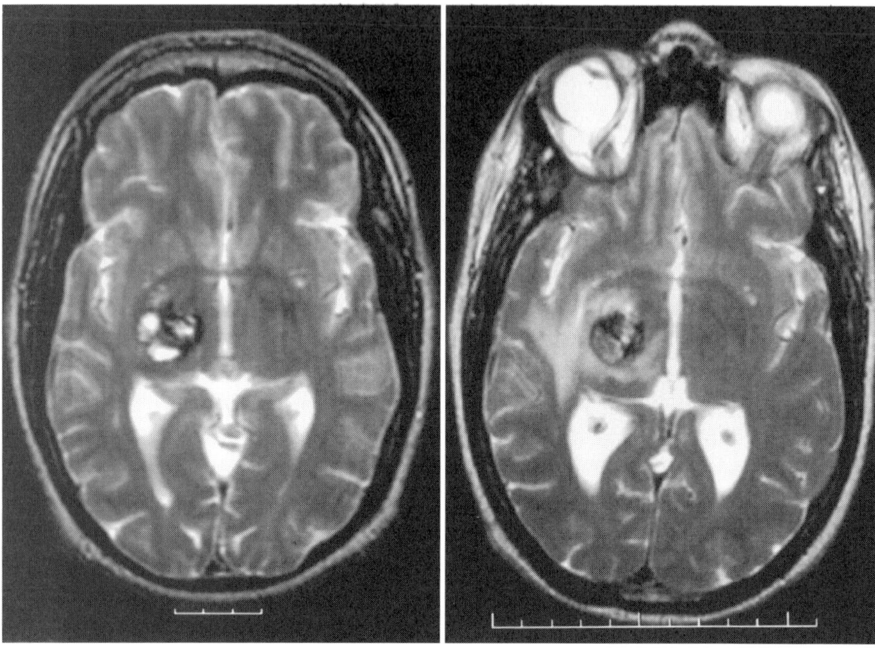

Figure 3. A 43-year-old man presented with left-sided weakness as a result of three prior hemorrhages from a right thalamic cavernous malformation, seen on axial T2-weighted MRI (**left**). The patient was treated with LINAC radiosurgery with a marginal dose of 15.0 Gy (isocenter dose 18.0 Gy). No additional hemorrhages were noted over a 3-year period following radiosurgery, but the patient developed radiation edema, seen on axial T2-weighted MRI (**right**).

ral course of hemorrhage from CMs is thus far not well enough characterized to allow differentiation between the two possibilities.

Complications

In all reported series, the selected doses were believed to produce a reasonably high rate of obliteration of the CM. This concern was balanced by a desire to minimize the probability of inducing adverse sequelae. Nevertheless, in the Stanford series, 12% of patients suffered permanent complications. Acute minor complications, consisting of transient seizures, nausea, or vomiting occurred in five of the earlier LINAC patients who had not been premedicated. Later patients were given prophylactic dexamethasone and promethazine hydrochloride, and did not experience these complications. All 47 helium ion patients were premedicated with oral dexamethasone; none had acute complications. Delayed complications included symptomatic radiation-induced edema (five patients, 8%) (Fig. 3); these patients were treated with marginal doses of 31.5 GyE to .85 cm^3, 18 GyE to 1.2 cm^3, 9 GyE to 15.2 cm^3, 18 GyE to 1.5 cm^3, and 15 GyE to 2.4 cm^3. Other complications included necrosis (one patient, 2%) and increased seizure frequency (one patient, 2%). Of the five patients with symptomatic radiation edema, worsening of headaches occurred in three and transient seizures in one. Three of the five symptomatic patients recovered fully to their previous condition. The one patient with histologically confirmed radionecrosis (marginal dose, 18 GyE; volume, 2.5 cm^3) had previously received whole brain radiation therapy (20 Gy) for treatment of childhood leukemia. Microsurgical resection of this patient's AOVM was performed 10 months after radiosurgery for progressive symptomatic worsening despite steroid therapy.

Duma et al reported an incidence of complications similar to the Stanford series when treating brainstem AOVMs (27% overall complications, 18% permanent).[53] In contrast, Kondziolka et al reported a lower incidence of permanent side effects when treating CMs (26% overall complications, 4% permanent).[35] The treatment risks from radiosurgery in this series are higher than those for high-flow AVMs located in similar critical locations.[54] This finding may be ascribable to the decreased ability to target AOVMs relative to angiographically visible AVMs, or alternatively, there may be a different biological response of AOVMs to radiosurgical treatment.

Role of Surgery

Surgical resection is the treatment of choice for CMs, especially for those located in easily accessible regions of the brain. However, some CMs are located in regions that pose an unacceptable surgical risk, and in these patients radiosurgery represents a potentially important alternative. The anatomical distribution of CMs in the published series reflects a selection bias for surgically inaccessible lesions.[7,35,47] This is consistent with the observation of Lobato et al that "deep location" CMs constitute a minority of operated cases.[5] Microsurgery also plays a role in managing patients with CMs who rehemorrhage after radiosurgery, who develop radiation necrosis, or in whom there is significant worsening of symptoms. We continue to favor surgical resection of CMs whenever possible, reserving radiosurgery for those CMs in surgically inaccessible or high-risk regions that have previously hemorrhaged.

Conclusion

Radiosurgery may produce a significant reduction in the risk of CM hemorrhage after a 2 or more year latency period. Most radiosurgical centers will consider a patient with a CM a candidate for radiosurgery if there is an MRI with radiographic characteristics of a CM, an unresectable location, and two or more clinical hemorrhages resulting in neurological deficits. Morbidity and mortality of this treatment appear to be acceptable given the risk of natural history of these lesions. Longer follow-up with larger numbers of patients and an improved understanding of the natural history of CMs will ultimately be required to elucidate the optimal management of this disorder.

References

1. Vanefsky MA, Norbash A, Snipes J, et al: A multivariate analysis of magnetic resonance characteristics and histopathology of angiographically occult vascular malformations. Stroke 1994;25:252.
2. Yasargil MG: Microsurgery. Vol IIIB. New York, Gerog Thieme Verlag, 1988, pp 415–418.
3. Martin N, Vinters H: Pathology and grading of intracranial vascular malformations. In Barrow DL (ed): Intracranial Vascular Malformations. Park Ridge, Illinois, American Association of Neurologic Surgeons, 1990, pp 1–30.
4. Johnson PC, Wascher TM, Golfinos J, et al: Definition and pathologic features. In Awad IA, Barrow DL (eds): Cavernous Malformations. Park Ridge, Illinois, American Association of Neurological Surgeons, 1993, pp 1–12.
5. Lobato RD, Perez C, Rivas JJ, et al: Clinical, radiological, and pathological spectrum of angiographically occult intracranial vascular malformations: analysis of 21 cases and review of the literature. J Neurosurg 1988;68:518–531.
6. Kondziolka D, Lunsford LD, Kestle JR: The natural history of cerebral cavernous malformations. J Neurosurg 1995;83:820–824.
7. Chang SD, Levy RP, Adler JR, et al: Stereotactic radiosurgery of angiographically occult vascular malformations: 14-year experience. Neurosurgery 1998; 43:213–221.
8. Steinberg GK, Chang SD, Gewirtz RJ, et al: Microsurgical resection of brainstem, thalamic, and basal ganglia angiographically occult vascular malformations. Neurosurgery 2000;46:260–271.
9. Kashiwagi S, van Loveren HR, Tew JM Jr, et al: Diagnosis and treatment of vascular brain-stem malformations. J Neurosurg 1990;72:27–34.
10. Rigamonti D, Dryer BP, Johnson BC, et al: The MRI appearance of cavernous malformations (angiomas). J Neurosurg 1987;67:518–524.
11. Aiba T, Tanaka R, Koike T, et al: Natural history of intracranial cavernous malformations. J Neurosurg 1995;83:56–59.
12. Steinberg GK, Chang SD: Surgical management of angiographically occult vascular malformations of the brainstem, thalamus, and basal ganglia. In Rengachary SS (ed): Neurosurgical Color Operative Atlas. Vol 8. Baltimore, William and Wilkins, 1999, pp 127–133.
13. Chang SD, Lopez JR, Steinberg GK: The use of electrophysiologic monitoring during resection of arteriovenous malformations and angiographically occult vascular malformations. J Neurosurg 1997;86:400A.
14. Fabrikant JI, Levy RP, Steinberg GK, et al: Charged-particle radiosurgery for intracranial vascular malformations. Neurosurg Clin N Am 1992;3:99–139.
15. Kida Y, Kobayashi T, Tanaka T: Treatment of symptomatic AOVMs with radiosurgery. Acta Neurochir Suppl (Wien) 1995;63:68–72.

16. Kondziolka D, Lunsford LD, Coffey RJ, et al: Stereotactic radiosurgery of angiographically occult vascular malformations: indications and preliminary experience. Neurosurgery 1990;27:892–900.
17. Levy RP, Steinberg GK, Fabrikant JI, et al: Stereotactic heavy-charged-particle radiosurgery for angiographically occult vascular malformations. In Lunsford LD (ed): Stereotactic Radiosurgery Update. New York, Elsevier, 1992, pp 177–183.
18. Levy RP, Fabrikant JI, Phillips MH, et al: Clinical results of stereotactic heavy-charged-particle radiosurgery for intracranial angiographically occult vascular malformations. In Steiner L (ed): Radiosurgery: Baseline and Trends. New York, Raven Press, 1992, pp 221–228.
19. Steiner L, Lindquist C, Adler JR, et al: Clinical outcome of radiosurgery for cerebral arteriovenous malformations. J Neurosurg 1992;77:1–8.
20. Steiner L: Radiosurgery in cerebral arteriovenous malformations. In Fein JM, Flamm ES (eds): Cerebrovascular Surgery. Vol 4. New York, Springer-Verlag, 1985, pp 1161–1215.
21. Steiner L: Treatment of arteriovenous malformations by radiosurgery. In Wilson CB, Stein BM (eds): Intracranial Arteriovenous Malformations. Baltimore, Williams and Wilkins, 1984, pp 295–313.
22. Steinberg GK, Chang SD, Levy RP, et al: Surgical resection of large incompletely treated intracranial arteriovenous malformations following stereotactic radiosurgery. J Neurosurg 1996;84:920–928.
23. Steinberg GK, Levy RP, Marks MP, et al: Vascular malformations: charged-particle radiosurgery. In Alexander E, Loeffler JS, Lunsford L (eds): Stereotactic Radiosurgery. New York, McGraw-Hill, 1993, pp 122–135.
24. Steinberg GK, Fabrikant JI, Marks MP, et al: Stereotactic heavy-charged-particle Bragg-peak radiation for intracranial arteriovenous malformations. N Engl J Med 1990;323:96–101.
25. Lunsford LD, Kondziolka D, Flickinger JC, et al: Stereotactic radiosurgery for arteriovenous malformations of the brain. J Neurosurg 1991;75:512–524.
26. Lunsford LD, Kondziolka D, Bissonette DJ, et al: Stereotactic radiosurgery of brain vascular malformations. Neurosurg Clin N Am 1992;3:79–98.
27. Levy RP, Fabrikant JI, Frankel KA, et al: Charged-particle radiosurgery of the brain. Neurosurg Clin N Am 1990;1:955–990.
28. Levy RP, Fabrikant JI, Frankel KA, et al: Stereotactic heavy-charged-particle Bragg peak radiosurgery for the treatment of intracranial arteriovenous malformations in childhood and adolescence. Neurosurgery 1989;24:841–852.
29. Leksell L: Stereotactic radiosurgery. J Neurol Neurosurg Psychiatry 1983; 46:797–803.
30. Friedman WA, Bova FJ: Linear accelerator radiosurgery for arteriovenous malformations. J Neurosurg 1992;77:832–841.
31. Colombo F, Pozza F, Chierego G, et al: Linear accelerator radiosurgery of cerebral arteriovenous malformations: an update. Neurosurgery 1994;34:14–20; discussion 20–21.
32. Colombo F, Benedetti A, Pozza F, et al: Linear accelerator radiosurgery of cerebral arteriovenous malformations. Neurosurgery 1989;24:833–840.
33. Betti OO, Munari C, Rosler R: Stereotactic radiosurgery with the linear accelerator: treatment of arteriovenous malformations. Neurosurgery 1989;24: 311–321.
34. Alexander E 3rd, Loeffler JS: Radiosurgery using a modified linear accelerator. Neurosurg Clin N Am 1992;3:167–190.
35. Kondziolka D, Lunsford LD, Flickinger JC, et al: Reduction of hemorrhage risk after stereotactic radiosurgery for cavernous malformations. J Neurosurg 1995;83:825–831.

36. Seo Y, Fukuoka S, Takanashi M, et al: Gamma Knife surgery for angiographically occult vascular malformations. Stereotact Funct Neurosurg 1995;64 (suppl 1):98–109.
37. Steinberg GK, Levy RP, Fabrikant JI, et al: Stereotactic helium ion Bragg peak radiosurgery for angiographically occult vascular malformations. Stereotact Funct Neurosurg 1990;57:64–71.
38. Gewirtz RJ, Crowley R, Levy RP, et al: Pathologic changes in surgically resected angiographically occult vascular malformations after radiation. J Neurosurg 1996;84:322.
39. Abe M, Kjellberg RN, Adams RD: Clinical presentations of vascular malformations of the brainstem: comparison of angiographically positive and negative types. J Neurol Neurosurg Psychiatry 1989;52:167–175.
40. Sze G, Krol G, Olsen WW, et al: Hemorrhagic neoplasms: MR mimics of occult vascular malformations. Am J Roentgenol 1987;149:1223–1230.
41. Wakai S, Ueda Y, Inoh S, et al: Angiographically occult angiomas: a report of thirteen cases with analysis of the cases documented in the literature. Neurosurgery 1985;17:549–556.
42. Drake CG: Cerebral arteriovenous malformations: considerations for and experience with surgical treatment in 166 cases. Clin Neurosurg 1979;26: 145–208.
43. Drake CG, Friedman AH, Peerless SJ: Posterior fossa arteriovenous malformations. J Neurosurg 1986;64:1–10.
44. Blakely EA, Ngo FQH, Curtis SB, et al: Heavy-ion radiobiology: cellular studies. In Lett JT (ed): Advances in Radiation Biology. Vol 11. New York, Academic Press, 1984, pp 295–389.
45. Adler JR, Cox RS, Kaplan I, et al: Stereotactic radiosurgical treatment of brain metastasis. J Neurosurg 1992;76:444–449.
46. Winston KR, Lutz W: Linear accelerator as a neurosurgical tool for stereotactic radiosurgery. Neurosurgery 1988;22:454–464.
47. Amin-Hanjani S, Ogilvy CS, Candia G, et al: Stereotactic radiosurgery for cavernous malformations: Kjellberg's experience with proton beam therapy in 98 cases at the Harvard cyclotron. Neurosurgery 1998;42:1229–1237.
48. Vanefsky MA, Cheng ML, Chang SD, et al: Correlation of magnetic resonance characteristics and histopathologic type of angiographically occult vascular malformations. Neurosurgery 1999;44:1174–1181.
49. Atlas SW: Intracranial vascular malformations and aneurysms: current imaging applications. Radiol Clin North Am 1988;26:821–837.
50. Del Curling O Jr, Kelly DL Jr, Elster AD, et al: An analysis of the natural history of cavernous angiomas. J Neurosurg 1991;75:702–708.
51. Robinson JR, Awad IA, Little JR: Natural history of the cavernous angioma. J Neurosurg 1991;75:709–714.
52. Zabramski JM, Wascher TM, Spetzler RF, et al: The natural history of familial cavernous malformations: results of an ongoing study. J Neurosurg 1994; 80:422–432.
53. Duma CM, Lunsford LD, Kondziolka D, et al: Radiosurgery for vascular malformations of the brain stem. Acta Neurochir Suppl (Wien) 1993;58:92–97.
54. Kjellberg RN, Hanamura T, Davis KR, et al: Bragg-peak proton-beam therapy for arteriovenous malformations of the brain. N Engl J Med 1983;309: 269–274.

Comment
Chapter 7

Fred G. Barker II, Sepideh Amin-Hanjani, Jay S. Loeffler

The role of radiosurgery in the treatment of CMs is an extremely controversial topic, for reasons that have been well outlined in this chapter. The source of the controversy is doubt about the efficacy of radiosurgery in reducing hemorrhage rates from CMs, which is not universally accepted. To date, there are no completed trials in which CM patients have been randomized to receive radiosurgery or observation. Because there are no plausible "surrogate markers" of treatment success (like arteriographic obliteration of AVMs), efficacy claims have relied on comparisons of the hemorrhage experience in treated groups with rates from various types of control groups (usually the same patients before treatment, or other untreated patients from the same or different institutions).

Unfortunately, the natural history of CMs is very poorly understood. The reported risk of hemorrhage from CMs has varied widely, from 0.25 to 57% per year–a 200-fold difference.[1–4] Some of the variability between studies seems to be the effect of patient-based risk factors, such as age, sex, history of prior hemorrhage, number of prior hemorrhages, and deep lesion location.[1,5–7] Variation between studies also results from differing assumptions about the period at risk for hemorrhage (the "denominator" in the equation of events observed divided by time spent at risk). Calculated hemorrhage risk differs when the risk interval is assumed to start at birth, at first presentation (with or without symptoms), or after a first hemorrhage. Finally, both "CM" and "hemorrhage" can be defined in different ways. Are all lesions with the characteristic MR appearance of CMs to be included, or just those that are known to be arteriographically occult, or should pathologic confirmation be required? Are all clinical events to be counted, or just those with radiographic proof of active hemorrhage? It is known that many clinical deteriorations in CM patients are not accompanied by imaging-detectable hemorrhage. How about clinically silent events that are seen on imaging studies to be acute hemorrhage? These important factors make comparisons between hemorrhage experience in different groups of patients extremely hard to interpret, and comparisons to "external" (literature-based) control hemorrhage rates[8] are simply inadequate.

How about comparisons to the treated group's own hemorrhage experience prior to treatment? The problem here is that the hemorrhage risk for an individual CM lesion seems to change over time. This change takes two forms. First, investigators have documented an apparently permanent increase in subsequent hemorrhage risk after the first clinically evident hemorrhage from a CM.[9] Second, CM hemorrhages have often been described as occurring in "clusters." Clusters of hemorrhage arise when a clinically evident hemorrhage is followed by a temporarily elevated risk of subsequent hemorrhage from that lesion. We have documented an elevated risk of subsequent hemorrhage in untreated CMs that persists for a little more than 2 years before lapsing back to a lower rate.[10] Most radiosurgical studies assume a 2- or 3-year "latency period" after CM radiosurgery before the risk of hemorrhage would be expected to decrease. Because most patients who undergo radiosurgery for CMs have suffered a hemorrhage shortly before referral for treatment, it is possible that the latency period and subsequent decrease in hemorrhage rates observed after radiosurgery could partly or wholly correspond to the spontaneous decrease in hemorrhage risk that occurs about 2 years after a preceding hemorrhage in untreated lesions.

Balanced against the questionable efficacy of radiosurgery for CMs is the very real risk of radiation-related complications. These have a characteristic appearance on MRI that distinguishes them from the spontaneous neurological declines that occur in some CM patients. Most investigators agree that the risk of radiosurgery complications is substantially higher for CM treatment than for treatment of an AVM with similar location and dose and treatment volume parameters, although the reason for this is not clear.[11,12] No group has yet succeeded in demonstrating a dose-efficacy relationship for CMs; thus, dose selection becomes rather arbitrary–neither the highest safe dose nor the lowest effective dose is known.

Many CMs are incidentally discovered and probably require no treatment. When treatment is indicated for lesions with progressive symptoms, or if the risk of rehemorrhage seems unacceptable, surgical removal is currently the unquestioned gold standard. Resection cures most patients with acceptable risk, even when lesions are located in deep or eloquent locations such as the thalamus or brainstem (the locations where treatment with either surgery or radiosurgery is most dangerous).[13,14] For the rare CM that truly fulfills the conditions outlined in this chapter (symptomatic hemorrhages and surgically inaccessible), radiosurgery may provide a benefit with acceptable risk, but this remains unproven. Both patients and physicians will be best served if radiosurgical treatment of CMs is limited to centers with a special interest in this topic, so that information to help future patients can be accrued.

References

1. Robinson JR, Awad IA, Little JR: Natural history of the cavernous angioma. J Neurosurg 1991;75:709–714.
2. Del Curling O, Kelly DL Jr, Elster AD, et al: An analysis of the natural history of cavernous angiomas. J Neurosurg 1991;75:702–708.

3. Kondziolka D, Lunsford LD, Flickinger JC, et al: Reduction of hemorrhage risk after stereotactic radiosurgery for cavernous malformations. J Neurosurg 1995;83:825–831.
4. Zabramski JM, Wascher TM, Spetzler RF, et al: The natural history of familial cavernous malformations: results of an ongoing study. J Neurosurg 1994;80:422–432.
5. Robinson JR Jr, Awad IA, Magdinec M, et al: Factors predisposing to clinical disability in patients with cavernous malformations of the brain. Neurosurgery 1993;32:730–736.
6. Aiba T, Tanaka R, Koike T, et al: Natural history of intracranial cavernous malformations. J Neurosurg 1995;83:56–59.
7. Porter PJ, Willinsky RA, Harper W, et al: Cerebral cavernous malformations: natural history and prognosis after clinical deterioration with or without hemorrhage. J Neurosurg 1997;87:190–197.
8. Karlsson B, Kihlstrom L, Lindquist C, et al: Radiosurgery for cavernous malformations. J Neurosurg 1998;88:293–297.
9. Maraire JN, Awad IA: Intracranial cavernous malformations: lesion behavior and management strategies. J Neurosurg 1995;37:591–605.
10. Barker FG 2nd, Amin-Hanjani S, Butler WE, et al: Temporal clustering of hemorrhages from untreated cavernous malformations of the central nervous system. Neurosurgery 2001;49:15–24.
11. Barker FG 2nd, Amin-Hanjani S, Butler WE, et al: Complication rates after radiosurgery for cavernous malformations (abstract). Neurosurgery 1998;43:670.
12. Pollock BE, Garces YI, Stafford SL, et al: Stereotactic radiosurgery for cavernous malformations. J Neurosurg 2000;93:987–991.
13. Amin-Hanjani S, Ogilvy CS, Ojemann RG, et al: Risks of surgical management for cavernous malformations of the nervous system. Neurosurgery 1998;42:1220–1228.
14. Steinberg GK, Chang SD, Gewirtz RJ, et al: Microsurgical resection of brainstem, thalamic, and basal ganglia angiographically occult vascular malformations. Neurosurgery 2000;46:260–271.

Chapter 8

Stereotactic Radiosurgery for Meningioma

Scott L. Stafford, Bruce E. Pollock, Robert L. Foote, Michael J. Link, Paula J. Schomberg

Introduction

Meningiomas account for approximately 15% of adult intracranial neoplasms and are rare in the pediatric population. These tumors originate from the arachnoid cap cells and generally exhibit benign histology.[1] Rhabdoid, papillary, and clear cell variants have been identified which often display a more aggressive clinical behavior despite their benign appearance.[2–4] Atypical and malignant meningiomas do occur,[5,6] and generally account for 15% and 4%, respectively, of tumors in large surgical series of primarily resected patients.[7,8] Patients with neurofibromatosis type 2 often develop meningiomas that can be multifocal.[9] Previous exposure to ionizing radiation can result in meningioma formation in 1 to 3% of patients after a latency interval of many years.[10] The median patient age in surgical series is typically in the mid 50s,[7,11,12] and there is generally a 1:2–3 male to female ratio. These tumors occur (in decreasing order of incidence) in the parasagittal falx, convexity, sphenoid wing, and other skull base locations.[7,11,13] Excellent reviews of the epidemiology of meningiomas can be found in the works of Black[14] and Wilson.[15]

Meningioma Management

Gross total resection, either a Simpson Grade I or II resection,[13] is considered the standard of care for meningioma patients. Recurrence rates after this degree of tumor removal ranges from 4% in clinical series,[7]

From Pollock BE (ed). *Contemporary Stereotactic Radiosurgery: Technique and Evaluation.* Armonk, NY, Futura Publishing Company, Inc.

to 24 to 32% for series published in the modern neuroimaging era.[12,16,17] However, some tumors cannot be completely excised due to their location and close relationship to critical neurovascular structures. Subtotal resection results in progression rates of 55 to 82% at 10 years.[7,12,16,18] Clinical deterioration for patients having subtotal resection generally is delayed compared to radiographic evidence of tumor progression as demonstrated by computed tomography (CT) of magnetic resonance imaging (MRI).[19] Surgical mortality rates between 1.5% and 16% have been published,[7,11,13,16,19–21] although mortality rates greater than 2% are rare in more recent series.

Advances in surgical techniques now allow gross total resection of tumors located in critical regions such as the cavernous sinus in up to 76% of patients.[22] However, the morbidity associated with this aggressive surgery is worth noting. The perioperative mortality rate was 5%. Major and minor complication rates occurred in 11% and 9.7% of patients, respectively, with worsening cranial nerve function in 6% of those patients presenting with initial dysfunction. A comparable series showed that gross total resection was accomplished in 61% of patients with tumors of the cavernous sinus.[23] The recurrence rate was 10% with a median follow-up of 33 months. The complications in this series included cerebral spinal fluid leak (21%) and cerebral infarction (5%). The perioperative mortality rate was 3%. Another skull base location where aggressive resection is frequently performed involves tumors originating in the petroclival region. A recent series reported that 32 of 41 patients (78%) had a gross total resection.[24] Of note, 24 of the 41 patients (59%) suffered a significant postoperative complication and one patient died. Further review of the literature yields an operative mortality ranging from 0 to 10%; new cranial nerve deficits develop in 20 to 50% of patients undergoing resection of clival meningiomas. Thus, it is clear that aggressive resection of skull base meningiomas can be accomplished. The question remains as to whether the morbidity and/or mortality associated with such surgery justifies its potential benefit.[25,26]

Postoperative external beam radiation therapy (EBRT) is an effective measure to reduce tumor progression rates for patients after subtotal resection of meningiomas.[27–29] The most recent update from the University of California at San Francisco showed improved progression-free survival for patients where CT or MRI was used for treatment planning (98% vs. 77%).[27] Morbidity was reported at 3.6%. Condra et al reported a progression-free survival rate of 76% and a cause-specific survival rate of 86% at 15 years in patients managed with surgery and EBRT.[17] In contrast, the progression-free survival and cause-specific survival rates in those managed by subtotal resection alone were 30% and 51%, respectively. Reported morbidity rates for postoperative irradiation vary from 3.6 to 10%.[7,27] No clear dose-response data is available in the dose ranges currently utilized (45–54 Gy).[12,17,18,27–29] Management of patients with malignant meningiomas remains challenging and the effect of postoperative EBRT on progression-free survival is not clear for this group of patients.[6,30–32]

With this data as a background, the role of radiosurgery in the management of menigiomas can be evaluated more completely.

Radiosurgery for Meningiomas

The treatment of meningiomas with radiosurgery was pioneered by Leksell's group in Sweden in 1976,[33] but did not come into general use until modern neuroimaging and computer treatment planning systems made accurate treatment planning feasible. Several factors make most patients with meningiomas good candidates for radiosurgery. First, most meningioma patients, especially those with skull base tumors, develop symptoms related to tumor location and not mass effect. In such patients, tumor resection does not guarantee symptom improvement, but rather, the goal of management becomes tumor control with minimal treatment-associated toxicity. For patients with large tumors and mass effect, surgical resection should be performed. Second, meningiomas typically image well with either CT or MRI, and are rarely invasive beyond their imaged borders. Thus, the optimal target volume for radiosurgery is readily determined.

Two different modalities using photons to effect treatment delivery have developed, and two centers in the USA employ protons in the radiosurgical management of these tumors. One photon delivery system is based on the introduction of the Leksell Gamma Knife® (Elekta Corp., Norcross, GA), and the other utilizes modified linear accelerators (LINACs). Early use of LINAC systems relied on a less conformal marginal dose distribution. However, the conformity in LINAC-based systems has improved with the advent of new treatment planning software and mini-multileaf hardware.

Results of Linear Accelerator Meningioma Radiosurgery

Tumor Control

Various peer-reviewed published data exist describing the use of LINAC-based radiosurgery for the treatment of menigiomas.[34–40] Most meningiomas treated with radiosurgery in these series are located in the skull base. The results of some of these series are summarized in Table 1. The mean tumor volume treated in these series ranged from 2.2 to 33 cm^3. The tumor marginal dose ranged from 10 to 50 Gy, typically encompassing the 80% isodose line. Local control was excellent and patients making

Table 1
Linear Accelerator Radiosurgery for Meningiomas*

First Author, Ref. No.	*No. of Patients*	*Age (yrs) Mean (range)*	*Tumor Marginal Dose (Gy) Mean (range)*	*Follow-up (mo) Mean (range)*	*Results*	*Complications*
Engenhart[34]	17	54 (41–74)	29 (10–50)	40 (1–60)	LC=100%, n=14 3 excluded due to death	35%
Hakim[35]	127	61.5 (20–88)	15 (9–20)	31 (1.2–79.8)	LC @ 5 yrs, 89% (benign) OS@ 5 yrs, 91% (benign) , 83% (atypical) , 25% (malignant)	4.7%
Chang[37]	55	55.1 (28–82)	18.3 (12–25)	48.4 (17–81)	LC@ 2 yrs, 98% Stable 69% Decreased size 19%	7.3%
Shafron[40]	70	55 (28–82)	12.7 (10–20)	23 (2–88)	LC=100% 56% unchanged 44% decreased	4.3%
Valentino[38]	72	53 (22–79)	37 (15–45) (maximum dose, 1–4 fractions)		LC=94%	0%

LC, local control; OS, overall survival.

up these series had a mixture of primary unresectable and subtotally resected tumors. Overall local control varied from an actuarial 5-year rate of 89% in one series,[35] to 98 to 100% in smaller series, with mean follow-up ranging from 23 to 48.4 months.[37,40] Of interest is the large series reported by Hakim et al in which survival and progression were subdivided into groups based on known histology.[35] The 5-year actuarial survival grouped by histology was: benign (89%), atypical (83%), and malignant (21%). The crude local failure rates were 6%, 8%, and 11%, respectively. Local control in these series was not analyzed with respect to whether previous surgery had a positive or negative influence on outcome.

Complications

With the available data in these series, it is difficult to distinguish strictly radiation-related complications because of numerous confounding factors. Acute minor complications were limited to transient signs of increased intracranial pressure, nausea, and pin site pain. Chronic serious complications varied from none in one series with 72 patients,[38] to as much as 30% in a series of 17 patients with tumors that were deemed unresectable.[34] However, most series reported a complication rate of approximately 5%. In the series by Engenhart et al, the tumor marginal dose utilized ranged from 10 to 50 Gy with a mean tumor marginal dose of 29 Gy.[34] The tumors averaged 4 cm in maximal dimension. In this paper, 5 of 17 patients (30%) suffered symptomatic radiation necrosis. This early experience led them to lower the tumor marginal dose for meningioma radiosurgery. Conversely, Shafron et al[40] managed 18 of 76 patients with a tumor marginal dose of 10 Gy. No patient in this low-dose group has been reported to sustain local failure. The mean tumor marginal dose for the entire series was 12.7 Gy and only two patients (3%) developed symptomatic radiation-related complications. As a result of these early reports, most centers have lowered radiation doses for meningiomas to minimize complications. Hopefully, such dose reduction schemes will not compromise long-term tumor growth control.

Results of Gamma Knife Meningioma Radiosurgery

Tumor Control

There are now many individual center peer-reviewed reports of patients treated with Gamma Knife radiosurgery for meningiomas.[8,41–50] Also, one multicenter study is evaluating radiosurgery in parasagittal meningiomas.[51] The largest of these series are summarized in Table 2. The mean tumor volume ranges from 4 to 16.8 cm^3. Local tumor control rates range from 89 to 100% with mean follow-up intervals extending to

Table 2
Gamma Knife Radiosurgery for Meningiomas

First Author, Ref. No.	*No. of Patients*	*Age (yrs) Mean (range)*	*Tumor Marginal Dose (Gy) Mean (range)*	*Follow-up (mo) Mean (range)*	*Results*	*Complications*
Kondziolka[8]	99	62 (12–84)	16 (9–25)	NS (60–120)	LF 4.9% Any failure 11.3%	4.8%
Hudgins[42]	100	61 (32–88)	15 (8–25)	36 (0.5–240)	LF: n=9, 5/9 dead of tumor 44 stable 47 decreased size Overall LC=91%	1 optic neuropathy 1 BS necrosis (after 2nd RS procedure) Transient 10%
Pendl[47]	97	NS (10–80)	13.8 (7–25)	18.5 (6–46)	LF: n=9, stable 56% decreased size 40%	4% pts worse
Morita[43]	88	56.3 (20–83)	16 (12–20)	35 (12–83)	LF=3% (n=2) 68% decreased size 30% stable size	5%
Liscak[49]	67	57 (19–82)	12 (10–14)	19 (2–60)	LF: n=0 48% stable 52% decreased size	4%
Nicolato[45]	50	56 (25–78)	18 (NS)	14 (4–31)	LF: n=3 (8%) 2 of 3 malignant tumors	Clincal outcome (13% worse)
Kondziolka[51]	203	59 (21–91)	15 (9–32)	42 (NS)	LF: n=22 (11%) PFS @ 5 yrs 93.4% no surgery 60% prior surgery 10/22 (p=0.08)	9.7%

BS, brainstem; LC, local control; LF, local failure; NS, not stated; PFS, progression-free survival; RS, radiosurgery; pts, patients.

more than 5 years. The two largest single series[42,50] had local control rates of 91% and 93% with average follow-up of 36 and 43 months, respectively. The multicenter study reported by Kondziolka et al[51] in 203 patients with mean follow-up of 3.5 years revealed only one factor that negatively influenced outcome. Without prior surgery, the 5-year local control rate was 93%, whereas, with previous surgery, the 5-year local control was only 60%. Prior exposure to EBRT could not be modeled because of insufficient events/numbers, and this confounding variable has not been well analyzed in other series. Other factors such as sex, age, marginal dose, and maximal dose had no impact on local control. The impact of previous surgery was also noted in Kondziolka et al's analysis of 99 patients treated at the Universtiy of Pittsburgh[8,52] in which only 1 of 36 patients (2.7%) having no previous surgery had local tumor progression. This finding may be due to either the limited number of patients having radiosurgery as primary management of their meningioma, or perhaps to a selection bias in patients who have failed previous surgery, predisposing them to a higher risk of recurrence. Nonetheless, as more meningioma patients are managed primarily with radiosurgery, the local failure patterns will need to be scrutinized further.

In our series, local failure occurred in 18 tumors from 3 to 94 months (median, 39 months) after radiosurgery and was heavily influenced by tumor histology. Exclusion of patients with atypical or malignant tumors showed that local control was no different for patients having no previous surgery compared with patients being treated for tumor recurrence after prior resection. However, the use of EBRT was associated with worse local control for these patients with benign tumors (n=180).

There is no clear evidence that small volume tumors (<7.5 cm^3) fail less often than larger volume tumors,[41–44,50,52] despite the data in patients in whom only parasagittal location was reported.[51] However, caution is needed in interpreting results across series and within series for this heterogenous patient population who have had a wide range of management approaches.

Complications

The reported chronic complications rate varies from 4 to 12%, and was found to be 9.7% in the combined series from the Meningioma Study Group.[51] In this series of patients treated for tumors of the falx, symptomatic brain edema occurred in 18 of 185 patients (10%) from 1 to 23 months after radiosurgery. Factors correlating with this complication were preexisting neurological dysfunction and previous surgery. Serious cases of brain or brainstem necrosis have been reported,[42,46,51] with one patient dying as a result. Cranial neuropathies after radiosurgery occur in approximately 3 to 8% of patients with skull base meningiomas. It appears that the special sensory nerves (optic, cochlear) are the most radiation sensitive, and the motor nerves are the most radioresistant. Frequently, cranial nerve deficits after radiosurgery will be transient.

Mayo Clinic Experience

Since the report by Morita et al[43] evaluating complications after skull base meningioma radiosurgery, we have continued to manage patients in a similar fashion with two exceptions. First, the number of isocenters of radiation used per procedure has increased to provide more conformal dose plans. Second, the radiation doses utilized are lower based on published local control rates and further follow-up of our own patients.

Between 1990 and 1998, we managed 190 patients with 206 meningiomas. The median age was 58 years (range, 20–90). There were 126 female patients. Prior surgery had been performed in 121 patients (59%). The location of treated tumors were skull base (71%), falcine (22%), and convexity (7%). The isodose line utilized for the tumor marginal dose was 50% in 191 lesions and varied from 33 to 90% in the other 15. The median tumor volume treated was 8.2 cm^3 (range, 0.5–50.5). The treated volume was greater than 7.5 cm^3 in 53% of lesions. The median tumor marginal dose was 16 Gy (range, 12–36).

Five-year progression-free survival was 93%, 68%, and 0% for benign (n=180), atypical (n=13), and malignant (n=9) tumors, respectively ($p<0.05$) (Fig. 1). Tumor progression occurred in 18 lesions at a median of 39 months after radiosurgery. In-field failure occurred for seven tumors,

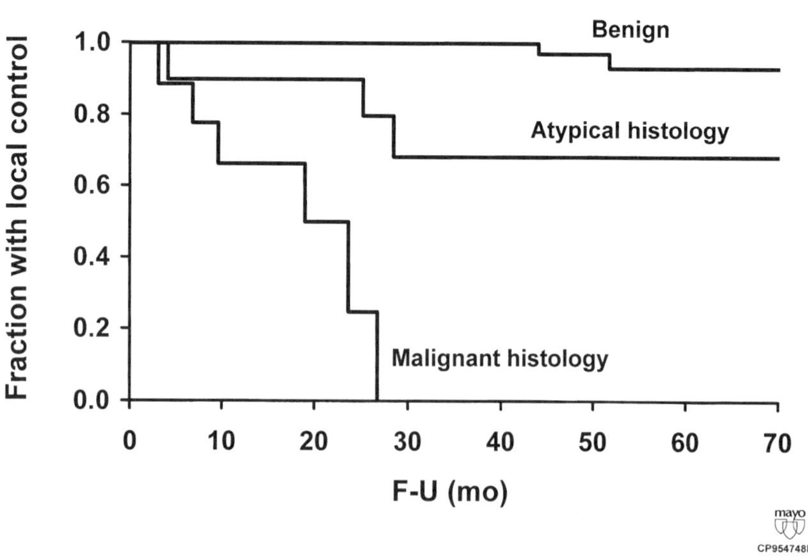

Figure 1. Progression-free survival of 190 patients treated at Mayo Clinic between 1990 and 1998.[50]

whereas the remaining failures developed either adjacent (n=2) to the irradiated volume (Fig. 2), or distant to the treated site. The tumors of two patients were reported to have progressed, but the available records were not adequate to classify the pattern of progression.

Complications occurred in 13% of patients but only resulted in a worsening long-term clinical outcome in six patients (3%). Complications

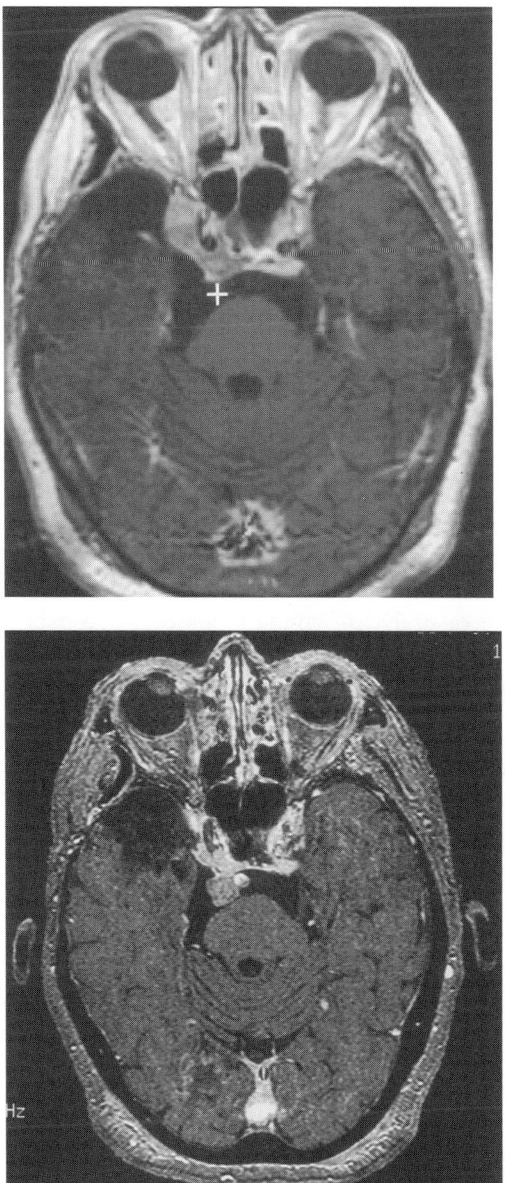

Figure 2. Marginal failure in a patient 75 months after radiosurgery of a recurrent right cavernous sinus meningioma. (**Top**) MRI at the time of the initial radiosurgery. (**Bottom**) MRI 75 months later shows tumor progression inferior to the previously irradiated volume.

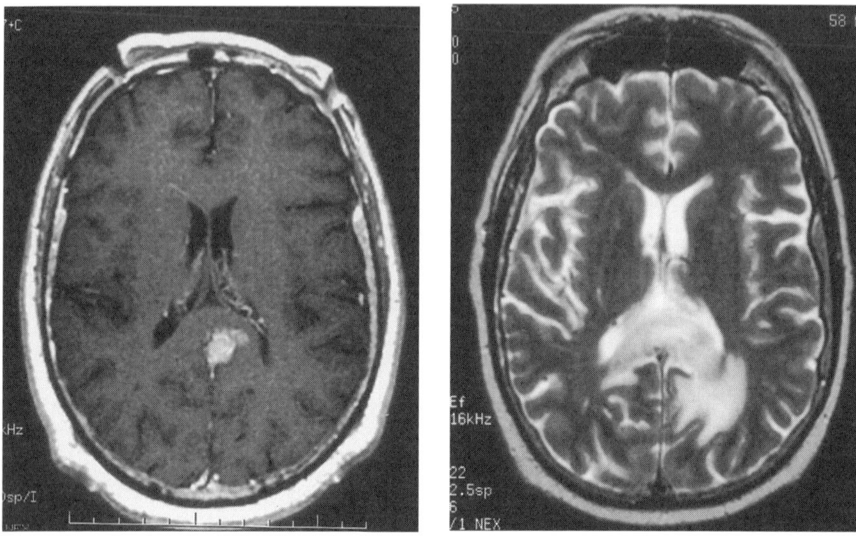

Figure 3. Patient with symptomatic edema after radiosurgery of a left falx meningioma. (**Left**) MRI at the time of radiosurgery. The patient was treated with 16 Gy to the 50% isodose line for a tumor volume of 10.8 cm^3. (**Right**) MRI 8 months after radiosurgery. The patient was treated with corticosteroids and made a complete recovery over several months.

included cranial nerve deficits (n=16), symptomatic edema (n=5), peritumoral cyst formation (n=2), and carotid stenosis (n=2). The cases of symptomatic edema developed 2 to 11 months after radiosurgery: all three patients who did not have prior EBRT made a complete recovery (Fig. 3). Two patients developed peritumoral cysts approximately 2 years after radiosurgery and both of these patients required further surgery.[50]

Radiation Tolerance of the Optic Apparatus

Much has been said regarding optic nerve tolerance and what dose should or should not be used to encompass any part of the optic apparatus. Tishler et al studied a combined group of patients treated with LINAC and Gamma Knife radiosurgery.[53] These investigators reported four cases of radiation optic neuropathy (RON) at doses of 9.7, 10.5, 12.5, and 21.9 Gy in a study of 62 patients from two institutions. Other cranial nerves did not appear to have a dose response related to the development of neuropathy. Moreover, there is some evidence that the length of an irradiated cranial nerve also relates to the risk of postradiosurgical cranial nerve deficit.[54] Hakim et al reported one patient with an RON after a tumor marginal dose of 15 Gy at the 70% isodose line using a 30-mm collimator.[35] Girkin et al reported four patients with an onset of RON ranging from 7 to 30 months after radiosurgery.[55] Based on these reports, most centers adhere to the guideline of delivering no more than 8 Gy to the optic apparatus.

Contrary to the assertion that 8 Gy or more carries a substantial risk of RON, Leber et al reported a series of patients having radiosurgery for cavernous sinus/parasellar region tumors.[56] The mean follow-up was 48 months. They found no cases of RON in 31 patients treated with doses less than 10 Gy, an approximately 30% risk for RON in 22 patients treated with 10 to 15Gy, and an 80% risk for RON if the dose exceeded 15 Gy. Morita et al reported no cases of RON with 59 patients receiving 8 Gy or more to some portion of the optic apparatus.[43] Since that report, our updated experience has found one case of RON occurring after the patient received 7 Gy to the optic nerve. Of note, this patient had previously undergone skull base resection and failed 58-Gy postoperative EBRT prior to treatment with radiosurgery.

It is our belief that radiation doses up to 12 Gy to a small portion of the optic apparatus will be well tolerated with an acceptable risk to the patient's vision. It is therefore vital that the treating physicians possess a clear understanding of the intracranial anatomy and the relation of the dose to surrounding normal tissues to optimize the results of radiosurgery.

Patient and Dose Selection for Meningioma Radiosurgery

Radiosurgery is being increasingly utilized in the management of meningioma patients. Obvious candidates would include patients with tumor progression/recurrence after subtotal resection, and patients who are unfit medically for surgical resection. However, radiosurgery as a primary management strategy for patients with meningiomas of the skull base may optimize patient outcomes compared to its use for patients having tumor removal. Another situation where primary radiosurgery may be indicated is for patients with tumors involving the falx that cannot be totally resected due to involvement of the superior sagittal sinus. Still, the relative short-term follow-up data available in most published radiosurgery series, and the heterogeneous groups treated, make comparing this approach to surgical resection impossible. Longer term follow-up information is needed before radiosurgery can be recommended for patients with resectable tumors.

Prescription dose selection must account for previous interventions such as surgery(s) and EBRT, as well as tumor location and proximity to adjacent critical structures. A sound understanding of the relevant literature which influences dose selection in a particular case based on the estimated risk of morbidity,[57–63] balanced against the chance of local control, is mandatory for successful management of these patients. Typically, the tumor margin dose has ranged from 10 to 20 Gy, prescribed to the 50 to 80% prescription isodose line depending on the radiation delivery system used.

Very little evidence of a dose response with regard to marginal dose and local control exists for meningiomas. One small series with limited follow-up reported that tumors of 4 of 12 patients treated with a marginal dose of 10 Gy or less failed within 1 year.[64] However, Shafron et al managed 10 patients with a marginal dose of 10 Gy and none have shown local failure to date.[40] Our current dose prescription guidelines for meningiomas varies primarily based on the tumor location. For skull base tumors, it is usually the radiation dose to adjacent cranial nerves that dictates our dose selection. Conversely, tumors along the falx are treated with doses that comply with known dose-volume predictions for radiation-related complications. Patients who have received prior EBRT typically receive lower radiation doses. As mentioned above, it appears that any single-fraction dose of 12 Gy or more achieves excellent local control, although short follow-up is a clear shortcoming for the majority of available data. Tumor margin doses less than 10 Gy are not indicated, given the available data.

References

1. O'Rahilly R, Miller F: The meninges in human development. J Neuropathol Exp Neurol 1986;45:588–608.
2. Perry A, Scheithauer BW, Stafford SL: Rhabdoid meningiomas. Am J Surg Pathol 1998;22:1482–1490.
3. Zorludemir S, Scheithauer BW, Hirose T, et al: Clear cell meningioma: a clinicopathologic study of a potentially aggressive variant of meningioma. Am J Surg Pathol 1995;19:493–505.
4. Pasquier B, Gasnier F, Pasquier D, et al: Papillary meningioma. Cancer 1986;58:299–305.
5. Perry A, Stafford SL, Scheithauer BW, et al: Meningoma grading an analysis of histologic parameters. Am J Surg Pathol 1997;21:1455–1465.
6. Perry A, Scheithauer BW, Stafford SL, et al: "Malignancy" in meningiomas. Cancer 1999;85:2046–2056.
7. Stafford SL, Perry A, Suman V, et al: Primarily resected meningiomas: outcome and prognostic factors in 581 Mayo Clinic patients, 1978 through 1998. Mayo Clin Proc 1998;73:936–942.
8. Kondziolka D, Levy EI, Niranjan A, et al: Long-term outcomes after meningioma radiosurgery: physician and patient perspectives. J Neurosurg 1999;91: 44–50.
9. Collins VP, Mordenskjold M, Dumanski JP: The molecular genetics of meningiomas. Brain Pathol 1990;1:19–24.
10. Modan B, Baidatz D, Mart H, et al: Radiation induced head and neck tumors. Lancet 1974;1:277–279.
11. MacCarty CS, Taylor WF: Intracranial meningiomas: experiences at the Mayo Clinic. Neurol Med Chir 1979;19:569–574.
12. Barbaro NM, Gutin PH, Sheline GE, et al: Radiation therapy in the treatment of partially resected meningiomas. Neurosurgery 1987;20:525–528.

13. Simpson D: The recurrence of intracranial meningiomas after surgical treatment. J Neurol Neurosurg Psychiatry 1957;20:22–39.
14. Black PM: Meningiomas. Neurosurgery 1993;32:643–657.
15. Wilson CB: Meningiomas: genetics, malignancy, and the role of radiation in induction and treatment. J Neurosurg 1994;81:666–675.
16. Mirimanoff RO, Dosoretz DE, Linggood RM, et al: Meningioma: analysis of recurrence and progression following neuorsurgical resection. J Neurosurg 1985;62:18–24.
17. Condra KS, Buatti JM, Mendenhall WM, et al: Benign meningiomas: primary treatment selection affects survival. Int J Radiat Oncol Biol Phys 1997;39: 427–436.
18. Taylor BW Jr, Marcus RB, Friedman WA, et al: The meningioma controversy: postoperative radiation therapy. Int J Radiat Oncol Biol Phys 1988;15:299–304.
19. Chan RC, Thompson GB: Morbidity, mortality, and quality of life following surgery for intracranial meningiomas. J Neurosurg 1984;60:52–60.
20. Adegbite AB, Khan MI, Paine KW, et al: The recurrence of intracranial meningiomas after surgical treatment. J Neurosurg 1983;58:51–56.
21. Yamashita J, Handa H, Iwaki K, et al: Recurrence of intracranial meningiomas, with special reference to radiotherapy. Surg Neurol 1980;14:33–40.
22. DeMonte F, Smith HK, Al-Mefty O: Outcome of aggressive removal of cavernous sinus meningiomas. J Neurosurg 1994;81:245–251.
23. De Jesus O, Sekhar LN, Parikh HK, et al: Long-term follow-up of patients with meningiomas involving the cavernous sinus: recurrence, progression, and quality of life. Neurosurgery 1996;39:915–920.
24. Kumar PP, Good RD, Patil AA, et al: Permanent high-activity iodine-125 in the management of petroclival meningiomas: case reports. Neurosurgery 1989;25:436–442.
25. Sekhar LN, Buchanan RI, Wright DC, et al: Benign tumors of the cavernous sinus: the case for agressive resection. Clin Neurosurg 1999;45:263–278.
26. Friedlander RM, Ojemann RG, Thornton AF: Benign tumors of the cavernous sinus: conservative surgery and adjuvant treatment. Clin Neurosurg 1999;45:279–282.
27. Goldsmith BJ, Wara WM, Wilson CB, et al: Postoperative irradiation for subtotally resected meningiomas. J Neurosurg 1994;80:195–201.
28. Haie-Meder C, Brunel P, Cioloca C, et al: Role of radiotherapy in the treatment of meningioma. Bulletin du cancer. Radiotherapie 1995;82:35–39.
29. Wara WM, Sheline GE, Newman H, et al: Radiation therapy of meningiomas. Am J Roentgenol Radiat Ther Nucl Med 1975;123:453–458.
30. Mahmood A, Caccamo DV, Tomecek FJ, et al: Atypical and malignant meningiomas: a clinicopatholigical review. Neurosurgery 1993;33:955–963.
31. Thomas HG, Dolman CL, Berry K: Malignant meningioma: clinical and pathological features. J Neurosurg 1981;55:929–934.
32. Jaaskelainen J, Haltia M, Servo A: Atypical and anaplastic meningiomas: radiology, surgery, radiotherapy, and outcome. Surg Neurol 1996;25:233–242.
33. Steiner L, Lindquist L, Steiner M: Meningiomas and Gamma Knife radiosurgery. In Al-Mefty O (ed): Meningiomas. New York, Raven Press, 1991, pp 263–272.
34. Engenhart R, Kimmig BN, Hover K, et al: Stereotactic single high dose radiation therapy of benign intracranial meningiomas. Int J Radiat Oncol Biol Phys 1990;19:1021–1026.
35. Hakim R, Alexander E 3rd, Loeffler JS, et al: Results of linear accelerator-based radiosurgery for intracranial meningiomas. Neurosurgery 1998;42:446–453.
36. Zamorano L, Saenz A, Matter A, et al: Radiosurgical treatment of meningiomas. Stereotact Funct Neurosurg 1997;69:156–161.

37. Chang SD, Adler JR: Treatment of cranial base meningiomas with linear accelerator radiosurgery. Neurosurgery 1997;41:1019–1027.
38. Valentino V, Schinaia G, Raimondi AJ: The results of radiosurgical management of 72 middle fossa meningiomas. Acta Neurochir 1993;122:60–70.
39. Rocher F, Sentenae I, Berger C, et al: Stereotactic radiosurgery: the Lyon experience. Acta Neurochir 1995;63:109–114.
40. Shafron DH, Friedman WA, Buatti JM, et al: Linac radiosurgery for benign meningiomas. Int J Radiat Oncol Biol Phys 1999;43:321–327.
41. Tanaka T, Kobayashi T, Kida Y: Growth control of cranial base meningiomas by stereotactic radiosurgery. Neurol Med Chir 1996;36:7–10.
42. Hudgins WR, Barker JL, Schwartz DE, et al: Gamma knife treatment of 100 consecutive meningiomas. Stereotact Funct Neurosurg 1996;66:121–128.
43. Morita A, Coffey R, Foote R, et al: Risk of injury to cranial nerves after gamma knife radiosurgery for skull base meningiomas: experience in 88 patients. J Neurosurg 1999;90:42–49.
44. Pendl G, Schrottner O, Eustcchio S, et al: Stereotactic radiosurgery of skull base meningiomas. Minim Invasive Neurosurg 1997;40:87–90.
45. Nicolato A, Ferraresi P, Foroni R, et al: Gamma knife radiosurgery in skull base meningiomas. Stereotact Funct Neurosurg 1996;66:112–120.
46. Hodes JE, Sanders M, Patel P, et al: Radiosurgical management of meningiomas. Stereotact Funct Neurosurg 1996;66:15–18.
47. Pendl G, Schrottner O, Friehs GM, et al: Stereotactic radiosurgery of skull base meningiomas. Stereotact Funct Neurosurg 1996;66:11–18.
48. Kurita H, Sasaki T, Kawamoto S, et al: Role of radiosurgery in the management of cavernous sinus meningiomas. Acta Neurol Scand 1997;96:297–304.
49. Liscak R, Simonova G, Vymazal JJL, et al: Gamma knife radiosurgery of meningiomas in the cavernous sinus region. Acta Neurochir 1999;141:473–480.
50. Stafford SL, Pollock BE, Foote RL, et al: Meningioma radiosurgery: tumor control, outcomes, and complications in 190 consecutive patients. Neurosurgery 2001;49:1029–1038.
51. Kondziolka D, Flickenger JC, Perez B: Judicious resection and/or radiosurgery for parasaggital meningiomas: outcomes from a multicenter review. Neurosurgery 1998;43:405–413.
52. Kondziolka D, Niranjan A, Lunsford LD, et al: Stereotactic radiosurgery for meningiomas. Neurosurg Clin N Am 1999;10:317–325.
53. Tishler RB, Loeffler JS, Lunsford LD, et al: Tolerance of cranial nerves of the cavernous sinus to radiosurgery. Int J Radiat Oncol Biol Phys 1993;27:215–221.
54. Linsky ME, Flickinger J, Lunsford LD: Cranial nerve length predicts the risk of delayed facial and trigeminal neuropathies after acoustic tumor stereotactic radiosurgery. Int J Radiat Oncol Biol Phys 1993;25:227–233.
55. Girkin C, Comey C, Lunsford L, et al: Radiation optic neuropathy after stereotactic radiosurgery. Ophthalmology 1997;104:1634–1643.
56. Leber K, Bergloff J, Pendi G: Dose-response tolerance of the visual pathways and cranial nerves of the cavernous sinus to stereotactic radiosurgery. J Neurosurg 1998;88:43–50.
57. Flickenger J, Kondziolka D, Lunsford LD: Dose and diameter relationships for facial, trigeminal, and acoustic neuropathies following acoustic neuroma radiosurgery. Radiother Oncol 1996;41:215–219.
58. Flickinger JC, Lunsford LD, Kondziolka D, et al: Radiosurgery and brain tolerance: an analysis of neurodiagnostic imaging changes after gamma knife radiosurgery for arteriovenous malformations. Int J Radiat Oncol Biol Phys 1992;23:19–26.

59. Larson DA, Flickenger JC, Loeffler JS: The radiobiology of radiosurgery. Int J Radiat Oncol Biol Phys 1993;25:557–561.
60. Maguire PD, Clough R, Friedman AH, et al: Fractionated external-beam radiation therapy for meningomas of the cavernous sinus. Int J Radiat Oncol Biol Phys 1999;44:75–79.
61. Shaw EG, Coffey RJ, Diapoli RP: Neurotoxicity of radiosurgery. Sem Radiat Oncol 1995;3:235–245.
62. Flickinger J, Schell MC, Larson DA: Estimation of complications for linear accelerator radiosurgery with the integrated logistic formula. Int J Radiat Oncol Biol Phys 1990;19:143–148.
63. Flickinger J: An integrated logistic formula for prediction of complications from radiosurgery. Int J Radiat Oncol Biol Phys 1989;17:879–885.
64. Ganz JC, Backlund FA: The results of gamma knife surgery of meningiomas, related to size of tumor and dose. Stereotact Funct Neurosurg 1992;61:23–29.

Comment

Chapter 8

Robert D. Strang, Ossama Al-Mefty

Introduction

In the preceding text, Stafford et al outline a carefully considered argument for using stereotactic radiosurgery as a primary and/or adjunctive treatment modality in the management of intracranial meningiomas. They cite the recurrence and complication rates of these benign, albeit formidable, lesions as a basis for accepting alternative treatment methods. However, the reader should be cautioned against extrapolating the results of select clinical series when considering the general treatment of meningiomas as a whole. In particular, most of the presented data regarding recurrence and complication rates of surgically managed meningiomas is related to lesions of the cavernous sinus and the petroclival region. These sites rank among the most unforgiving and technically challenging regions in all of neurosurgery. Certainly, the authors do not mean to equate surgical resection of sphenopetroclival meningiomas with that of convexity meningiomas. In addition, some of the tumors treated surgically in these series were not candidates for radiosurgery based on size, configuration, location, clinical presentation, or a combination thereof. Finally, some of the cited surgical series were older, and, as such, may not have benefited from some of the more recent, evolving advances in microsurgical and skull base technique. Nevertheless, Stafford et al do present an important perspective with regard to the multidisciplinary treatment of meningiomas. Their viewpoint is strengthened by the inclusion of their own straightforward and honest radiosurgical data.

Role of Radiation Treatment in the Management of Meningiomas

In this chapter, the authors state, and we agree, that microsurgical resection of meningiomas and their dural attachments "is the standard of care for meningioma patients." This is particularly true in cases of larger lesions where immediate decompression of the neural elements is required. Clearly, larger lesions presenting with mass effect, brainstem compression, or progressive neurological deficit should be treated with surgical resection. For small asymptomatic meningiomas, close follow-up with serial neurological assessments and neuroimaging is a valid treatment option, particularly in older patients or those with significant medical comorbidities. However, some meningiomas, especially those arising from the cranial base, have been considered high risk or inoperable based on location alone. Consequently, several new treatment options, including radiotherapy and radiosurgery, have been introduced. It is important to point out, however, that anatomy-based microneurosurgery[1] and the development of advanced skull base techniques[2–11] have led not only to a greater understanding of these lesions, but also to increasingly improved outcomes.

Conventional fractionated external beam radiation therapy has been available on a large scale longer than radiosurgery and, therefore, longer term follow-up data exists in the treatment of benign meningiomas. Its implementation began primarily as an adjunctive treatment to surgical resection in those lesions where complete resection had not been achieved. The authors state that, "postoperative external beam radiation therapy is an effective measure to reduce tumor progression rates for patients after subtotal resection of meningiomas," and they have used this rationale as a basis for employing radiosurgery as a primary treatment option for meningiomas. However, the importance of even longer follow-up periods cannot be overstated. Radiation therapy does not result in the cure of skull base meningiomas, but rather it delays their symptomatic recurrence. Mathiesen et al found that, while the 10-year mortality rate was lower in patients treated with radiation therapy, there was no difference in survival at 20-year follow-up.[12] They therefore concluded that the role of radiation therapy in the management of skull base meningiomas is one of palliation in unresectable tumors.

Although radiotherapy has been reported to result in fewer cranial neuropathies than radiosurgery,[13] it has the distinct disadvantage of including nondiseased neural structures in the treatment plan. This may not be as much of a concern in the treatment of malignant disease, but the serious long-term side effects of radiation therapy in the treatment of benign brain tumors has been well documented.[14,15] Therefore, stereotactic delivery of high-dose ionizing radiation in single-fraction radiosurgery has been regarded as an attractive alternative to conventional radiotherapy as an adjunct to, or replacement for, microsurgical resection. In contrast to surgical resection, the treatment goal of radiosurgery is not eradication of the tumor, but rather "tumor control." The definition of this ideal varies between reports. Some reports define "progression-free survival" or "control" as lack of tumor growth[16–20]; others use a measure of "clinical tumor control" as defined by no requirement for surgical resection.[21] Based on these definitions, radiosurgical series report control rates ranging from 98 to 100% for short-term follow-up of 2 years.[17,20] This control drops to 92 to 95% at 35 months and 86.7% at 96 months.[16,22] Although no strict definitions of control are given in the preceding chapter, Stafford et al do report tumor progression in 18 of 206 meningiomas (9%) at a median of 39 months after radiosurgery. Radiosurgical results must, however, be interpreted with caution given the natural history and slow growth of meningiomas. During an average follow-up period of 47 months, Olivero et al found that only 22% of meningiomas demonstrated any detectable growth on neuroimaging.[23] The growth rate ranged from 0.2 cm over 180 months to 1 cm over 12 months and all patients remained asymptomatic. This translates to a progression-free survival rate of 78% and a clinical control rate of 100% for these untreated lesions over the 47-month follow-up period. Indeed, our own series of nonsurgically treated patients shows similar results with a 90% progression-free survival rate and a 100% clinical control rate over 47.3 months. Therefore, it remains unclear which meningiomas have realistically benefited from radiosurgery and which have merely followed the natural course of a slow-growing, histologically benign lesion. Perhaps for this reason, the radiosurgical literature has begun reporting tumor shrinkage rates with increasing frequency. Depending on the length of the follow-up period, decreased tumor volume has been reported in 23 to 68% of radiosurgically treated meningiomas.[16,17,20–22] However, it remains clear that the goal of radiosurgery is tumor control and not reduction of tumor volume. This is especially relevant since reduction in tumor size does not necessarily correlate with improvement of clinical symptoms; nor does early tumor shrinkage portend long-term tumor control.[16,21,24] Moreover, the cytoreductive effect of radiosurgery cannot match the outcomes of microsurgery, which, for any surgical series, will result in tumor volume reduction rates of 100%.

Pitfalls of Radiosurgery

The concept of radiosurgery as a minimally invasive treatment option compared with open microsurgical resection has also been enticing. Certainly, in the short term, the effects of radiosurgery are far less evident than those seen with open surgery; this is true for both its desired results as well as its complications. This philosophy is particularly important to heed when treating meningiomas because extended survivals are reasonable to expect by virtue of their slow-growing, benign nature. Some of the earlier radiosurgical literature reported significant neurological morbidity associated with treatment. Engenhart and colleagues reported delayed brain edema and radiation necrosis in 38% of patients.[25] This was probably secondary to considerably higher maximum doses to tumor volume than those that are currently in use today, and the authors allude to this. Over the past decade, significant advances in treatment planning, neuroimaging, and software applications have allowed for safer delivery of radiosurgical doses. In current studies, the rates of brain edema and radiation necrosis have dropped to 6 to 7%.[17,18] In this chapter, Stafford et al report a 3% rate of symptomatic brain edema. Nevertheless, despite recent advances, the neurological morbidity from radiosurgical treatment of meningiomas remains significant (Fig. I). Present series report treat-

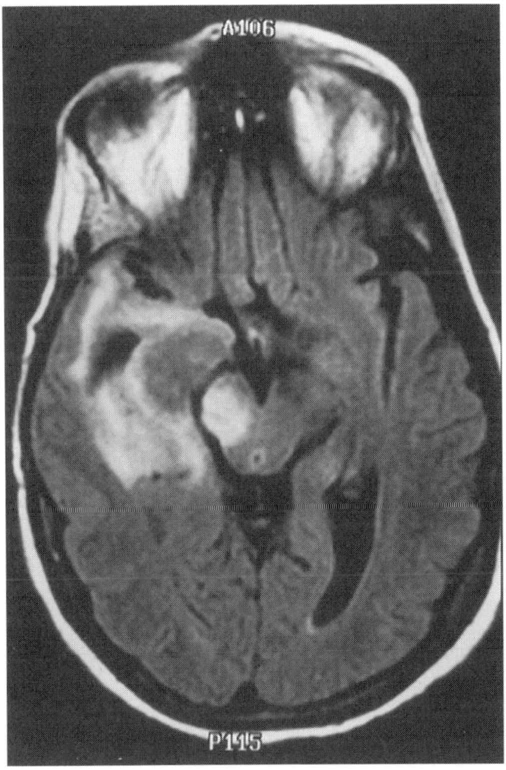

Figure 1. MRI showing severe temporal lobe edema in a patient treated with Gamma Knife radiosurgery. Note the involvement of the adjacent mesencephalon.

ment-related neurological deficits in 8.8 to 19.4% of patients.[16,20–22,26] The majority of deficits were related to cranial neuropathy and many patients were affected more than once. The authors' results are certainly consistent, with a 13% complication rate reported in this chapter. Clearly, radiosurgery should not be considered as noninvasive, and patients need to be counseled as to the potential risks and benefits of this and other treatment modalities prior to definitive management.

Advantages of Microsurgery

It may be argued that microsurgical resection of meningiomas has several distinct advantages over radiosurgery as a primary treatment option. First, microsurgical resection offers the possibility of obtaining tissue for definitive histologic diagnosis. Although some have considered meningiomas to have highly characteristic, if not pathognomonic, features on neuroimaging, the literature is replete with reports of various lesions mimicking meningiomas. Cavernous malformations, metastatic lesions, lymphoma, hemangiopericytoma, and inflammatory lesions are among the possible diseases that may resemble meningiomas.[27–29] It is imperative that the correct diagnosis be made because most nonmeningiomatous skull base lesions have better operative outcomes with a greater potential for total resection and cranial nerve recovery when compared to meningiomas.[27] Perhaps more importantly, some disease processes, such as sarcoidosis, do not respond to radiosurgery. Treatment with this modality may result in diagnostic delays and, thus, delays in the delivery of definitive care. Even when meningioma is, in fact, the correct diagnosis, it must be remembered that only 90% are considered truly benign.[30,31] The remaining 10% are made up of atypical or frankly malignant variants, both of which may require adjuvant therapy. Moreover, 2% of recurrent meningiomas have dedifferentiated to a more aggressive form,[31] so that even prior histologic ev-

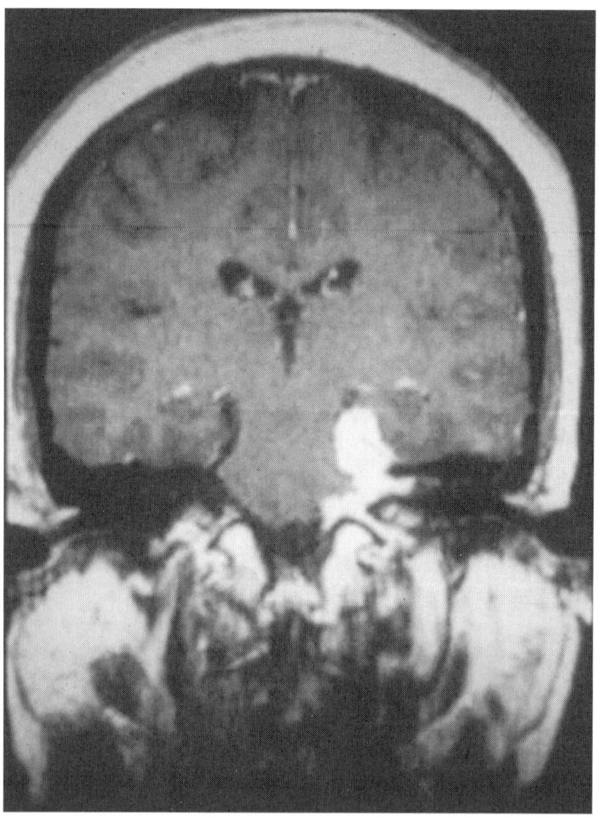

Figure II. (**A**) Coronal post-contrast T1 MRI revealing a homogeneously enhancing lesion involving the left petrous apex. Preoperative diagnosis was meningioma. Caseating granuloma was found at surgery. *(Continued.)*

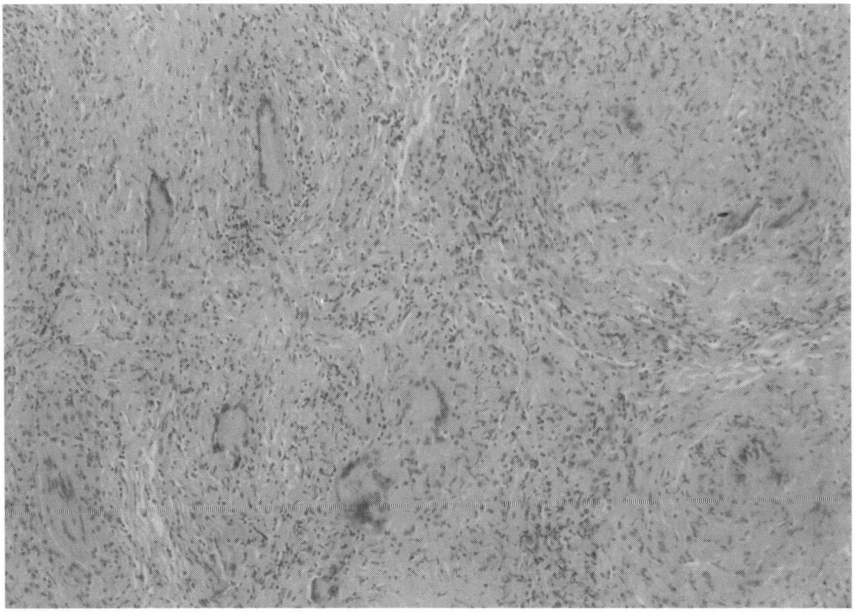

Figure II. (**B**) Hematoxylin and eosin preparation demonstrates nodular arrangements of epithelioid histiocytes. Note the formation of giant cells.

idence of benignity does not necessarily exclude present aggressive behavior. With these facts in mind, it is surprising that many radiosurgical centers are willing to treat these lesions without a tissue diagnosis. Just a decade ago such treatment was a rare occurrence.[25] However, there has been an increasing trend to treat based on radiographic criteria alone. During the past 2 years, several of the larger radiosurgical series have reported treating 37 to 44% [16,21,22] of patients without histologic confirmation of benign meningioma. In our surgical series of small (<2.5 cm) skull base meningiomas (i.e., meningiomas that would have been considered ideal radiosurgical targets), 2 of 30 patients (7%) were found at surgery to have nonmeningiomatous lesions. One patient had a cavernous malformation arising in the cavernous sinus that was completely excised with microsurgical technique. The other was found to have a caseating granuloma involving the petroclival region (Fig. II) and appropriate medical therapy was initiated. Radiosurgery would not have been considered to be an ideal primary treatment option in either of these cases. At best, misdiagnosis leads to delay in the delivery of definitive care; at worst, it may lead to a detrimental outcome for the patient.

In addition to offering tissue for histologic diagnosis, open surgery provides immediate decompression of compromised neurovascular structures. Indeed, some failures of radiosurgery have been attributed not to tumor growth, but to a failure to provide timely relief of symptoms.[21] This is particularly important when pain is the initial presenting symptom. Of all skull base meningiomas, those arising from Meckel's cave and the petroclival region have the highest propensity to present with pain. We have found surgical management for these meningiomas to be most rewarding as it results in rapid and dramatic reduction of pain. Samii et al have corroborated our observations and they have reported resolution of facial pain in 100% of patients operated for such lesions.[32]

Conclusion

When considering the various options for the treatment of meningiomas, several salient points exist. Surgical resection of meningiomas remains the gold standard for the treatment of these lesions. Modern microsurgical and skull base techniques have resulted in improved safety and efficacy, reaffirming the role of surgical resection as the primary therapeutic option in the management of meningiomas. Although radiosurgery may be considered for select patients (particularly the elderly or those with significant medical disease), its unproven long-term efficacy precludes it from being considered as a primary, first-line treatment standard for all meningiomas. Indeed, the preceding chapter also suggests that radiosurgery may be an inappropriate treatment for atypical and malignant meningiomas. Finally, we believe that nonsurgical management of asymptomatic lesions is a valid treatment option in carefully selected patients, and its results, to date, are comparable with those of radiosurgery.

References

1. Yasargil MG. Microneurosurgery: Vol I. New York, Thieme Medical Publishers, 1994, pp 26.
2. Kawase T, Shiobara R, Toya S: Anterior transpetrosal-transtentorial approach for sphenopetroclival meningiomas: surgical method and results in 10 patients. Neurosurgery 1991;28:869–876.
3. Samii M, Tatagiba M, Carvalho GA. Retrosigmoid intradural suprameatal approach to Meckel's cave and the middle fossa: surgical technique and outcome. J Neurosurg 2000;92:235–241.
4. Seoane E, Rhoton AL: Suprameatal extension of the retrosigmoid approach: microsurgical anatomy. Neurosurgery 1999;44:553–560.
5. Sekhar LN, Schessel DA, Bucur SD, et al: Partial labyrinthectomy petrous apicectomy approach to neoplastic and vascular lesions of the petroclival area. Neurosurgery 1999;44:537–552.
6. Tedeschi H, Rhoton AL: Lateral approaches to the petroclival region. Surg Neurol 1994;41:180–216.

7. Al-Mefty O, Fox JL, Smith RR: Petrosal approach for petroclival meningiomas. Neurosurgery 1988;22:510–517.
8. Bricolo AP, Turazzi S, Talacchi A, et al: Microsurgical removal of petroclival meningiomas: a report of 33 cases. Neurosurgery 1992;31:813–828.
9. Al-Mefty O: Clinoidal meningiomas. J Neurosurg 1990;73:840–849.
10. Pieper DR, Al-Mefty O: Management of intracranial meningiomas secondarily involving the infratemporal fossa: Radiographic characteristics, pattern of tumor invasion, and surgical implications. Neurosurgery 1999;45:231–238.
11. Day JD: Cranial base surgical technique for large sphenocavernous meningiomas: technical note. Neurosurgery 2000;46:754–759.
12. Mathiesen T, Lindquist C, Kihlstrom L, et al: Proposed grading system to predict the extent of resection and outcomes for cranial base meningiomas. Neurosurgery 1996;39:2–9.
13. Nutting C, Brada M, Brazil L, et al: Radiotherapy in the treatment of benign meningioma of the skull base. J Neurosurg 1999;90:823–827.
14. Al-Mefty O, Kersh JE, Routh A, et al: The long-term side effects of radiation therapy for benign brain tumors in adults. J Neurosurg 1990;73:502–512.
15. Sekhar LN, Patel S, Cusimano M, et al: Surgical treatment of meningiomas involving the cavernous sinus: evolving ideas based on a ten year experience. Acta Neurochir 1996;65(suppl):58–62.
16. Morita A, Coffey RJ, Foote RL, et al: Risk of injury to cranial nerves after Gamma Knife radiosurgery for skull base meningiomas: experience in 88 patients. J Neurosurg 1999;90:42–49.
17. Chang SD, Adler JR: Treatment of cranial base meningiomas with Linear accelerator radiosurgery. Neurosurgery 1997;41:1019–1027.
18. Kondziolka D, Lunsford LD, Coffey RJ, et al: Stereotactic radiosurgery of meningiomas. J Neurosurg 1991;74:552–559.
19. Connell PP, Macdonald RL, Mansur DB, et al: Tumor size predicts control of benign meningiomas treated with radiotherapy. Neurosurgery 1994;44:1194–1200.
20. Duma CH, Lunsford LD, Kondziolka D, et al: Stereotactic radiosurgery of cavernous sinus meningiomas as an addition or alternative to microsurgery. Neurosurgery 1993;32:699–705.
21. Kondziolka D, Levy EI, Niranjan A, et al: Long-term outcomes after meningioma radiosurgery: physician and patient perspectives. J Neurosurg 1999; 91:44–50.
22. Subach BR, Lunsford LD, Kondziolka D, et al: Management of petroclival meningiomas by stereotactic radiosurgery. Neurosurgery 1998;47:437–445.
23. Olivero WC, Lister JR, Elwood PW: The natural history and growth of asymptomatic meningiomas. A review of 60 patients. J Neurosurg 1995;83:222–224.
24. Valentino V, Schinaia G, Raimondi AJ: The results of radiosurgical management of 72 middle fossa meningiomas. Acta Neurochir 1993;122:60–70.
25. Engenhart R, Kimmig BN, Hover KH, et al: Stereotactic single high dose radiation therapy of benign intracranial meningiomas. Int J Radiat Oncol Biol Phys 1990;19:1021–1026.
26. Tishler RB, Loeffler JS, Lunsford LD, et al: Tolerance of cranial nerves of the cavernous sinus to radiosurgery. Int J Radiat Oncol Biol Phys 1993;27:215–221.
27. Eisenberg MB, Al-Mefty O, DeMonte F, et al: Benign nonmeningeal tumors of the cavernous sinus. Neurosurgery 1999;44:949–955.
28. O'Sullivan MG, van Loveren HR, Tew JM: The surgical resectability of meningiomas of the cavernous sinus. Neurosurgery 1997;40:238–247.
29. Aziz KMA, van Loveren HR: Primary lymphoma of Meckel's cave: mimicking trigeminal schwannoma. Case report. Neurosurgery 1999;44:859–863.

30. Salazar OM. Ensuring local control in meningiomas. Int J Radiat Oncol Biol Phys 1998;15:501–504.
31. Rohringer M, Sutherland GR, Louw DR, et al: Incidence and clinicopathological features of meningioma. J Neurosurg 1989;71:665–672.
32. Samii M, Carvalho GA, Tatagiba M, et al: Surgical management of meningiomas originating in Meckel's cave. Neurosurgery 1997;41:767–775.

Chapter 9

Stereotactic Radiosurgery for Vestibular Schwannoma

Jean Régis, Pierre Hughes Roche, Christine Delsanti, Outouma Soumare, Jean Marc Thomassin, William Pellet

Introduction

Since the first quarter of the 20th century when Walter Dandy developed an operation for the complete extirpation of vestibular schwannomas (VS),[1] surgeons have achieved an admirable success rate in dealing with such tumors. Vestibular schwannomas typically are slow growing, allowing the nervous system to compensate for the enlarging mass. As a result, these tumors can become rather large without symptoms other than hearing loss, tinnitus, or unsteadiness. Improved neuroimaging permits early tumor recognition and excellent treatment results are now available to VS patients. Consequently, conservative management with serial imaging is generally proposed for the elderly or patients in poor medical condition. For such patients, most tumors remain unchanged or grow very slowly over short follow-up intervals.[2]

Radiosurgery, as conceived by Lars Leksell, is a neurosurgical technique used to manage a variety of neurosurgical pathologies.[3] Although the Gamma Knife developed by Leksell uses ionizing radiation, he believed that this was a neurosurgical device, and not a tool for radiotherapy. Radiosurgery provides a maximum dose inside the target volume with a "lethal" effect on the concerned tissues. However, the radiation falls off very rapidly outside the prescribed dose plan. Although the use of radiosurgery began nearly 50 years ago, it is still controversial for several

This work was supported by Assistance Publique des Hôpitaux de Marseille and by the French Ministry of Health (PHRC 1994).

From Pollock BE (ed). *Contemporary Stereotactic Radiosurgery: Technique and Evaluation.* Armonk, NY, Futura Publishing Company, Inc. © 2002.

reasons. First, unlike ordinary surgical instruments, the machines are very expensive and must be set up in a special environment, typically outside the operating room. Second, radiosurgery relies on a multidisciplinary team including neurosurgeons, physicists, radiotherapists, and neuroradiologists. Third, every neurosurgeon cannot have such a tool placed at his disposal. This often creates an environment of competition between those with access to this technology and physicians who are unable or unwilling to offer to patients the option of radiosurgery.

The debate regarding the role of radiosurgery in the management of VS patients has been especially brisk. Vestibular schwannomas (formerly referred to as acoustic neuromas) appeared as a logical indication for Gamma Knife, and the first VS patient underwent radiosurgery in June 1968.[4,5] During this same period the introduction of the operative microscope, improved anesthesia, and utilization of new surgical approaches allowed experienced surgeons to completely remove these tumors with preservation of the facial nerve in the majority of cases.[6] Neuro-otological surgical teams initially were indifferent to radiosurgery, which was inaccessible to most patients. Moreover, radiosurgery at that point was unproven for benign tumors like schwannomas. However, in the 1980s, the team from Stockholm,[7] and later from the University of Pittsburgh,[8,9] began to publish reports showing the results of VS radiosurgery. It was at this juncture that opponents to radiosurgery became more vocal. Critics of radiosurgery stated that patients would be at risk for the long-term complications reported after conventional radiotherapy, such as delayed brain necrosis,[10] radiation-induced neoplasms,[11] and cranial nerve neuritis.[12] Other concerns involved the lack of tumor removal, and also that irradiated tissues would make microsurgery more difficult for the patients that fail radiosurgery.[13,14] The radiosurgical experience refutes such claims and provides increasing data that this less invasive and more functionally conservative technique may be the preferable treatment.[15–17] Currently, only those who are opposed on principle still put forward these arguments.

The modalities currently used for stereotactic radiosurgery (SRS) include photon devices such as the Gamma Knife and modified linear accelerators (LINACs), or proton and heavy-ion charged particles generated in cyclotron.[18] However, only centers using the Gamma Knife have reported on large series: Stockholm (669 cases),[5,19] Pittsburgh (273 cases),[16] Charlottesville (200 cases),[20] and Prague (122 cases).[21] Authors using the other devices have reported primarily small series with short follow-up.[22,23]

Thanks to the conviction and to the efforts of Professor Robert Sedan, it was possible to acquire a Gamma Knife in Marseille in 1992. At that time, our otoneurosurgical team had operated on 600 VS patients and we had evaluated the long-term functional results obtained by our microsurgery patients.[24,25] We created in an "otoneurosurgical-radiosurgical"

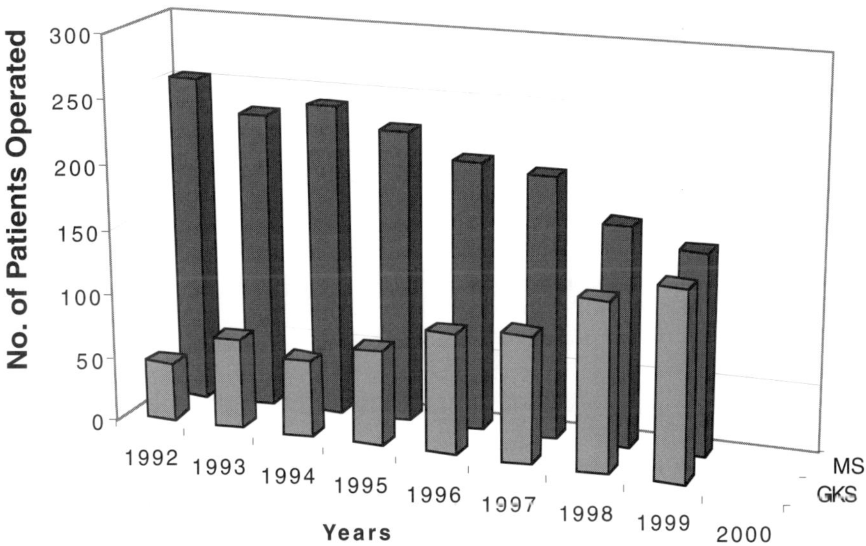

Figure 1. Vestibular schwannoma surgery for patients with small- to medium-sized tumors in France between 1992 and 2000. Note that, in only 8 years, half of the patients had radiosurgery (GKS) and the trend suggests that more patients will have radiosurgery than microsurgery (MS) in the future.

team in Marseille and, since 1992, the first author has operated radiosurgically on 707 VS cases. We are now performing radiosurgery on half the total number of small- to medium-sized VS operated in France (Fig. 1). Our series includes 52 patients (7%) with neurofibromatosis type 2 (NF2), and 80 patients (11%) with recurrent tumors after prior surgical resection. Of 575 sporadic VS patients primarily treated with radiosurgery, a minimum 3-year follow-up has been obtained for 382 patients (66%). The number of patients with 5-, 6-, and 7-year follow-up are 212, 144, and 77, respectively.

The authors of this report are a multidisciplinary team including a group of otoneurosurgeons and ear, nose, throat surgeons. Our goal is to evaluate the functional outcomes for patients undergoing either SRS or microsurgery for small- to medium-sized VS, and to use this to clarify the role of each of these surgical techniques.

Rationale of Vestibular Schwannoma Radiosurgery

Recognition of the efficacy of SRS requires an evaluation of natural history of untreated tumors. Linskey compiled 199 patients from 10 series in the literature with untreated VS.[26] During an average duration of the neuroimaging follow-up of 2.6 years (range, 0.25–16), 38% of tumors increased in size, 59% were unchanged, and 3% decreased. Compared to patients having radiosurgery, they concluded that SRS provided a benefit in tumor control. Likewise, in a series of NF2 patients who had SRS unilaterally, comparison of the treated and untreated sides showed a higher rate of tumor reduction or stability on the treated side.[27] In our series, we compared tumor size at the time of evaluation and SRS. Over a mean interval of only 7 months, 254 tumors enlarged (36.4%). The mean growth was 1.1 mm. This data should be kept in mind regarding follow-up after SRS.

The aim of VS surgery is to prevent the functional consequences due to growth of the untreated tumor, rather than improvement of preoperative symptoms, regardless of the technique used.[28–31] Microsurgery achieves this goal by extirpation of the lesion whereas SRS accomplishes the goal by stopping the tumor's growth. Radiosurgery provides a biological treatment as the tumor, converted to a lump of postmitotic schwann cell remnants, is no longer capable of growing. Several years of follow-up are usually required to demonstrate the efficacy of SRS. In fact, the tumor volume frequently does not decrease during the first years after the procedure. However, most patients are more concerned about how they feel and look than a persistent imaging abnormality on magnetic resonance imaging (MRI).[32,33] Still, some patients simply cannot bear the thought of having a mass inside their head. For such patients, microsurgery will remain the best treatment.

Radiobiology of Vestibular Schwannoma Radiosurgery

Apoptosis and obliteration of tumor vasculature have been evoked to account for the ability of SRS to prevent tumor growth.[34] Undoubtedly, double-strand breaks in the DNA directly from the radiation, or indirectly by the action of free radicals, certainly are critical. If only one strand is broken, the other one will serve as a template allowing DNA repair. Single-strand injury is thus inadequate, and if many cells are so damaged, the irradiated tissue will be unaffected and radiosurgery will be a failure. On the contrary, if both strands are broken the cells will die more or less rapidly or, perhaps, stay in an irreversible growth arrest state. Therefore, the effectiveness of SRS relates mostly to the radiation dose and the cell sensitivity to ionizing radiation.

Early attempts at VS radiosurgery utilized doses of 50 Gy or more in the middle of the target volume.[5,7] This provided rapid necrosis of the tumor, but with frequent injury to the adjacent cranial nerves. Doses were progressively reduced to 26 or 28 Gy which improved the morbidity of the procedure but has not reduced the rate of tumor growth control.[15,16] It appears that this dose range continues to provide sufficient DNA injury, or perhaps, radiation-induced apoptosis as outlined by Tsuzuki et al.[35] Damage to cell membranes, mitochondria, or vascular insult may also contribute to the apoptotic effect of SRS.[36] Decreased intratumoral bloodflow has been shown after VS SRS by thallium-201 chloride single photon emission computed tomography.[37]

The radiation sensitivity of cells correlates with the degree of DNA condensation: condensed DNA is more likely to collide with passing radiation particles. As DNA is in the most condensed state during metaphase, it can be understood that tissues with an increased proliferative index (neoplasms) are more radiosensitive than tissues that are not actively dividing (normal tissue). Thus, dose fractionation permits more cells to be exposed to radiation during a sensitive state, while still permitting nearby normal cells to repair between sessions. However, for tumors with low mitotic activities (i.e., schwannomas, meningiomas) that mimic normal tissues, there is little theoretical benefit to dose fraction.[38–41] Thus, it must be emphasized that SRS is a procedure made to destroy an intracranial volume with a high dose of ionizing radiations in a single session. This is fundamentally different than stereotactic radiotherapy, which delivers radiation over multiple sessions. To quote Linskey,[42] "fractionated radiotherapy relies on differences in radiosensitivity and repair capability between normal and neoplastic tissue, . . . whereas radiosurgery relies on the physical parameters of accuracy of targeting and steepness of radiation fall-off at the edge of the treatment volume,. . ., the dose utilized (being) high enough to affect all normal and neoplastic tissue within the treatment volume." Vestibular schwannoma as slow-growing neoplasms are late-responding tissues to ionizing radiations. Thus, they are relatively resistant to low fractionated doses from which they may recover. For these reasons, long-term control of VS is more likely after a single, high dose of radiation compared to smaller, fractionated dose schemes.

Technical Considerations

Imaging and Anatomical Considerations

Vestibular schwannomas tend to have irregular surface contours and are in close relation to the brainstem and cranial nerves. Accurate depiction of the three-dimensional tumor volume requires high-resolution imaging in all three anatomical planes for precise target selection and dose planning. After head frame application we perform MRI and CT scans. Magnetic resonance imaging is performed after phantom testing and includes an axial T2-weighted sequence (0.5-mm contiguous slices) and a postgadolinium axial T1-weighted volume acquisition (1-mm contiguous slices). High-resolution contrast-enhanced CT (axial 1-mm contiguous slices) is performed with bony and parenchymal algorithms. The CT imaging ensures stereotactic accuracy and permits correction of any MRI distortion.[43,44]

Vestibular schwannoma generally arises from the inferior branch of the vestibular nerve and generally invades this nerve initially. It then quickly invades the cochlear nerve which can become indistinguishable from the tumor.[45–49] Only the facial nerve preserves its continuity and is simply flattened on the convexity of the schwannoma. When the tumor becomes large, it threatens other cranial nerves in the posterior fossa and the pons. The very close relationship between the tumor and these nervous elements emphasizes the need for truly conformal dose planning.

Dosimetry

Improved computer software has been the major factor permitting truly conformal dose plans. The irregular shape of most VS usually requires multiple radiation isocenters for optimal dose planning (Fig. 2). After stereotactic imaging, fusion of the MR sequences with the bony CT scan is, in our experience, very important to evaluate distortion in the x, y, and z directions (Fig. 3). The microsurgery experience has shown that the most common location for the VIIth nerve is the anterior middle third (more rarely the anterior-superior portion), and for the VIIIth nerve, the anterior-inferior portion.[31,50] A determination of the individual relationship between these nerves and the tumor is valuable, with adjustments in the dosimetry based on these findings. Long TR imaging is extremely helpful for determining the topography of the nerves in the cistern; the

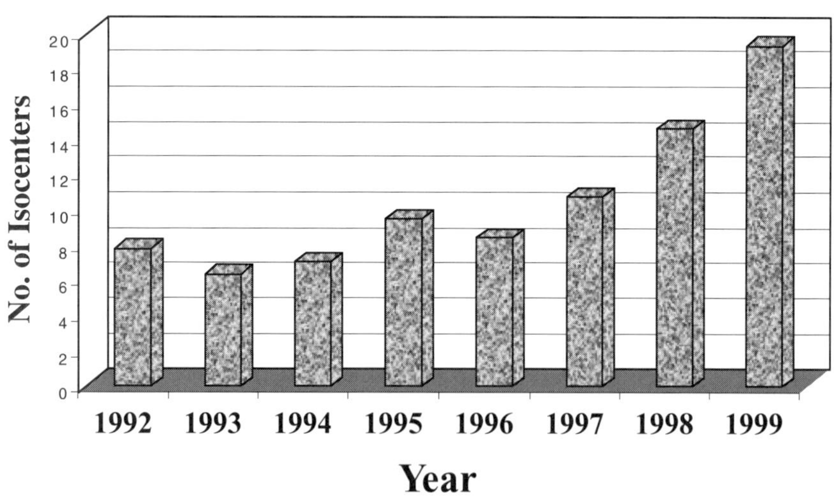

Figure 2. Evolution of the number of isocenters, over 8 years of practice. The introduction of advanced dose-planning software (1997), and more recently the introduction of the automatic positioning system (2000), has dramatically increased the number of isocenters used to improve the conformality of our dose plans.

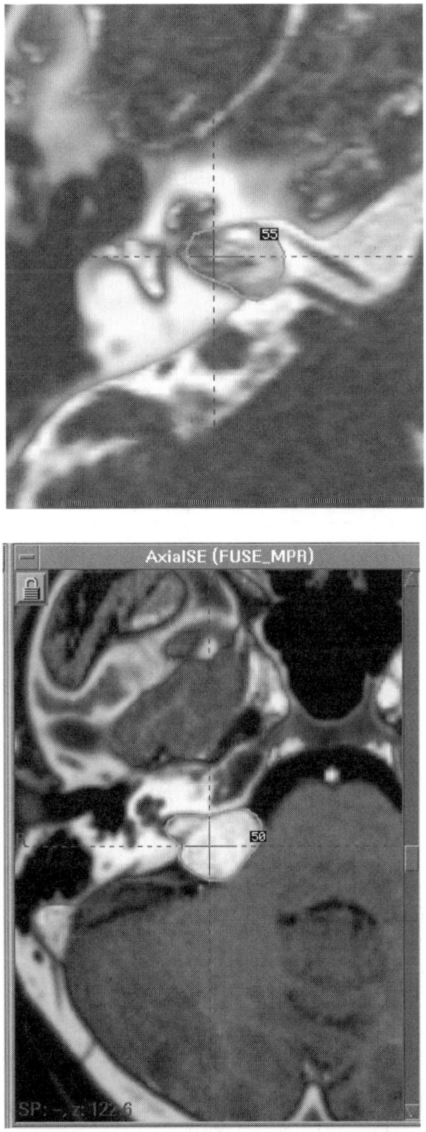

Figure 3. Axial images used for dose planning. (**Top**) Fusion of bone window CT and a three-dimensional postgadolinium MRI showing the 50% isodose line. (**Bottom**) High-resolution T2-weighted MRI of a right Grade II tumor fused with the CT. This sequence allows localization of the facial nerve anteriorly and the vestibulocochlear nerve inferiorly.

postgadolinium volume acquisition is mandatory for delineation of the intracanalicular portion. A combination of radiation isocenters with beam diameters of 4, 8, 14, and 18 mm are used to create a conformal dose plan. For lesions very close to the brainstem, we sometimes block selective beam channels to specially shape the isodose gradient fall-off. Dose selection is based mainly on the prescription isodose volume. Since our first treated case in July 1992, we have followed the recommendations of Noren,[5,51] and have used marginal doses between 12 and 14 Gy. For very large tumors we typically use 10 Gy (9 Gy in one case). Recurrent tumors in deaf patients with facial palsy may receive doses as high as 16 Gy at the margin. The vast majority of the patients have been discharged from the hospital on the day after the radiosurgery.

The Marseille Experience

Tumor Control

Progressive tumor regression is generally only observed after several years (Fig. 4). In most cases, there is some enlargement in tumor size over the 6 months following SRS. Mean diameter augmentation is 0.3 mm (range, −3.3 to +5.2 mm) for patients with good results and 1.7 mm for our failures. In 78% of cases, a distinct loss of the central tumor contrast enhancement was also noticed at 6 months. At 1 year, most of the tumors are the same size as the day of treatment and continue to decrease with time. This early loss of contrast enhancement and a slight growth in volume is thus to be expected and should not be interpreted as a sign of failure or a justification for a microsurgical approach. We consider an increase of 20% of the initial volume at 2 years as a sign of failure. At last follow-up, MRI revealed that 38% of tumors were smaller (mild volume decrease, 21%; major volume decrease, 17%), 58% were unchanged, and 4% were larger. Fourteen patients (1.8%) have required additional treatment to date (microsurgery, 11; repeat SRS, 3). All failures occurred before 3 years. Noren showed, in a group of patients followed over several decades, that all the patients who were considered to be under control at 5 years were still so after 20 years.[5] Therefore, we can reasonably expect that sustained tumor growth will involve less than 5% of patients, even when analyzed using life table methods.

Patients with cystic VS represent a difficult problem as complications occurring after SRS include a high failure rate due to extratumoral cyst requiring surgery, and hydrocephalus. In our series, we treated patients with 23 cystic VS. No patient had NF2 and it was the first treatment for all patients. Preoperatively, cystic VS were larger (Grade I, 0%; Grade II, 43.5%; Grade III, 52%; Grade IV, 4.5%; compared to Grade I, 5.5%; Grade II, 53%; Grade III, 31%; Grade IV, 6.5%),[52] and more patients had pre-

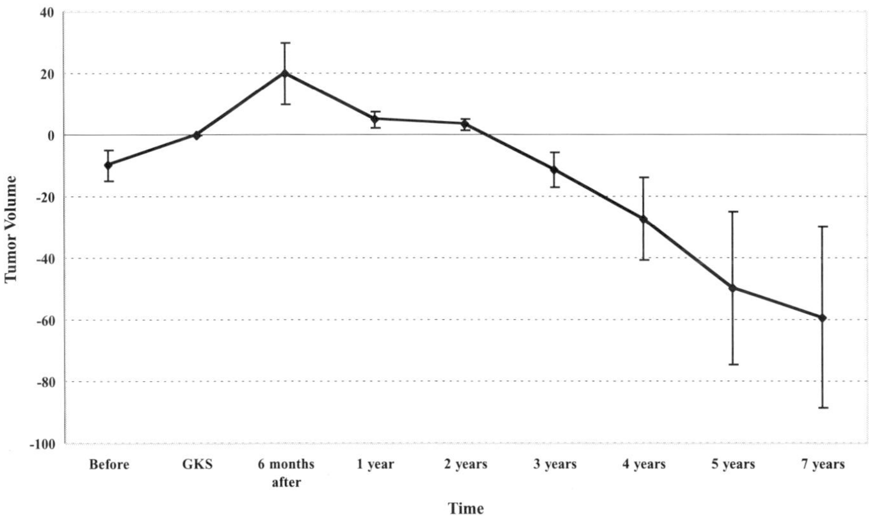

Figure 4. Average tumor volume and time before and after radiosurgery (GKS). The size of the lesion on the treatment day (in mm^3) is the reference volume. Variations in size are expressed as percent of this size. This figure shows that the average tumor volume increases over time before radiosurgery and during the first 2 years after the procedure.

served functional hearing preoperatively compared to noncystic VS (61% vs. 39%). After SRS two patients developed transient trigeminal neuropathies. No patient had facial weakness. Nine of 14 patients (64%) retained functional hearing. No extratumoral macrocyst or hydrocephalus appeared, but three patients required another treatment because of an increased volume (microsurgery in two cases, SRS in one case). Thus compared to noncystic VS, the failure rate appears to be increased (13% vs. 2%).

Complications

Trigeminal neuropathy appeared in 1.6% of the patients after SRS. Among the first 100 cases the incidence of facial numbness was 5%; for the next 600 patients the incidence was 0.7%. Facial weakness occurred in eight patients after SRS (Grade II, n=2; Grade III, n=5; Grade V, n=1).[53] The facial weakness completely recovered in seven patients. The incidence of facial weakness has also decreased since 1992. Three of the first 100 patients (3%) developed facial weakness compared to only five among the next 600 patients (0.8%). Hearing improved in 3% of cases, was stable in 71%, and became nonfunctional in 17%. Nine percent of patients became deaf. Such improved results reflect not only our learning curve, but also improved imaging and dose-planning techniques.

In our experience, hydrocephalus was diagnosed before SRS in 28 patients (4%): 19 patients had sporadic VS and had not undergone previous microsurgery. Shunting was performed preoperatively in seven cases and postoperatively in five cases. During the follow-up period, ventricular enlargement occurred in 20 patients without preoperative hydrocephalus. For these patients, shunting was performed in seven, from 6 to 36 months after SRS. Thus, the incidence of new hydrocephalus requiring shunting after SRS was 1%, quite similar to the experience after either microsurgery or the natural history of untreated tumors.

Neurofibromatosis 2

Patients with NF2 represent a distinct management problem. Compared with the results of patients with unilateral sporadic VS, the results of surgical resection are poor in terms of hearing preservation, facial nerve function, and recurrence rate.[54] Although the mechanism of the gene failure affecting schwannomin is currently understood, therapeutic trials have not reached the "in vivo step." In this situation, radiosurgery may be a significant alternative to microsurgery. We recently reviewed our preliminary results for this patient group. Between July 1992 and December 1997, 27 NF2 patients (35 tumors) underwent SRS and had more than 1 year of follow-up. The median age was 28 years (range, 14–65 yrs); 15 patients (56%) harbored the severe form of the disease (Wishart phenotype) while 12 patients (44%) were classified under the Gardner mild phenotype of NF2. For the eight patients having bilateral treatment, SRS was done as a single procedure in four cases and was two-staged in four cases. Twelve patients had undergone prior surgery. Nine patients had recurrent tumors and three documented enlargement of known residual tumor. Tumors ranged from Grade II to IV.[52] We treated 9 Grade II tumors, 19 Grade III tumors, and 7 Grade IV tumors. Tumor volume ranged from 0.4 to 14.4 cm^3 (mean, 3.9 cm^3). The mean peripheral dose was 13 Gy (range, 10–18); most patients were treated at the 50% isodose line.

The median clinical and radiological follow-up time was 32 months (range, 6–70 mos). Hydrocephalus occurred in one patient 4 months after simultaneous treatment of bilateral Grade IV tumors, requiring an emergency ventriculoperitoneal drainage. No trigeminal neuralgia or lower cranial nerve neuropathy was observed. After SRS, facial nerve function deteriorated in three patients (9% of the treated tumors). In two cases, worsening occurred at 6 and 12 months after the treatment and recovered under steroid therapy. In both cases, high peripheral doses (17 and 18 Gy, respectively, on Grade II tumors) were delivered in a deliberate strategy of tumor control, since preoperative hearing was poor. The third case de-

Table 1
Facial Nerve Status Before and After Radiosurgery for Patients with Neurofibromatosis Type 2 (n=35)*

	Grade After Radiosurgery					
Grade Before Radiosurgery	**I**	**II**	**III**	**IV**	**V**	**VI**
I	22			1		
II		5				
III			2			
IV						
V						
VI						5

*Facial grade according to the House-Brackmann scale.[53]

veloped a permanent facial palsy 19 months after SRS of a Grade III tumor. The delivered dose at the tumor margin was 11 Gy. The rate of permanent radiation-induced facial nerve weakness was 3% (Table 1). Hearing results are available on 35 ears with a median of 30 months of follow-up (Table 2). The overall hearing preservation rate was 67%, and preservation of useful hearing (Gardner-Robertson Classes I and II)[55] was obtained for 8 of 14 ears (57%). In NF2 patients, in whom hearing is often impaired on both sides, it seems reasonable to include Class III in the category of useful hearing. Preservation of Classes I to III was possible in 14 of 17 ears (82%). In one case, permanent hearing deterioration occurred at 4 years after SRS associated with tumor growth from an ipsilateral petroclival meningioma. In most cases, hearing deterioration occurred in the 2-year period following SRS. However, one patient lost hearing suddenly at 24 hours after SRS.

Table 2
Hearing Before and After Radiosurgery for Patients with Neurofibromatosis Type 2 (n=35)*

	Class After Radiosurgery				
Class Before Radiosurgery	**I**	**II**	**III**	**IV**	**V**
I	6		2		
II		2	1	2	1
III			3		
IV				3	1
V					15

*Hearing according to the Gardner-Robertson scale.[55]

Twenty-six of 35 tumors (74%) were controlled at last follow-up. Retrospective analysis of the major failure cases (more than 20% increasing volume) showed that three patients underwent the treatment during the initial period of our experience, with a CT scan planification and a reduced number of isocenters used. Moreover, two of them had very questionable indication for this treatment since they harbored bilateral Grade IV tumors. Three patients underwent a subsequent microsurgical removal. In one case, a clinical deterioration occurred 4 months after SRS (compressive axial signs and hydrocephalus). In the two other cases, because of deafness, implantation of a cochlear nucleus implant was done during the same procedure. In both cases, surgeons (from another team) did not consider that the SRS entailed additional surgical difficulty.

Our results are comparable to the literature and appear inferior to those obtained for sporadic VS. Several explanations are possible to explain these differences. In NF2 patients, we treated larger tumors (mean volume of 4 cm^3 vs. 1.2 cm^3 for sporadic VS). Also, to preserve any residual hearing or avoid brainstem damage in cases of bilateral treatment, we sometimes used reduced doses. Target definition was often obscured by previous microsurgery. Finally, whether those schwannomas have the same radiosensitivity as sporadic VS remains debatable.

Because of the heterogeneity of each patient, SRS of NF2 patients should take into account the following parameters: tumor growth and size (proof of tumor growth, and tumor volume <10 cm^3), degree of hearing loss (especially in case of a single hearing side, watchful waiting seems preferable), and NF2 subtype (in case of a severe form, our opinion is to recommend the less invasive treatment). Another question is the suitable timing for bilateral treatment. Our opinion is that for bilateral growing tumors with some hearing from each ear, a 2-year interval between the two procedures is desirable if the tumor volume remains compatible with SRS. Indeed, it is debatable whether to risk simultaneous bilateral hearing loss. However, our experience confirms that SRS compares favorably with microsurgery of VS in NF2 patients. The advantage of SRS relates to the significant number of patients in whom we can preserve functional hearing. Yet, SRS should be restricted to small- and medium-sized growing tumors. Treatment strategy of NF2 patients should be planned by multidisciplinary experienced teams with the ability to perform both microsurgery and SRS.

Microsurgery or Radiosurgery

Tumor Control

Tumor recurrence after microsurgery is not as rare as some authors commonly claim. To accurately estimate the rate, follow-up must be very long for these benign neoplasms. In a series of 228 patients we followed up to 10 years after microsurgery, 3% recurred at 3 years, 7% at 6 years, and 9% at 10 years. Of note, 97% of these tumors were thought to have been totally removed. Thus, in our microsurgical series operated by translabyrinthine approach we found a recurrence rate after complete resection of 9%. The average time until tumor recurrence was 8 years after surgery. This is in agreement with the findings of the Acoustic Neuroma Registry (1579 patients operated by microsurgery between 1989 and 1994) in which 8% of the patients had persistent or recurrent tumors on postoperative imaging.[56] Cerullo et al reported a 9% recurrence rate in a series of 55 patients in whom a gross-total tumor removal was achieved.[57] Mazzoni et al found an 11% recurrence rate in 46 patients followed by MRI more than 3 years after microsurgery.[58] The overall rate was 8% in his total population (104 patients operated between 1975 and 1993). Tumor recurrence in this series was experienced from 1 to 7 years after surgery. In comparison, with the currently used reduced doses delivered at the tumor margin (10–12 Gy), we do not have long-term data about tumor control rate. However, unlike some centers, our policy has been to use these low doses since the very beginning of our experience. Thus, despite the use of "low doses" our tumor control rate remains above 97% and is constant for the population with more than 3-years of follow-up. As a result, based on our data, the probability for additional surgery is not different if the first treatment was SRS or microsurgery.

We previously reported the functional outcomes of 178 VS patients after surgical resection.[25] This study clearly showed that even in a population with acceptable objective results (House-Brackmann Grades I–II, 66%), the postoperative functional deterioration and worsening of the quality of life reported by the patients were surprisingly high. To evaluate and compare the functional outcome of patients after VS SRS, we designed a prospective study with identical methodology as in the microsurgery series. Our aim was to evaluate postoperative outcomes from a patient's perspective. This aspect must be added to the "objective evaluation" performed by physicians for a valid comparison between the two treatments[32]; this has not been investigated in previous studies. For statistical analysis, only patients with Grade II or III tumors were considered.[52] Objective results and questionnaires were compared for the first 100 consecutive SRS patients with more than 4-years of follow-up to 110 microsurgery patients fulfilling the inclusion criterions. The results are outlined in Table 3. Patients who underwent SRS were less likely to have facial weakness or spasm, eye difficulties, facial numbness, or feeding troubles. The SRS patients were also more likely to maintain functional hearing and be able to return to their prior work. No difference was detected in regards to tinitus, vertigo, or imbalance. In order to express the results in a condensed manner, we organized the questions and answers from the patient questionnaire into six groups

Table 3
Comparison of Functional Outcomes After Microsurgery and Radiosurgery

Complaint	*Microsurgery (%)*	*Radiosurgery (%)*
Parameters significantly different		
Facial palsy	47	0
Hemispasm	27	3
Loss of functional hearing	62.5	30
Ocular troubles	83	27
Hypoesthesia	29	4
Feeding troubles	16	9
No return to work	34	1
Parameters with no significant difference		
Tinnitus	40	50
Vertigo	68	63
Imbalance	22	26

corresponding to different sectors of complaints: facial palsy, facial spasm, ocular disturbance, facial hypesthesia, eating troubles, and coordination. Overall, 98% of SRS patients had zero to two complaints (Fig. 5). The mean time off from work was 7 days after SRS compared to 130 days after microsurgery.

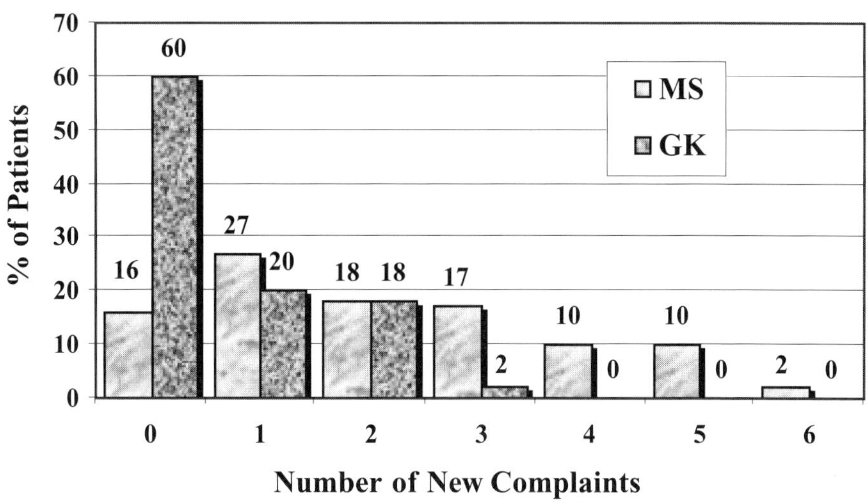

Figure 5. Comparison of the global sensorimotor functioning index of patients after radiosurgery (GK) or microsurgery (MS). Patients are grouped according to the number of new complaints they develop after surgery. Note that 98% of radiosurgery patients have zero to 2 new complaints, whereas only 61% of microsurgery patients have that many new complaints.

There are some necessary methodological problems and assumptions in this study that need to be pointed out. The main criticism is that patients were not randomized to the two treatments. However, the SRS and microsurgery populations were equivalent in terms of preoperative parameters. Also, patient estimates are extremely subjective. Still, we feel it is crucial to integrate such subjective data into our results for VS patients because objective neurological and otological examinations tend to underestimate the true functional outcomes of patients.[24,25,33,58] Nonetheless, the functional outcomes we documented are clearly better after SRS than microsurgery for VS patients. It can also be argued that the microsurgery comparison group had poor results, and thus the study design favored SRS. As outlined in Table 4, the results of Pellet et al are quite comparable to the best available data in the literature.[25,28–31,54,59–62] Obviously, there is an evident learning curve with both microsurgery and SRS. This needs to be taken into account when comparing series from different historical periods.[63]

Concerns Regarding Radiosurgery

Cancer Genesis

The incidence of malignant VS is low. A review of the literature shows only eight case reports. Of these eight patients, two patients had NF2, whereas six patients had sporadic VS. As the relation between malignancy and radiation exposure is well known for NF2 patients, these will not be discussed further. For the six patients with sporadic VS, two were discovered at the time of first surgery.[64,65] The other four patients had undergone either surgical resection (n=2),[66,67] radiosurgery (n=1),[68] or both microsurgery and SRS (Kurita, personal communication). Of note, in all three patients who had previous microsurgery, the pathology showed benign VS at the time of the first operation. In cases having initial SRS, as no histologic specimens are available, it is not possible to assess if the lesion was already malignant at that time. The delay between microsurgery and the diagnosis of malignancy was 10 and 11 months compared to 5 and 6 years for the two patients having SRS. Thus, the available data do not allow us to draw any conclusion. The only evidence is that the risk of secondary neoplasm in a VS following microsurgical resection or radiosurgery seems to be very low indeed. Of course very extensive follow-up is required for further understanding of this uncommon phenomenon. However, the risk of malignant change following radiation appears to be outweighed by the many advantages of radiosurgery and should not provide a deterrent to offering the alternative of radiosurgery even to young patients.

Table 4
Objective Results of Vestibular Schwannoma Microsurgery Compared to the Marseille Radiosurgery Experience

Author(s), Year	*No. of Patients*	*Facial Preservation* (%)*	*Hearing Preservation† (%)*	*CSF Leak (%)*	*Lower Cranial Nerve Deficit (%)*	*Mortality (%)*
Hardy et al, 1989[59]	100	29	ND	13	5	3
Fischer et al, 1992[54]	102	66	29	3	ND	2.9
Ebersold et al, 1992[60]	256	64	24	11	2	1
Glasscock et al, 1993[61]	161	ND	35	13	ND	0
Pellet et al, 1993[25]	178	66	37.5	7.5	3	1.8
Gormley et al, 1997[62]	179	77	38	15	2	1
Samii et al, 1997[28–30]	1000	59	40	9.2	5.5	1.1
Marseille GK series	770	99	74	0	0	0

CSF, cerebrospinal fluid; ND, not discussed; GK, Gamma Knife.
*House-Brackmann Grade I or II.[53]
†Gardner-Robertson Class I or II.[55]

Difficulty of Microsurgery After Failed Radiosurgery

Even if the rate of failed VS SRS is low (<3%), the number of treatment failures will increase with the number of patients having SRS. Thus, an important issue is to know whether or not SRS makes microsurgery more difficult in those failed cases. Some authors have claimed that this was undeniably the case.[14] Based on the limited experience, many surgeons present this as an argument against the role of SRS as primary management when asked by patients. In this section, we provide the data from our own series of operated cases after failed SRS and also analyze the findings in the literature.

Since July 1992, more than 770 VS patients have undergone SRS, including 52 NF2 patients (7%). Data from a minimum of 3-year follow-up have been obtained for 382 patients, and at last follow-up, MRI has shown a major tumor growth in 14 patients (3.7%) with unilateral VS. Eleven patients underwent microsurgery, whereas three underwent additional SRS because of suboptimal previous dosimetry. Among the 11 operated patients, four underwent microsurgery at our center. The other seven patients were treated at different centers from which they were initially referred for SRS. Unfortunately, data regarding indication for surgery, difficulties of the procedure, and postoperative course were not systematically brought to our knowledge. Two additional patients with NF2 also had microsurgery at our center after failed SRS. Thus, at our center, six VS were resected after prior SRS by the same surgeon (W. Pellet) with a previous surgical experience of more than 700 operated VS. In all cases the translabyrinthine approach was used. This route was justified by both tumor size (>2 cm in the cerebellopontine angle in all cases), and the fact that no patient had functional hearing preoperatively.

In the four patients with sporadic VS, the indication for microsurgery was evidence of sustained tumor growth (>20%) after a minimum 2-year follow-up documented by serial MRI. In one of these four cases, the surgery was more difficult compared to a typical VS removal. It was noted that the arachnoid membranes were thickened, and the tumor was adhered to the brainstem and facial nerve. In the three other cases, the procedure appeared to be uneventful even if some changes in tumor consistency and bleeding were observed. Total removal was achieved in all cases documented by postoperative MRI. Preservation of the anatomical continuity of the facial nerve was also achieved in all cases. At discharge, the House-Brackmann facial grading was I or II in three cases, and III for the patient with the increased surgical difficulty. For the two NF2 patients having later microsurgery, surgery was performed at 6-month follow-up in one case. This patient had undergone a bilateral radiosurgery for Grade IV tumors. She presented developed hydrocephalus at 3 months requiring ventriculoperitoneal drainage. Her neurological status worsened, due to significant brainstem compression. The side with worse hearing was selected for microsurgery. Operative difficulties were encountered, due to the tumor volume and adherence to the brainstem and cranial nerves, but are also usually found in other cases of NF2 patients during a first hand surgery. Complete tumor removal was achieved. Despite anatomical preservation of the facial nerve, the patient had a Grade IV weakness at last follow-up. On the other side, the tumor volume remains unchanged 8 years after SRS. The other patient was operated at 3-year follow-up for a sustained tumor growth. The surgery was described as uneventful, removal was complete, and facial nerve Grade II was obtained.

In 1995, the House Ear Clinic, Los Angeles, CA, published its experience with microsurgery after failed SRS and concluded categorically that SRS made later surgical resection more difficult.[14] Briefly, five patients were described who had prior SRS with various devices without modern imaging or treatment planning. At surgery, the anatomical features were obscured and all the patients had poor outcomes. However, all five patients had one or more features that would make surgical resection more difficult, even if they had not undergone SRS (tumor size, NF2, prior microsurgery). Thus, the data provided in this report are difficult to interpret and, in our opinion, are only of historical interest. More recently, Pollock et al reported 13 patients with sporadic VS operated after SRS in the modern era (2.9% of treated cases).[69] Six patients had undergone microsurgery before SRS. In three cases, the indication for microsurgery was increased symptoms without tumor growth. Of the 10 cases with documented tumor growth, the mean volume increase was 124%. This apparently dramatic increase from 2.5 to 5.6 cm^3 means, in fact, that the mean tumor diameter increased from 16 to 22 mm, if we assimilate the volume of the tumor to a unique sphere. Thus, it seems clear that additional watchful waiting of a subgroup of these patients would have permitted the avoidance of further microsurgery. Total removal was obtained in only seven cases, and additional difficulties were observed in 8 of the 13 patients (62%). Loss of the peritumoral arachnoid plane, tumor fibrosis, and adjacent scarring were the source of the surgical difficulties. Poor results with regard to facial nerve preservation, one brainstem infarction and two cases of lower cranial nerve deficits were noted. However, only three of the seven patients (43%) who had not undergone previous microsurgery were believed to have tumors more difficult to resect. Another team has operated on four patients after SRS (T. Fukushima, unpublished data). In one case, the patient was operated soon after SRS due to a dramatic increase in tumor size. Surgery was uneventful and outcome was favorable. In the three other cases, microsurgery was delayed but also justified by a significant volume increase. In each case, dissection of the facial nerve was considered more difficult due to adherence between the tumor and nerves. It was also noted that the facial nerve was unexpectedly fragile for these three patients.

It is impossible to conclude, based on present information, whether prior SRS makes later microsurgery more difficult. The only way to provide a reliable answer will be to collect more data in a formal prospective fashion. However, the limited anecdotal experiences described may allow us to make some general recommendations. First, if it appears that the facial nerve dissection is especially difficult, then leaving a shell of tumor may improve the patient's facial nerve outcome. This difficulty happens more frequently if surgery is performed early after SRS. Second, and more important, the best way to reduce morbidity is to properly select which patients actually require microsurgery. The documentation of sustained tumor growth on serial imaging should be required, with a minimum follow-up of 1 or 2 years after SRS, if possible. Thus, increasing symptoms or new symptoms (facial numbness or weakness) without evidence of tumor growth should not lead to microsurgery. Indeed, we do not have enough understanding of tumor kinetics after SRS, but some tumors clearly enlarge at first and then later stabilize or decrease, sometimes years after the treatment.

When SRS fails to stop the tumor from growing, our tendency is to immediately recommend microsurgery. However, three patients in our experience underwent a second SRS for continued tumor growth. Obviously, the analysis of the initial dose plan is critical to determine if repeat SRS is reasonable. In cases where the patient was treated during the first period with crude imaging (CT) and dosimetry, if the tumor increase occurs from a previously untreated part, then a second SRS can be proposed. Other factors that could lead us to perform repeat SRS would include small tumor size, preservation of useful hearing, or the patient's desire to avoid open surgery. To date, all three patients are under control and no patient has developed subsequent clinical worsening. Thus, if we include these three patients as controlled with SRS, then only 1.9% of our patients with sporadic VS (7 of 362 patients with more than 3 years follow-up) have required further resection.

Radiosurgery to Preserve Hearing

Initially, our strategy was to treat Grade I VS only if hearing was poor (below Class II),[55] or if there was clear enlargement on serial imaging. This strategy was based on the assumption that the radiosurgery was more likely to impair hearing than the "wait and see" approach. In order to address the question of which strategy was more likely to result in the preservation of useful hearing, we reviewed our Grade I patients managed with SRS or conservative therapy. In this study, 91 Grade I patients were managed with serial imaging (n=54) or SRS (n=37). With a mean follow-up of 4 years (range, 1.2–12 years), 39 of 54 patients (72%) in the conservative arm showed tumor enlargement. Thirty-eight patients became either Grade II or III; one patient's tumor enlarged to a Grade IV. This patient underwent later microsurgery via a translabyrinthine approach. For the other 38 patients, SRS was proposed. Of the patients having initial SRS, no patient has demonstrated later tumor growth (Fig. 6). Also, patients having SRS were more likely to preserve useful hearing compared to no treatment (Fig. 7). Twelve of 14 patients (86%) retained useful hearing after SRS; none of the 10 tumors receiving doses less than 14 Gy have lost useful hearing. Thus, if preservation of useful hearing and the absence of further tumor interventions are desirable, it should be noted that SRS achieved this in 86% of cases compared to only 20% with conservative therapy. Based on these results, our recommendation has dramatically changed and we now advise early SRS for Grade I patients and preserved useful hearing.

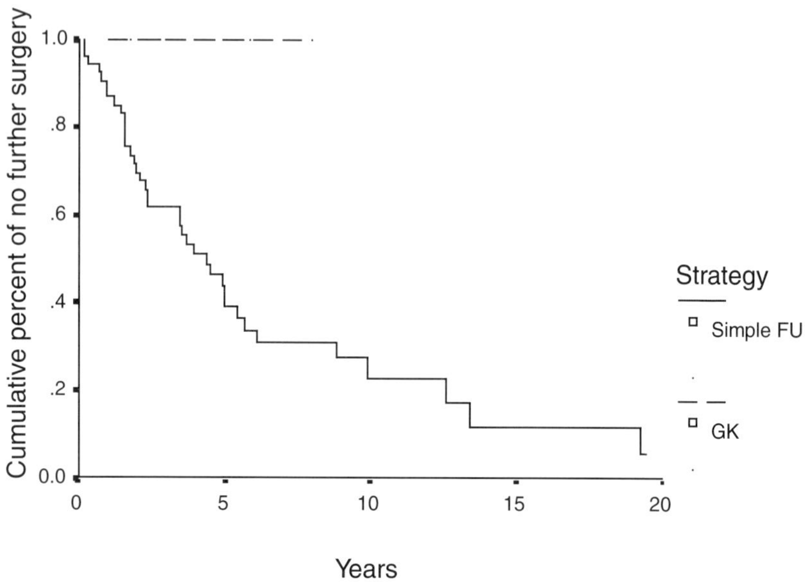

Figure 6. Requirement for further surgery with observation (Simple FU) or radiosurgery (GK) in patients with Grade I tumors. No failures have been observed for the radiosurgical patients compared to 65% of patients needing surgery within 5 years in the observation group.

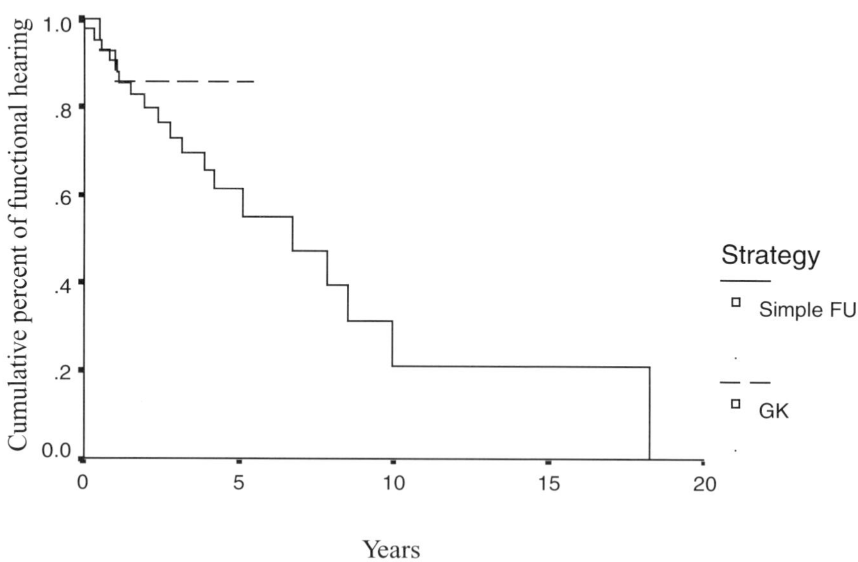

Figure 7. Preservation of functional hearing with observation (Simple FU) or radiosurgery (GK) in patients with Grade I tumors. At 5-year follow-up, the probability of preservation of functional hearing is 83% after radiosurgery and only 45% for simple observation.

Conclusions

In spite of the great advances in the microsurgical removal of VS, significant morbidity remains a possibility. The tumors are now detected much earlier and, frequently, patients with newly diagnosed VS have minimal symptoms and normal hearing. For these patients, selection of the best management option often presents a therapeutic dilemma. From an ethical point of view, patients should be informed of all the available surgical techniques. Thus, it is incumbent upon physicians to provide up-to-date information regarding radiosurgery and to consider it among the treatment modalities currently available for patients who do not wish to have microsurgical removal. We believe that VS patients should be managed by multidisciplinary surgical teams including neurosurgeons and otolaryngologists, in collaboration with radiation oncologists and physicists.

Indication for VS radiosurgery is, first, *a question of conviction*; one must first be convinced that use of this technology is reasonable. According to its innovative status, it was appropriate that early users await confirmation of its theoretical possibilities. We believe that reported results, based on a sufficient number of patients who have been followed for an adequate length of time, are now available and conclusive. The low risk of radiosurgery and its limited disruption of patients' lives are convincing arguments to choose this method whenever it is possible.

It is also *a question of frame of mind* regarding neurosurgeons and otolaryngologists, especially those who do not have this technology at their own disposal. Indeed, they are required to entrust their patients to another team or, a more constructive and more enriching alternative, cooperate with the team performing SRS. Regardless of this choice, it is an important decision and particularly difficult for those who have made VS surgery their speciality. Such individuals may feel they have "the most to lose" and, consequently, are the most reluctant to accept SRS. Moreover, as authorities on VS surgery, they argue against SRS and their opinions are highly regarded. It must be cautioned that opinions regarding SRS should be based on firsthand experience, rather than "prejudiced" interpretation of the literature.

Last, indications for VS radiosurgery are *a question of common sense.* Management of these benign tumors must recognize that both microsurgery and SRS provide excellent outcomes. However, all would agree that in the setting where neither method is firmly supported with overwhelming evidence, then the less invasive and less dangerous option should be preferred by both physicians and their patients.

Acknowledgments: The authors wish to thank Mr. Gouvernet, Ms. G. Kassapian, and Mr. Porcheron for their greatly appreciated help.

References

1. Dandy W: Operation for total removal of cerebellopontine (acoustic) tumors. Surg Gynecol Obstet 1925;41:129–148.
2. Deen HG, Ebersold MJ, Harner SG, et al: Conservative management of acoustic neuroma: an outcome study. Neurosurgery 1996;39:260–266.
3. Leksell L: The stereotaxic method and radiosurgery of the brain. Acta Chir Scand 1951;102:316–319.
4. Leksell L: A note on the treatment of acoustic tumors. Acta Chir Scand 1969;137:763–765.
5. Noren G: Gamma knife radiosurgery for acoustic neurinomas. In Gildenberg PL, Tasker RR (eds): Textbook of Stereotactic and Functional Neurosurgery. New York, McGraw-Hill, 1996, pp 835–844.
6. Brackmann D, Hitselberger W, Beneke J: Acoustic neuromas: middle fossa and translabyrinthine removal. In Smith RR (ed): Microneurosurgery. St Louis, Mosby, 1987, pp 311–314.
7. Noren G, Arndt J, Hindmarsh T: Stereotactic radiosurgery in cases of acoustic neurinoma: further experience. Neurosurgery 1983;13:12–22.
8. Kamerer DB, Lunsford LD, Moller M: Gamma knife: an alternative treatment for acoustic neurinomas. Ann Otol Rhinol Laryngol 1988;97:631–635.
9. Linskey ME, Lunsford LD, Flickinger JC: Radiosurgery for acoustic neurinomas: early experience. Neurosurgery 1990;26:736–745.
10. Valk P, Dillon W: Radiation injury of the brain. Am J Neuroradiol 1991;12: 45–62.
11. Al-Mefty O, Kersh JE, Routh A, Smith RR: The long-term side effects of radiation therapy for benign brain tumors in adults. J Neurosurg 1990;73:502–512.
12. Guy J, Mancuso A, Beck R, et al: Radiation-induced optic neuropathy: a magnetic resonance imaging study. J Neurosurg 1991;74:426–432.
13. Brackmann D, Kwartler JA: Treatment of acoustic tumors with radiotherapy. Arch Otolaryngol Head Neck Surg 1990;116:161–162.
14. Slattery WH III, Brackmann D: Results of surgery following stereotactic irradiation for acoustic neuromas. Am J Otol 1995;16:315–319.
15. Flickinger JC, Kondziolka D, Lunsford LD: Dose and diameter relationships for facial, trigeminal and acoustic neuropathies following acoustic neuroma radiosurgery. Radiother Oncol 1996;41:215–219.
16. Flickinger JC, Kondziolka D, Pollock BE, Lunsford LD: Evolution in technique for vestibular schwannoma radiosurgery and effect on outcome. Int J Radiat Oncol Biol Phys 1996;36:275–280.
17. Kondziolka D, Lunsford L, McLaughlin M, Flickinger J: Long-term outcomes after radiosurgery for acoustic neuromas. N Engl J Med 1998;339:1426–1433.
18. Luxton G, Petrovich Z, Jozsef G, et al: Stereotactic radiosurgery principles and comparison of treatment methods. Neurosurgery 1993;32:241–259.
19. Noren G: Long-term complications following gamma knife radiosurgery of vestibular schwannomas. Stereotact Funct Neurosurg 1998;70(suppl 1):65–73.
20. Prasad D, Steiner M, Steiner L: Gamma surgery for vestibular schwannoma. J Neurosurg 2000;92:745–759.
21. Liscak R, Novotny J, Urgosik D, et al: Statistical analysis of risk factors after gamma knife radiosurgery of acoustic neurinomas. In Kondziolka D (ed): Radiosurgery. Basel, Karger, 1999, pp 205–213.
22. Martens F, Verbeke L, Piessens M, Van Vyve M: Stereotactic radiosurgery of vestibular schwannomas with a linear accelerator. Acta Neurochir Suppl (Wien) 1994;62:88–92.
23. Mendenhall W, Friedman W, Buatti J, Bova F: Preliminary results of linear

accelerator radiosurgery for acoustic schwannomas. J Neurosurg 1996;85: 1013–1019.
24. Pellet W: Stereotactic radiosurgery for acoustic neurinomas and petrous apex and cerebellopontine angle meningiomas. Crit Rev Neurosurg 1991;1:331– 342.
25. Pellet W, Emram B, Cannoni M, et al: Les resultats fonctionnels de la chirurgie des neurinomes de l'acoustique unilateraux. Neurochirurgie 1993; 39:24–41.
26. Linskey ME: Stereotactic radiosurgery for acoustic tumors. Neurosurg Clin N Am 1992;3:191–205.
27. Linskey ME, Lunsford LD, Flickinger JC: Tumor control after stereotactic radiosurgery in neurofibromatosis patients with bilateral acoustic tumors. Neurosurgery 1992;31:829–838.
28. Samii M, Mathies C: Management of 1000 vestibular schwannomas (acoustic neuromas): surgical management and results with an emphasis on complications and how to avoid them. Neurosurgery 1997;40:11–23.
29. Samii M, Matthies C: Management of vestibular schwannomas (acoustic neuromas): hearing function in 1000 tumor resection. Neurosurgery 1997;40: 248–262.
30. Samii M, Matthies C, Tatagiba M: Management of vestibular schwannomas (acoustic neuromas): auditory and facial nerve function after resection of 120 vestibular schwannomas in patients with neurofibromatosis. Neurosurgery 1997;40:696–706.
31. Sampath P, Rini D, Long D: Microanatomical variations in the cerebellopontine angle associated with vestibular schwannomas (acoustic neuromas): a retrospective study of 1006 consecutive cases. J Neurosurg 2000;92:70–78.
32. Hudgins WR: Patients' attitude about outcomes and the role of gamma knife radiosurgery in the treatment of vestibular schwannomas. Neurosurgery 1994;34:459–463.
33. Wiegand DA, Fickel V: Acoustic neuroma the patient 's perspective: subjective assessment of symptoms, diagnosis, therapy, and outcome in 541 patients. Laryngoscope 1989;99:179–187.
34. Linskey ME, Martinez AJ, Kondziolka D, et al: The radiobiology of human acoustic schwannoma xenografts after stereotactic radiosurgery evaluated in the subrenal capsule of athymic mice. J Neurosurg 1993;78:645–653.
35. Tsuzuki T, Tsunoda S, Sakaki T, et al: Tumor cell proliferation and apoptosis associated with the Gamma Knife effect. Stereotact Funct Neurosurg 1996;66 (suppl 1):39–48.
36. Fukuoka S, Oka K, Seo Y, et al: Apoptosis following gamma knife radiosurgery in a case of acoustic schwannoma. Stereotact Funct Neurosurg 1998; 70(suppl 1):88–94.
37. Seo Y, Fukuoka S, Nakagawara J, et al: Effect of Gamma Knife radiosurgery on acoustic neurinomas: assessment by 99mTc-DTPA-human serum albumin- and 201TlCl-single photon emission computed tomography. Stereotact Funct Neurosurg 1996;66(suppl 1):93–102.
38. Andrews DW, Silverman CL, Glass J, et al: Preservation of cranial nerve function after treatment of acoustic neurinomas with fractionated stereotactic radiotherapy: preliminary observations in 26 patients. Stereotact Funct Neurosurg 1996;64:165–182.
39. Colin P, Scavarda D, Delemer B, et al: Fractionated stereotactic radiotherapy: results in hypophyseal adenomas, acoustic neurinomas, and meningiomas of the cavernous sinus. Cancer Radiother 1998;2:207–214.
40. Poen J, Golby A, Forster K, et al: Fractionated stereotactic radiosurgery and preservation of hearing in patients with vestibular schwannoma: a preliminary report. Neurosurgery 1999;45:1299–1305.

41. Varlotto J, Shrieve D, Alexander E III, et al: Fractionated stereotactic radiotherapy for the treatment of acoustic neuromas: preliminary results. Int J Radiat Oncol Biol Phys 1996;36:141–145.
42. Linskey ME: Stereotactic radiosurgery versus stereotactic radiotherapy for patients with vestibular schwannoma: a Leksell gamma knife society 2000 debate. J Neurosurg 2000;93(suppl 3):90–95.
43. Walton L, Hampshire A, Forster DM, Kemeny AA: A phantom study to assess the accuracy of stereotactic localization, using T1-weighted magnetic resonance imaging with the Leksell stereotactic system. Neurosurgery 1996;38: 176–178.
44. Walton L, Hampshire A, Forster DM, Kemeny AA: Stereotactic localization with magnetic resonance imaging: a phantom study to compare the accuracy obtained using two-dimensional and three-dimensional data acquisitions. Neurosurgery 1997;41:131–137.
45. Forton G, Moeneclaey L, Declau F, Marquet J: The involvement of the cochlear nerve in neurinomas of the eighth cranial nerve. Arch Otorhinolaryngol 1989;246:156–160.
46. Luetje CM, Whittaker CK, Callaway LA: Histological acoustic tumor involvement of the eighth nerve and multicentric origin in the eighth nerve. Laryngoscope 1983;93:1133–1139.
47. Neely J, Hough J: Histologic findings in two very small intracanalicular solitary schwannomas of the eighth nerve. Ann Otol Rhinol Laryngol 1986;95: 460–465.
48. Neely JG: Is it possible to totally resect an acoustic neuroma and preserve hearing? Otolaryngol Head Neck Surg 1984;92:162–167.
49. Ylikoski J, Palva T, Collan Y: Eighth nerve in acoustic neuromas. Arch Otolaryngol 1978;104:532–537.
50. Ryu H, Tanaka T, Yamamoto S, et al: Magnetic resonance cisternography used to determine precise topography of the facial nerve and three components of the eighth cranial nerve in the internal auditory canal and cerebellopontine cistern. J Neurosurg 1999;90:624–634.
51. Noren G, Greitz D, Hirsch A, Lax I: Gamma knife surgery in acoustic tumours. In Steiner L (ed): Radiosurgery: Baseline and Trends. New York, Raven Press, 1992, pp 141–148.
52. Koos WT, Day JD, Matula C, Levy D: Neurotopographic considerations in the microsurgical treatment of small acoustic neurinomas. J Neurosurg 1998;88: 506–512.
53. House JW, Brackmann DE: Facial nerve grading system. Otolaryngol Head Neck Surg 1985;93:146–147.
54. Fischer G, Fischer C, Remond J: Hearing preservation in acoustic neurinoma surgery. J Neurosurg 1992;76:910–917.
55. Gardner G, Robertson JH: Hearing preservation in unilateral acoustic neuroma surgery. Ann Otol Rhinol Laryngol 1988;97:55–66.
56. Wiegand D, Ojeman R, Fickel V: Surgical treatment of acoustic neuroma (vestibular schwannoma) in the United States: report from the Acoustic Neuroma Registry. Laryngoscope 1996;106:58–66.
57. Cerullo LJ, Grutsch JF, Heiferman K: The preservation of hearing and facial nerve function in a consecutive series of unilateral vestibular nerve schwannoma surgical patients. Surg Neurol 1993;39:485–493.
58. Mazzoni A, Calabrese V, Moschini L: Residual and recurrent acoustic neuroma in hearing preservation procedures: neuroradiologic and surgical findings. Skull Base Surg 1996;6:105–112.
59. Hardy DG, Macfarlane R, Baguley D, Moffat DA: Surgery for acoustic neurinoma: an analysis of 100 translabyrinthine operations. J Neurosurg 1989;71: 799–804.

60. Ebersold MJ, Harner SG, Beatty CW, et al: Current results of the retrosigmoid approach to acoustic neurinoma. J Neurosurg 1992;76:901–909.
61. Glasscock ME III, Hays JW, Minor LB, et al: Preservation of hearing in surgery for acoustic neuromas. J Neurosurg 1993;78:864–870.
62. Gormley W, Sekhar L, Wright D, et al: Acoustic neuromas: results of current surgical management. Neurosurgery 1997;41:50–60.
63. Pollock B, Lunsford LD, Noren G: Vestibular schwannoma management in the next century: a radiosurgical perspective. Neurosurgery 1998;43:475–481.
64. Best P: Malignant triton tumour in the cerebellopontine angle: report of a case. Acta Neuropathol (Berl) 1987;74:92–96.
65. Kudo M, Matsumoto M, Terao H: Malignant nerve sheath tumor of acoustic nerve. Arch Pathol Lab Med 1983;107:293–297.
66. Han D, Kim D, Chi J, et al: Malignant triton tumor of the acoustic nerve: case report. J Neurosurg 1992;76:874–877.
67. McLean C, Laidlaw J, Brownbill D, Gonzales M: Recurrence of acoustic neurilemoma as a malignant spindle-cell neoplasm: case report. J Neurosurg 1990;73:946–950.
68. Comey CH, McLaughlin M, Jho H, et al: Death from a malignant cerebellopontine angle triton tumor despite stereotactic radiosurgery: case report. J Neurosurg 1998;89:653–658.
69. Pollock BE, Lunsford LD, Kondziolka D, et al: Vestibular schwannoma management. Part II. Failed radiosurgery and the role of delayed microsurgery. J Neurosurg 1998;89:949–955.

Comment
Chapter 9

Rick A. Friedman, Derald E. Brackmann

In the preceding chapter, Régis et al outline their experience with vestibular schwannoma (VS) radiosurgery over the past several years. Although the described results are quite good, we continue to have reservations regarding the use of radiosurgery to manage patients with this benign tumor. In this commentary, we present the argument as to why surgical excision should be considered the treatment of choice for the majority of patients with VS.

In the earlier part of the 20th century, many patients with VS presented with debilitating neurological sequelae.[1] In 1967, Olivecrona reported facial paresis at the time of tumor diagnosis in 54.7% of his patients.[2] This fact, combined with the emphasis placed on preservation of life, certainly explain Dandy's statement in 1941 that "paralysis of the facial nerve must usually be accepted as a necessary sequel of the operation."[3] In 1950, Pennybacker and Cairns, in their review of 130 cases of VS, stated that "complete facial paralysis seems a small price to pay for relief from an acoustic tumour."[4]

Neural preservation in VS surgery, like surgical mortality, has undergone tremendous evolution over the past century. With the introduction of the operating microscope and the revival of the middle cranial fossa and translabyrinthine approaches by William House in 1961, mortality rates dropped dramatically, and the focus of VS removal shifted to the preservation of neural function. Patients undergoing VS surgery today expect that they will survive surgery; as such, they are most concerned with preservation of facial function and, when appropriate, auditory function.

The total number of VS removed at the House Ear Clinic now approaches 5000. With experience and refinements of technique, the results have progressively improved. The following is an up-to-date review of our past and present series with regard to postoperative outcomes.

Middle Cranial Fossa Approach

Hearing preservation is the major reason we use this approach in appropriately selected patients. Our hearing preservation rates described in five series from 1989 to the present demonstrate preservation of hearing to within 15 dB speech reception threshold and 15% word recognition score in 59% to 71% of operated patients.[5–8] Our most recently published series demonstrated 60% Class A or B hearing according to the reporting guidelines of the American Academy of Otolaryngology–Head and Neck Surgery, and we have seen the same success in the management of NF2.[5,9] These results compare favorably with those of recently reported Gamma Knife immediate post-treatment hearing preservation results.[10] We recently reviewed the duration of hearing preservation postoperatively and found 89% of patients retained useful hearing with a minimum of 5 years of postoperative follow-up. This is in sharp contrast to the radiation therapy literature demonstrating significant hearing deterioration over time.

The middle cranial fossa approach has, in the past, been described as an approach placing the facial nerve at undue risk. This has not been our experience. Our most recent reviews demonstrate excellent postoperative facial nerve function (House-Brackmann Grade I or II) in over 94% of our patients.[7,8]

The middle cranial fossa approach provides an unobstructed view of the entire internal auditory canal and its contents. This allows complete tumor removal under direct vision. In a review of 500 cases with several years of follow-up, we identified only one case of residual tumor (0.2%).

We have not seen a permanent neurological complication following this approach. A single patient experienced a postoperative seizure that responded to Dilantin. After 1 year of seizure prophylaxis, the Dilantin was stopped and no further seizures have occurred. We feel that our low rates of complications are the result of short temporal lobe retraction times (average, 90 minutes).

Translabyrinthine Approach

A recent review from our database of VS cases provides data from 1302 patients who underwent a translabyrinthine approach between 1982 and 1993. Their mean age was 50.0 years; 46% were male and 54% were female. Tumor size varied from 0.5 to 6.5 cm, with a mean size of 2.4 cm. Operating time averaged 3.3 hours. Three (0.2%) deaths occurred in this series.

Data on long-term (6 months) facial nerve function as determined by the House-Brackmann scale were available on 889 cases, with a mean follow-up time of 2.1 years. Of these, 58.2% had a Grade I function; 12.6%, Grade II; 13.2%, Grade III; 7.8%, Grade IV; 3.3%, Grade V; and 5.1%, Grade VI. In this same group of patients undergoing surgery since the advent of facial nerve monitoring (1988), 59% were Grade I; 15.4%, Grade II; 9.3%, Grade III; 7.7%, Grade IV; 4.2%, Grade V; and 4.5%, Grade VI. The vast majority of the poor facial nerve outcomes occurred in larger (>4 cm) tumors. When comparing the risk of facial nerve paralysis in comparable tumors (<3.0 cm), the surgical risks in our hands are only a few percent greater when compared to the most recent Gamma Knife reports cited above.

Postoperative Follow-up

In our experience, VS rarely recur after translabyrinthine removal. Our recurrence rate for unilateral tumors removed through the translabyrinthine approach treated between 1961 and 1995 was 0.3%.[11] The average interval to recurrence was 10 years. Based upon these findings we have recommended a single gadolinium-enhanced MRI 5 years postoperatively.

Stereotactic Irradiation

Radiosurgery is a term originally popularized by Leksell referring to a procedure that delivers three-dimensional stereotactic external beam irradiation to a specified tissue volume in a single session. This term is now applied to various techniques, including gamma units using ^{60}Co photons, protons, helium ions, and neutron beams, and modified LINAC units. Stereotactic external beam irradiation differs from conventional external beam radiation therapy in several important ways: (1) treatment of small tissue volumes in the range of 1 to 30 cm^3; (2) a single fraction of radiation is typically delivered. Some institutions are exploring fractionated therapy, but, for the treatment of VS, long-term data with significant numbers of patients is lacking; and (3) high-dose gradients at field edges minimize dose deposition outside the target volume. Since its introduction in 1969, the gamma unit has been used to treat VS based upon these principles. With the initial use of high marginal doses and CT planning, the complications reported from experienced centers far exceeded those reported from microsurgical centers of excellence.[12] However, with the improved technology of MRI for treatment planning, and the gradual empirical reduction in marginal dosing, the complication rates have reached levels comparable to those reported by those centers.

As discussed previously, the evolution of goals in the treatment of VS has shifted from solely the preservation of life, to include the preservation of function (facial and auditory). Now, the goal of any form of intervention that is chosen should be lifelong control.

The concern over the management of these benign tumors with stereotactic irradiation lies partially in this principle of lifelong control. Studies have clearly demonstrated a dose-response relationship with single-fraction radiation. This relationship, at the current doses employed to the tumor margin, does not demonstrate complete cell kill. This fact is based upon the fundamentals of radiation-induced cell death. Irradiated cells are the most sensitive to injury during metaphase. Benign tumors have few cells in this phase of the cell cycle in comparison to malignant tumors. The ultimate result of irradiation is DNA damage secondary to the direct effects of the gamma rays, or strand breaks from oxygen radicals that are generated. There are also indirect tumor effects that result from radiation-induced damage to nutrient vessels. The cells with damaged DNA either undergo apoptosis (programmed cell death) due to the load of DNA strand breaks, or they undergo cell cycle arrest. The total and marginal doses currently prescribed have been done so empirically, with insufficient biological evidence that the cells will all undergo apoptosis. These cells will not remain in cell cycle arrest indefinitely. They will either enter an apoptotic pathway, or they will harbor radiation/repair-induced mutations that will allow them to reenter the cell cycle and grow.

The time that it will take to see the fraction of tumors with cells reentering the cell cycle can only be estimated, as there is no long-term (20–30 years) follow-up. All of the irradiated VS seen at our institution, and in the literature, demonstrate enhancement up to a decade after treatment, suggesting that a significant fraction of cells have not undergone apoptosis.

As dosing has recently undergone significant reduction in an effort to reduce complications, a brief review of current data from experienced centers is provided. Flickinger et al recently provided data on 199 patients receiving Gamma Knife radiotherapy (median marginal dose, 13 Gy) for their VS with a median follow-up of 30 months.[13] The range of follow-up with the number of patients at each year was not provided. Additionally, the authors state that they had "more than one year MR follow-up" in 147 patients. Of those followed, to their knowledge, five patients (3.4%) have required microsurgical removal for continued tumor enlargement. In this same group of patients they identified MR evidence of 1 to 2 mm of tumor growth in nearly 10%.

In a recent series of patients treated with Gamma Knife (marginal doses of approximately 13 Gy), Prasad et al reviewed 95 patients with 5 to 10 years of follow-up and found tumor growth in 6.3%.[14] When analyzing their complications, they noted that, despite hearing preservation in many of the patients immediately after treatment, approximately 60% lost their preserved hearing over time. These figures support those of the Marseilles experience outlined in this chapter. We also agree with the Marseilles group that cystic tumors should be considered for microsurgery due to the risk of postirradiation complications.

We believe that all of these series lack sufficient follow-up. This is best illustrated by the experience with radiotherapy in another benign intracranial neoplasm, pituitary adenomas. In a study of radiotherapy for nonfunctional pituitary adenomas, Breen and co-authors demonstrated actuarial tumor control rates of 77.6 ± 6.3% and 64.7 ± 12.9% at 20 and 30 years, respectively.[15] From these studies it is clear that, to completely assess tumor "control" with radiotherapy, several decades of follow-up on these newer dosing strategies will be required. As mentioned above, these irradiated tumor cells may reenter the cell cycle due to induced mutations, potentially in genes regulating growth control resulting in neoplasia. The authors of this chapter suggest, in contrast to the findings of

Breen et al, that radiation failures will occur early. This has not been our experience in the 30 cases of microsurgical management of radiation failures performed at our institution. We have seen several cases of failure beyond 3 to 5 years.

As described above, radiation-induced mutations can occur in other growth control genes leading to neoplasia. Studies in primates exposed to single-dose radiation, similar to those given with Gamma Knife for VS, demonstrated a 50% incidence of malignant brain tumor in the decade following irradiation.[16] In a study of neoplasia in patients receiving radiation therapy for adenotonsillar hyperplasia, approximately one-third developed thyroid gland tumors and many were malignant.[17] In this same cohort of patients, there were 66 neural tumors (2.2%), 67 salivary tumors (2.3%), and 93 carcinomas (3.1%) of multiple tissue types. In a follow-up study of 3013 of this same cohort receiving 7.5 Gy in three divided doses over 3 weeks, 85 neural tumors were identified in 70 patients (2.3%).[18] This included 15 meningiomas, 27 cranial nerve schwannomas, and one malignant neural sheath tumor. The incidence of VS in this group of patients was 0.7%, nearly 1000-fold greater than the normal population. One of the most striking features of this study was that new tumors were identified more than 30 years after the initial treatment. This underscores the need for long-term follow-up, not only for regrowth of the treated VS, but also for the appearance of radiation-induced neoplasia. To date, there have been several reports in the literature of malignant tumors appearing after radiation therapy for VS.[19–22] Based upon the findings of Breen et al described earlier for radiated pituitary adenomas, an actuarial rate for developing a radiation-induced neoplasm of 2.7 ± 1.9% at 10 and 30 years, and the data cited above, we will likely be seeing similar results after VS radiation therapy.

Conclusions

Based upon our current rates of hearing preservation, facial nerve functional preservation, and cure (over 99%), we recommend microsurgery for those patients undergoing therapy for their VS. We strongly recommend against radiation therapy for NF2 based on our results and the unknown effects of irradiation in a condition known to result from a mutation in a growth control gene.[19]

As no mode of therapy is without risk, we thoroughly discuss tumor observation with patients that have this as an option. Until studies demonstrating long-term tumor control (a minimum of three decades) with less than the expected rate of malignant transformation (approximately 3%) are available, we will only recommend radiation therapy for patients requiring treatment who are not surgical candidates either by personal choice or infirmity. Often, these are older patients.

References

1. Cross JP: Unilateral neurilemmomas of the eighth cranial nerve: then and now. Am J Otol 1981;3:28–34.
2. Olivecrona H: Acoustic tumors. J Neurosurg 1967;26:6–13.
3. Dandy WE: Results of removal of acoustic tumors by the unilateral approach. Arch Surg 1941;42:1026–1033.
4. Pennybacker JB, Cairns H: Results in 130 cases of acoustic neurinoma. J Neurol Neurosurg Psychiatry 1950;13:272–277.
5. Brackmann DE, Owens RA, Friedman RA, et al: Prognostic factors for hearing preservation in vestibular schwannoma surgery. Am J Otol 2000;21:417–424.
6. Shelton C, Brackmann DE, House WF, Hitselberger WE: Middle fossa acoustic tumor surgery: results in 106 cases. Laryngoscope 1989;99:405–408.
7. Brackmann DE, House JR 3rd, Hitselberger WE: Technical modifications to the middle fossa craniotomy approach in removal of acoustic neuromas. Am J Otol 1994;15:614–619.
8. Slattery WH 3rd, Brackmann DE, Hitselberger W: Middle fossa approach for hearing preservation with acoustic neuromas. Am J Otol 1997;18:596–601.
9. Brackmann DE, Fayad JN, Slattery WH, et al: Early proactive management of vestibular schwannoma in neurofibromatosis type 2. Neurosurgery 2001;49:274–283.
10. Niranjan A, Lunsford D, Flickinger JC, et al: Dose reduction improves hearing preservation rates after intracanalicular acoustic tumor radiosurgery. Neurosurgery 1999;45:753–765.
11. Shelton C: Unilateral acoustic tumors: how often do they recur after translabyrinthine removal? Laryngoscope 1995;105:958–966.
12. Noren G, Greitz D, Hirsch A, Lax I: Gamma knife surgery in acoustic tumors. Acta Neurochir Suppl 1993;58:104–107.
13. Flickinger JC, Kondziolka D, Niranjan A, Lunsford D: Results of acoustic neuroma radiosurgery: an analysis of 5 years' experience using current methods. J Neurosurg 2001;94:1–6.
14. Prasad D, Steiner M, Steiner L: Gamma surgery for vestibular schwannoma. J Neurosurg 2000;92:745–759.
15. Breen P, Flickinger JC, Kondziolka D, Martinez AJ: Radiotherapy for nonfunctional pituitary adenoma: analysis of long-term tumor control. J Neurosurg 1998;89:933–938.
16. Beir V: Health effects of exposure to low levels of ionizing radiation. National Academy Press, Washington D.C.
17. Schneider AB, Shore-Freedman E, Ryo UY, et al: Radiation-induced tumors of the head and neck following childhood irradiation. Medicine 1985;64:1–15.
18. Sznajder L, Abrahams C, Parry DM, et al: Multiple schwannomas and meningiomas associated with irradiation in childhood. Arch Intern Med 1996;156:1873–1878.
19. Baser M, MacCollin M, Sujansky E, et al: Malignant nervous system tumors in patients with neurofibromatosis type 2. Presented at the 1996 FASEB Summer Research Conference on Neurofibromatosis, Snowmass, CO, June 29, 1996.
20. Wiet RJ, Micco AG, Bauer GP: Complications of the Gamma Knife. Arch Otolaryngol Head Neck Surg 1996;122:414–416.
21. Fagan P, Chang P, Turner J: Triton tumour: letter to the editor. J Neurosurg 1999;90:987–989.
22. Shamisa A, Bance M, Nag S, et al. Glioblastoma multiforme occurring in a patient treated with gamma knife surgery. J Neurosurg 2001;94:816–821.

Chapter 10

Stereotactic Radiosurgery for Pituitary Adenoma

Alex M. Landolt, Nicoletta Lomax, Stefan G. Scheib

Introduction

Pituitary adenomas are typically slow growing, benign tumors. The tumor growth fraction usually ranges from 0.1 to 1%, with rare tumors having indices up to 4%.[1] This low-growth fraction places pituitary adenomas among tumors with a late response to radiation (meningiomas, schwannomas). As a result, pituitary adenomas have a low α/β ratio rendering them excellent candidates for single-fraction treatment.[2] The first large series of pituitary adenoma patients to be treated with stereotactic radiosurgery were published by the groups in Berkley, CA (Lawrence) and Boston, MA (Kjellberg), who used heavy charged particle irradiation (helium and proton beams) taking advantage of the Bragg-peak effect.[3,4] However, proliferation of charged particle irradiation has been restricted by the cost and limited availability of this technology. We will therefore not discuss this topic further despite new interest that has developed recently. Stereotactic radiosurgery of tumors of the sella region gained popularity with the introduction and widespread usage of the Leksell Gamma Unit, further fueled by a number of favorable reports for this patient group. By the end of 1999, 9790 patients suffering from pituitary adenomas underwent radiosurgery with the Gamma Knife, as shown in a recent survey of the International Leksell Gamma Knife Society. This represents about 10% of all Gamma Knife procedures worldwide. Only few reports exist on stereotactic linear accelerator (LINAC) irradiation used either in a single session (stereotactic radiosurgery), or repeatedly in fractions (stereotactic radiotherapy).

From Pollock BE (ed). *Contemporary Stereotactic Radiosurgery: Technique and Evaluation.* Armonk, NY, Futura Publishing Company, Inc. © 2002.

We will present the indications, technique, results, and complications of Gamma Knife radiosurgery of secreting and nonsecreting pituitary adenomas based on 111 pituitary adenoma patients treated in Zürich since the autumn of 1994. We will also present a review of the literature concerning the results of the Gamma Knife and stereotactic LINAC radiosurgery and radiotherapy. Practical aspects regarding the management of patients with pituitary adenomas will be emphasized.

Gamma Knife Treatment of Pituitary Adenomas

Indications for Gamma Knife Treatment

Gamma Knife treatment must be considered as a therapeutic option for every patient with a recurrent pituitary adenoma and, particularly, for all patients with residual adenoma after surgical resection because the results of repeat surgery are often not successful.[5] The Gamma Knife is used only in exceptional cases as the primary treatment for patients who reject anesthesia or open surgery. Open surgery is generally preferred because it can cure instantaneously, whereas radiosurgery becomes effective only after a latency of 1 to 2 years. Medical reasons to use stereotactic radiosurgery as a primary tool have become progressively rare since the introduction of the modern, potent, antisecretory drugs that can successfully prepare for open surgery patients who previously might have been considered unfit for an open procedure. Table 1 outlines the role of radiosurgery relative to medical treatment and tumor removal. In this therapeutic cascade, the rank of radiosurgery as a therapeutic option is based on the adenoma's endocrine type and represents the mainstream of our own therapeutic approach. Table 2 shows the distribution of endocrine diagnoses managed by the senior author with either microsurgery or radiosurgery from 1973 to 2000.

Table 1
Therapeutic Cascade Generally Used for Treating Pituitary Adenomas*

Treatment	*Acromegaly*	*Cushing's Disease*	*Prolactinomas*	*Nonsecreting Adenomas*
1st choice	Microsurgery	Microsurgery	Dopamine agonists	Microsurgery
2nd choice	Stereotactic radiosurgery	Stereotactic radiosurgery	Microsurgery	Stereotactic radiosurgery
3rd choice	Octreotide	Ketoconazole Mitotane	Stereotactic radiosurgery	Repeat surgery
4th choice	Dopamine agonists	Adrenalectomy		

*Used by the author.

Table 2
Distribution of Endocrine Types in Personal Microsurgical and Gamma Knife Series

Diagnosis	*Microsurgical Series**	*Gamma Knife Series***
Acromegaly	25.2%	38.7%
Nonsecreting adenomas	25.7%	28.8%
Prolactinoma	38.0%	22.5%
Cushing's disease	8.8%	6.3%
Nelson's syndrome	1.8%	2.7%
TSH-adenoma	0.5%	0.9%
Total number	1260	111

TSH, thyroid-stimulating hormone.
*Entire series of first author, 1973–Spring 2000.
**Entire series of first author, 1994–Spring 2000.

Adenoma Size and Extension

The volume of intracranial tumors thought to be manageable with radiosurgery is limited to 22.4 mL (corresponding to a sphere with a diameter of about 35 mm), if a reference (maximum) dose of 50 Gy is used, because of the dose-volume effect.[6] However, when treating suprasellar tumor extensions, the limiting factor is usually not tumor volume, but rather, the proximity of the tumor to the optic nerve and the chiasm, where the dose is constrained to 8 to 9 Gy. Experience has shown that for recurrent pituitary adenomas this tumor volume is rarely exceeded unless there is an extensive skull base invasion. In such cases, we try to reduce the irradiated adenoma volume as much as possible by performing decompressive surgery initially. Staging tumors in this fashion allows improved endocrine control, and reduces the radiation dose to the hypothalamus and optic pathways due to the smaller treatment volume. The target volumes in our series of 111 cases range between 0.8 and 18.5 mL (median, 2.0 mL); 94.5% of the cases were less than or equal to 8.5 mL. The main endocrine groups (acromegaly, prolactinomas, nonsecreting adenomas) had similar target volumes, whereas Cushing's disease deviates towards smaller prescription isodose volumes and patients with Nelson's syndrome had larger target volumes (Fig. 1).

In comparison to stereotactic radiosurgery, fractionated radiotherapy has the disadvantage of a high rate of delayed hypopituitarism secondary to the effects of radiation on the hypothalamus and neuroendocrine centers.[7,8] The focused nature of radiation delivery used by the Gamma Knife permits a significant reduction in the radiation exposure to adjacent structures such as the hypothalamus, while maintaining a high radiation dose to the tumor. For example, we have noted a significant reduction in

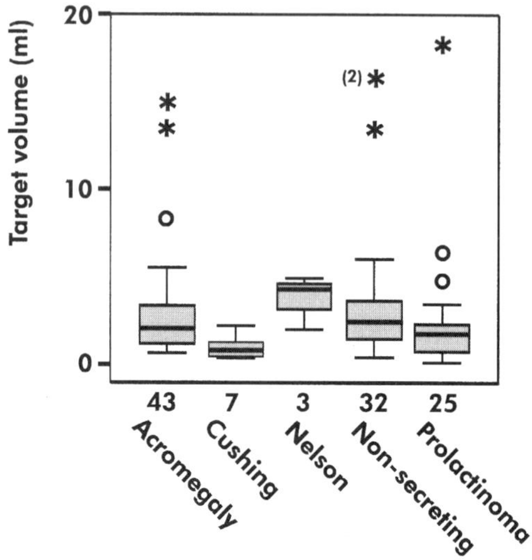

Figure 1. Box plot of target volume of individual endocrine types of 110 Gamma Knife-treated pituitary adenomas. The single case of a thyroid-stimulating hormone-secreting adenoma is omitted. The circles represent outliers (1.5–3 box heights above the box), the asterisks represent far outliers (more than 3 box heights above the box).

the dose delivered to the median eminence in our series of prolactinomas by reducing the volume of the Gamma Knife-treated targets.[9] The median dose received in patients with targets less than 1.7 mL was approximately 4 Gy, compared to a dose of more than 6 Gy for patients with tumors greater than 1.7 mL ($p=0.01$). This fact, in conjunction with the radiation sensitivity of the optic system, reinforces the need to debulk large adenomas prior to radiosurgery.

Radiosurgical Dose Planning

We utilize both magnetic resonance imaging (MRI) and computed tomography (CT) for dose planning. Other centers work with MRI images only.[10] The CT scan is used primarily for definition of the optic nerves in the area of the orbital apex, for delineation of scar tissue originating from the fat transplants in the sella and sphenoid sinus, and as a control for possible minor MRI distortions. The CT images have a thickness of 1 mm and are contrast enhanced. For MRI, a volume acquisition with a fast speed gradient echo (3D/TE 2.2/Fr, flip angle 20°) is obtained. The section thickness is 1.0, spaced 0 mm, and the matrix 256, Nex 3, FOV = 26 cm.

The dose is typically prescribed to an isodose that closely conforms to the tumor using multiple small radiation isocenters; this is most frequently the 50% isodose line. The 100% isodose (reference dose point) is at the dose maximum. We use a reference dose that is as high as possible while still limiting the dose to the optic nerves and the chiasm. The most frequently used reference dose is 50 Gy (77.2% of our cases). However, higher doses have been used in 9.6%, lower doses in 13.2% of our series of 111 patients (range, 16–70 Gy). The dose applied to the optic apparatus is carefully evaluated during the planning procedure. For routine planning and also for scientific purposes, we outline not only the target, but also the optic nerves, chiasm, and optic tracts. This can be done easily, if the x/y-plane of the stereotactic frame is aligned parallel to the optic nerves. This forward tilting of the stereotactic headframe facilitates volumetric evaluation of the optic apparatus.

The three-dimensional dose distribution is obtained by filling the target volume with multiple isocenters (shots) to conform the prescription isodose volume (PIV) as closely as possible to the target volume (TV). The volume within the target receiving at least the prescription isodose is termed $TV_{(PI)}$. The target coverage is calculated as the fraction of the target volume receiving at least the prescription isodose ($TV_{(PI)}/TV$). The mean coverage for all our pituitary patients is 0.9. The conformity index is calculated as ($TV_{(PI)}/PIV$) and has values ranging from 0 to 1, with 1 being the ideal case. The mean conformity index value for all our pituitary patients is 0.76. To achieve this degree of conformality, we typically use high shot numbers (median, 12 shots) and small collimator sizes (4 and 8 mm). This is necessary because recurrent and persisting pituitary adenomas after unsuccessful surgery usually have irregular outlines.

Plugging of individual beams is done to produce a steeper dose gradient towards the optic apparatus (Fig. 2). This decreases the radiation dose to the optic nerves and is particularly important if the gap between the upper tumor surface and the optic nerves is narrow. The plug positions are calculated by the planning system. Plugging for protection of the brainstem is rarely necessary. The review of our 111 patients shows that we used between 0 and 100 (mean, 22) plugs per shot. Only 15% of our patients needed no plugs. As mentioned previously, forward tilting of the stereotactic frame increases the radiation dose to the lenses requiring additional beam blocking. However, this forward tilting helps to keep the gamma angle close to 90° when we align the upper surface of the 9-Gy isodose within the steepest dose fall-off parallel to the optic nerves. We used in our series of 111 treatments a gamma angle of 70 to 110° (mean, 90°) in 96% of the cases. This position is more comfortable for the patient treated with the B model of the Gamma Knife.

Acromegaly

Acromegaly, in our institution and in reports from most other centers, is the most frequent indication for Gamma Knife treatment of pitu-

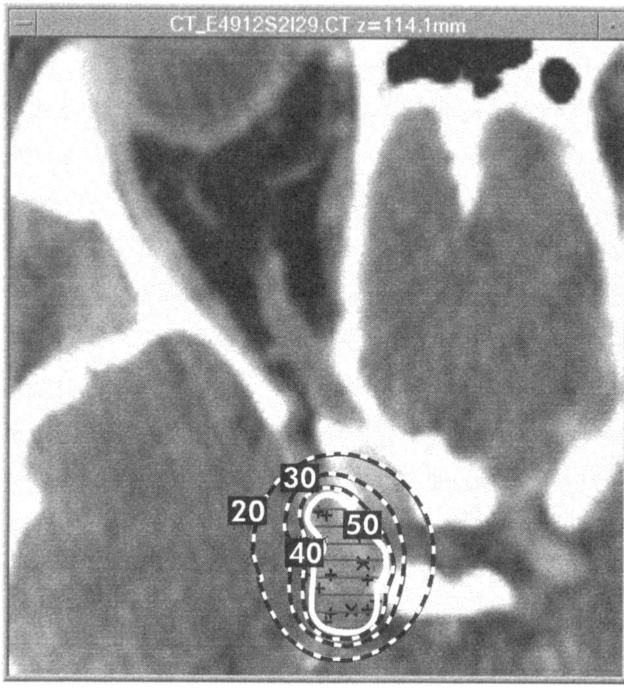

A

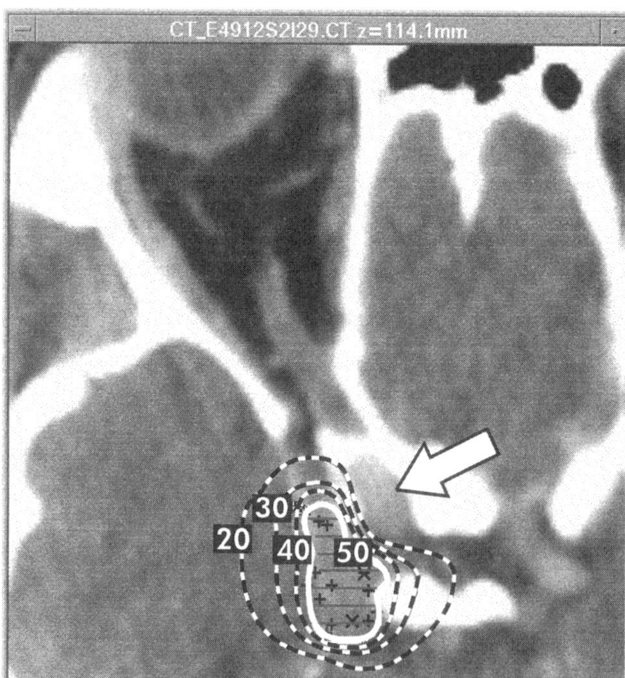

B

Figure 2. Axial CT dose plan showing radiation exposure of optic nerve without (**A**) and with (**B**) plugging of 92 gamma sources. *(Continued.)*

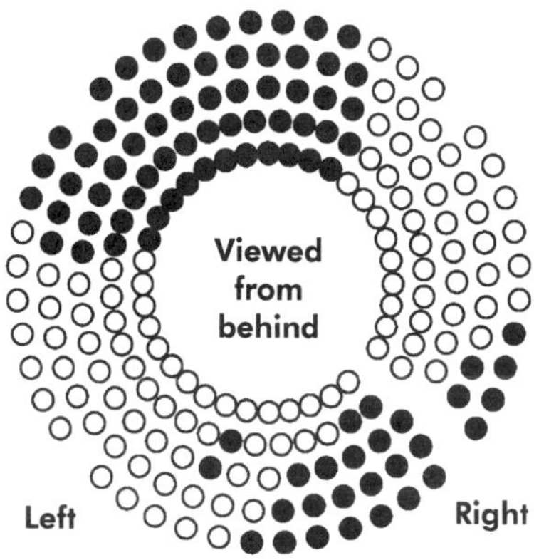

C

Figure 2. (**C**) Plug pattern used for this patient. Note the displacement of the isodose curves (50%, 40%, 30%, 20%) in B, corresponding to 25, 20, 15, and 10 Gy and the reduction of the radiation exposure to the optic nerve in the optic canal (arrow) to less than 10 Gy. The tumor mass delineated by the 50 percentile is marked by horizontal hatches. The + and x signs indicate projections and positions of isodose centers (total number, 14).

itary adenoma patients. Table 3 outlines the published experience with Gamma Knife radiosurgery for growth hormone-producing tumors.[11-26] Unfortunately, comparison of these studies is difficult. Most studies present endpoints obtained after different periods of time disregarding the dynamic nature of hormone parameter normalization that can only be represented by a cumulative distribution function (Kaplan-Meier estimate).[27] Moreover, the definition of "normal" differs and does not necessarily follow the definitions as described by endocrinologists. It is now accepted that normalization of insulin-like growth factor I (IGF-I) is a more important parameter than growth hormone, because the later is quite labile and single values are not significant. The oral glucose tolerance test (OGTT) is actually the "gold standard," but it cannot be checked regularly at short intervals. A high cutoff point of "normal growth hormone," however, has to be judged with caution and is often associated with a high success rate. The radiation doses used vary and the technique of target definition, particularly in older reports using the Kula system, is rather imprecise. Review of the 175 patients reported in the literature shows that normalization of the age-adjusted IGF-I level is more difficult to achieve than reduction of the growth hormone alone. Series considering IGF-I have generally lower success rates (range, 20–71%) than the others using only growth hormone values (range, 29–100%). This is despite rather similar prescribed margin and maximum radiation doses between these series.

Table 3

Gamma Knife Treatment of Acromegaly: Review of the Literature*

First Author (Year)	*Criteria for Cure*	*Margin Dose (Gy)*	*Maximal Dose (Gy)*	*Follow-up (years)*	*No. of Patients*	*Percent "Normal"*
Thorén (1991)[11]	GH <5 ng/mL	?	17–70	1–20.8	21	29
Stephanian (1992)[12]	?	15–>25	28–60	1	4	75
Ganz (1993)[13]	<2.5 ng/mL	10–25	?	>1.5	4	25
Pollock (1994)[14]	GH <5 ng/mL	?	20–60	>1.5	8	38
Motti (1996)[15]	?	12–22	?	0.5–1	2	50
Martinez (1998)[16]	GH <7 ng/mL IGF-I normal**	15–30	50–80	2.2–3.8	7	71
Pan (1998)[17]	<12 ng/mL	11–39	27–70	2–3	12	100
Lim (1998)[18]	<2 ng/mL	30–35	60–70	0.25–4.5	16	38
Ikeda (1998)[19]	?	25–30	50–60	0.25–5.2	5	80
Morange-Ramos (1998)[20]	GH <5 ng/mL IGF-I normal**	12–35	?	0.5–2.5	15	20
Witt (1998)[21]	?	9.6–30	20–60	?	14	64
Hayashi (1999)[22]	?	23.9	?	>0.5	22	41
Kim (1999)[23]	?	18–40	35–80	?	13	38
Laws (1999)[24]	IGF-I normal**	>18	?	>0.5	36	25
Mokry (1999)[25]	GH and IGF-I normal	9–25	19–50	0.5–6	10	40
Landolt (2000)[26]	GH <5 ng/mL IGF-I normal**	25	50	0.3–3.7	31	32

GH, growth hormone; IGF-I, insulin-like growth factor I.

*Only the most recent publication is included if an author has published several reports.

**Age and sex-dependent.

We previously compared two groups of acromegalic patients, one treated with fractionated radiotherapy (n=50, 40 Gy/20 fractions), with 16 patients having Gamma Knife radiosurgery and demonstrated improved outcomes after radiosurgery (Fig. 3).[27] The mean time to normalization of growth hormone and IGF-1 values was reduced from 7.8 years with fractionated radiotherapy to 1.4 years with the Gamma Knife. In that study, no correlation was noted between a reduction in tumor size on follow-up MRI and endocrine results; 4 of 6 patients with normal IGF-I values had decreased tumor size compared to 3 of 6 patients who continued to suffer from acromegaly. The extent of shrinkage, in our patients, is

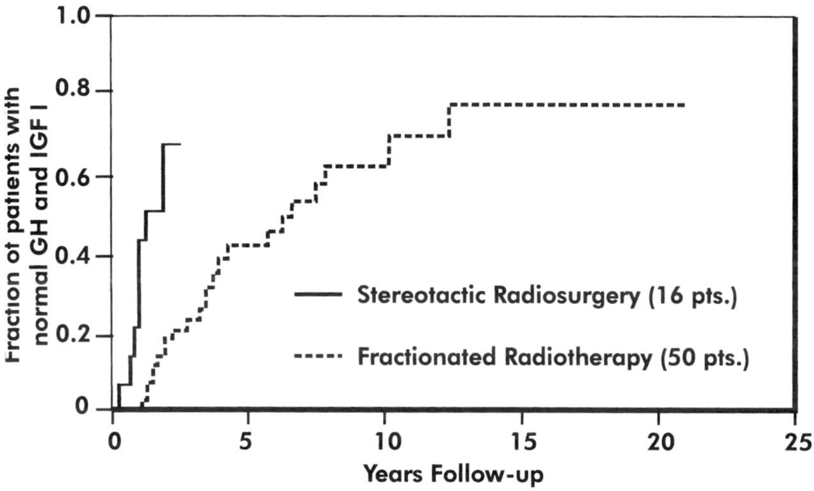

Figure 3. Cumulative distribution function (Kaplan-Meier estimate) of 50 acromegalic patients treated with fractionated radiotherapy and 16 acromegalic patients treated with the Gamma Knife. The comparison of the two curves with a log-rank test shows a significant difference (significance, $p=0.0001$.) Reprinted from Landolt et al[27] with permission of the Journal of Neurosurgery.

always modest (Fig. 4). Thus, our experience differs from other authors. Tumor reductions between 50 and 100% have been described.[13,16,18,20] Younger patients seemed to be more radiosensitive.

We have found recently, that treatment of the adenomas with the antisecretory drug octreotide during the radiation exposure impairs the results of Gamma Knife radiosurgery (Fig. 5).[26] The use of octreotide, particularly its long-acting formula is becoming increasingly popular.[28] We think that this effect of octreotide occurs because the drug reduces the metabolic activity of the tumor, analogous to pentobarbital in normal brain,[29] or as hypoxia and hypothermia in other tissues.[30] The reduction of the metabolic activity increases the radioresistence of the adenoma. Our observations have led us to change our management of acromegalic patients undergoing radiosurgery.[26] Currently, we perform radiosurgery only during an octreotide gap. The last injection of microencapsulated long-acting octreotide is given about 4 months before the Gamma Knife procedure. Three daily injections of 100 mg of the short-lasting formula are started 6 weeks later and continued until 2 weeks before radiosurgery. This allows a short gap in octreotide treatment (about 2 weeks). Octreotide is restarted immediately after radiosurgery with the usual precautions.

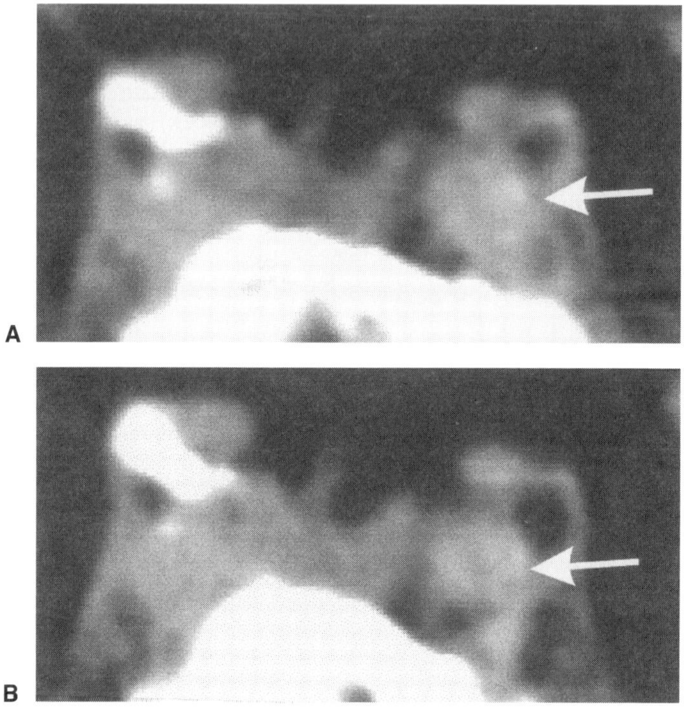

Figure 4. Acromegaly: adenoma remnant in left cavernous sinus (**A**) after transsphenoidal microsurgery. (**B**) The same patient 1 year after Gamma Knife. Growth hormone and IGF-I were normalized. Note shrinkage of tumor. The tumor is indicated with arrows.

Corticotropic Adenomas

Cushing's Disease

We have been able to collect reports concerning 122 patients treated with the Gamma Knife for Cushing's disease (Table 4).[13–25,31–33] The results as a whole appear favorable because 58% of the patients reported could be "cured." However, the criteria used for defining "cure" vary considerably. The pronounced variation in the radiation dose used does not allow recommendations for treatment dose to be established. One long-term study following 18 patients for periods of 12 to 22 years has been recently published.[33] The patients, however, cannot necessarily be compared with other, more recently treated groups because of the lack of accurate target localization (lack of modern imaging techniques) and the use of much higher target doses (60–230 Gy given in 1–4 treatment sessions). An overall success rate of 83% was found. The most pronounced drop in urinary cortisol occurred within the first 3 months after treatment. However, a further fall in adrenocorticotrophic hormone (ACTH; corticotropin) could be found even after more than 10 years.

We have treated six patients with Cushing's disease. One patient was treated twice. Two suffered from small tumor remnants; one had a large tumor localized in both cavernous sinuses. The adenoma could not be seen in three patients. A reference (maximum) dose of 50 Gy was used in all patients with the exception of one patient in whom a dose of 70 Gy was given. The 50% isodose was used as prescription dose for all patients. Two patients were cured 1 and 2 years after the treatment. Three are controlled with slowly decreasing doses of ketoconazole. One patient did not respond and was also resistant to medical treatment with ketoconazole. This patient underwent a second Gamma Knife to a larger target 2 1/2 years after the first procedure. Almost 1 year later, the patient is improving and the disease is being controlled with metopirone.

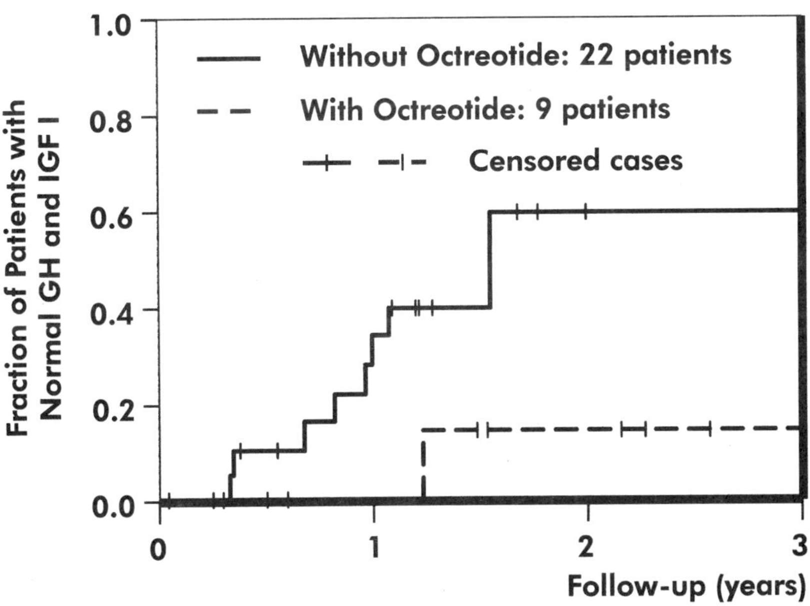

Figure 5. Cumulative distribution function (Kaplan-Meier estimate) showing endocrine control in 31 acromegalic patients treated with Gamma Knife radiosurgery while receiving, or not receiving, simultaneous octreotide medication. (A log-rank test shows a significant difference of the two curves, significance, p=0.042). Reprinted with permission from Landolt et al.[26]

Table 4
Gamma Knife Treatment of Cushing's Disease: Review of the Literature

First Author (Year)	*Criteria for Cure*	*Margin Dose (Gy)*	*Maximal Dose (Gy)*	*Follow-up (years)*	*No. of Patients*	*Percent "Normal"*
Rähn (1980)[31]	1	50–70%*	60–100	1–5	18	55
Ganz (1993)[13]	2	25	50–83	>1.5	4	50
Pollock (1994)[14]	3	?	20–60	>1.5	11	73
Seo (1995)[32]	4	20, 35	?	2	2	50
Motti (1996)[15]	5	12–22	?	>0.5	2	50
Martinez (1998)[16]	6	11–36	22–60	?	3	100
Pan (1998)[17]	7	23–34	30–43	1	4	100
Lim (1998)[18]	?	30–35	60–70	2	4	25
Ikeda (1998)[19]	?	12.5–35	25–70	–5	8	62
Morange-Ramos (1998)[20]	8	14–35	?	2.5	6	66
Witt (1998)[21]	?	9.6–30	20–60	?	21	43
Hayashi (1999)[22]	?	23.9	?	>0.5	10	10
Kim (1999)[23]	?	18–40	35–80	?	8	62
Laws (1999)[24]	5	>18	?	>0.5	39	59
Mokry (1999)[25]	?	10–20	20–44	0.5–6	3	33
Höybye (2001)[33]	9	?	60–100**	12–22	18	83

Definition of "cure": (1) Urine-free cortisol <330 nmol/24 hrs; (2) Urine-free cortisol <650 nmol/24 hrs; (3) ACTH <80 pg/mL; urine-free cortisol <90mg/24 hrs; (4) ACTH <4.8 pg/mL, serum cortisol <15.5 g/100mL; (5) "Normal" 24-hr urine-free cortisol; (6) ACTH <10 g/L, urinary cortisol <650 nmol/24 hrs; (7) "Normal ACTH"; (8) Urine-free cortisol < 90 g/24 hrs, ACTH and plasma cortisol in "normal" range; (9) ACTH <11 pmol/L, "normal" urine-free cortisol.

*Isodose at surface.

**Dose of first treatment; in entire series up to 4 treatments with total doses up to 230 Gy.

The difficulty in target definition is nicely demonstrated by our experience in treating patients with Cushing's disease. We define the target, as in other endocrine adenoma types, whenever possible, as the remaining adenomatous tissue visible on MRI scans. This, however, was impossible in three of our patients. The adenomas may have been too small, or may have been obscured by the scar formation from previous microsurgical intervention. Two possible solutions exist for the problem: (1) definition of the target according to the findings of the previous surgery including the adjacent cavernous sinus, or (2) inclusion of the entire "normal" pituitary gland together with the cavernous sinus into the target area. This second principle was used successfully in one of our patients (Fig. 6). The recurrent symptoms of the patient disappeared 2 years after treatment and the patient does not show any endocrine deficits 3 years after radiosurgery.

Nelson's Syndrome

Reports describing the results of treating patients suffering from the Nelson syndrome are rare: only two reports presenting 12 patients are

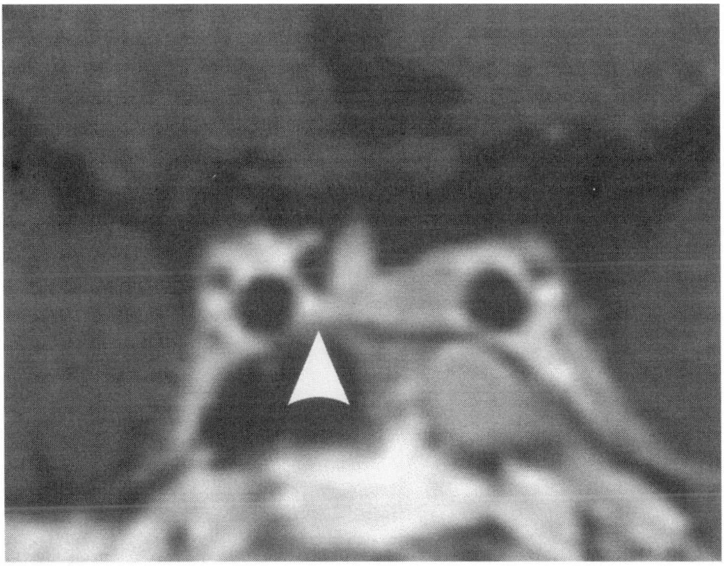

A

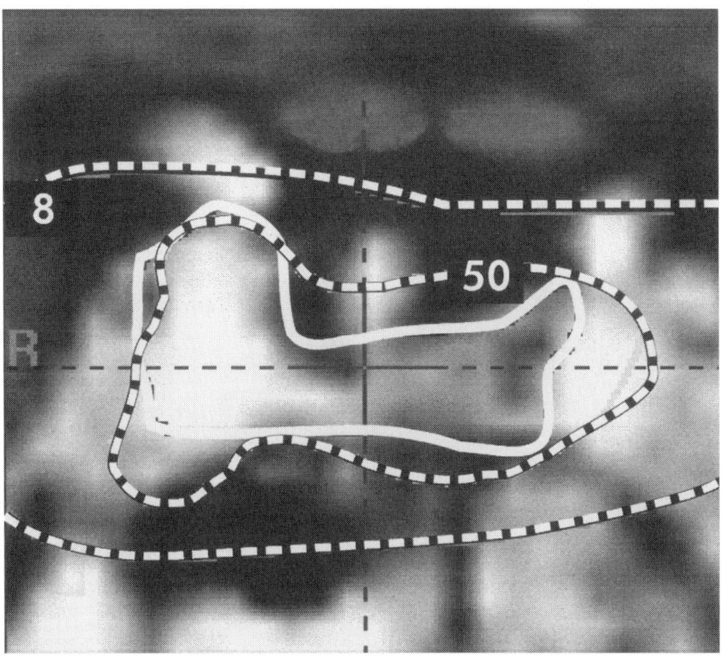

B

Figure 6. Coronal MRI in patient suffering from recurrent Cushing's disease (**A**) The arrowhead points to the site of the previous adenoma location. The Gamma Knife dose plan (**B**) shows the outline of the entire pituitary gland (white line) and the 50th and 8th percentiles.

available.[13,24] To this, we can add only three personal observations. Evaluation of the endocrine result of therapy is difficult in patients with Nelson's syndrome because adrenalectomized patient have elevated ACTH values unless they are suppressed with cortisone substitution. Only one patient with a final ACTH of less than 60 pg/mL was observed by Laws and Vance.[24] Ganz et al described two patients treated with the Gamma Knife (maximum dose, 50 and 70 Gy) whose tumors decreased in size. This was accompanied by a lowering of the ACTH. A third patient irradiated with 50 Gy showed no improvement.[13]

Our first patient, a 47-year-old woman, 17 years after adrenalectomy for Cushing's disease, 16 years after transsphenoidal surgery, 13 years after transcranial adenomectomy, and 12 years after fractionated radiotherapy (total dose, 52 Gy), underwent Gamma Knife treatment in 1997 because of a slow enlargement of the remaining pituitary adenoma. A reference dose of only 40 Gy (prescription dose of 20 Gy to the tumor margin) was used because of the previous radiotherapy. The ACTH values and the tumor size have remained unchanged over 3 years. The second patient, a 40-year-old woman, 22 years after adrenalectomy for Cushing's disease and 15 years after first time transsphenoidal surgery, had to undergo repeat transsphenoidal decompression in 1997 because the tumor recurrence had become too large for Gamma Knife treatment. The patient suffered after the surgical reexploration from gonadotroph and somatotroph insufficiency. The 1.9-mL remaining adenoma volume was treated 3 months after decompression with a reference dose of 50 Gy (25 Gy to the tumor margin). The tumor's proliferation index (MIB-1 expression) was 0.9% at the time of the reoperation. One year later, the tumor volume had decreased by 21% and the ACTH level had decreased (after 25-mg cortisone) from greater than 1800 ng/L to 302 ng/L, but was not yet normal. Her skin pigmentation had decreased visibly. Although not hormonally normal, we consider this as a success due to the usual biological behavior of Nelson adenomas.

The third patient, a 61-year-old woman suffered from a malignant ACTH-secreting pituitary tumor. She underwent fractionated pituitary irradiation in 1947 at the age of 13 years. Adrenalectomy was done at the age of 23 years because of persistent disease. A second pituitary irradiation (dose unknown) was done at the age of 25 years. Subtotal transsphenoidal resections of the invasive adenoma had to be done three times, at the age of 45, 60, and 61 years because of visual deterioration caused by tumor growth. The Gamma Knife treatment (reference dose, 50 Gy; marginal dose 16 Gy) was done in 1995 at the age of 61 years. However, a fourth, unsuccessful transsphenoidal decompression was necessary because of progression of the visual deficit 4 months after radiosurgery. The patient became blind and died 2 years later in a nursing home. Histologic examination of the two tumor biopsies obtained 5 months before and 4 months after the Gamma Knife treatment showed a pituitary adenoma

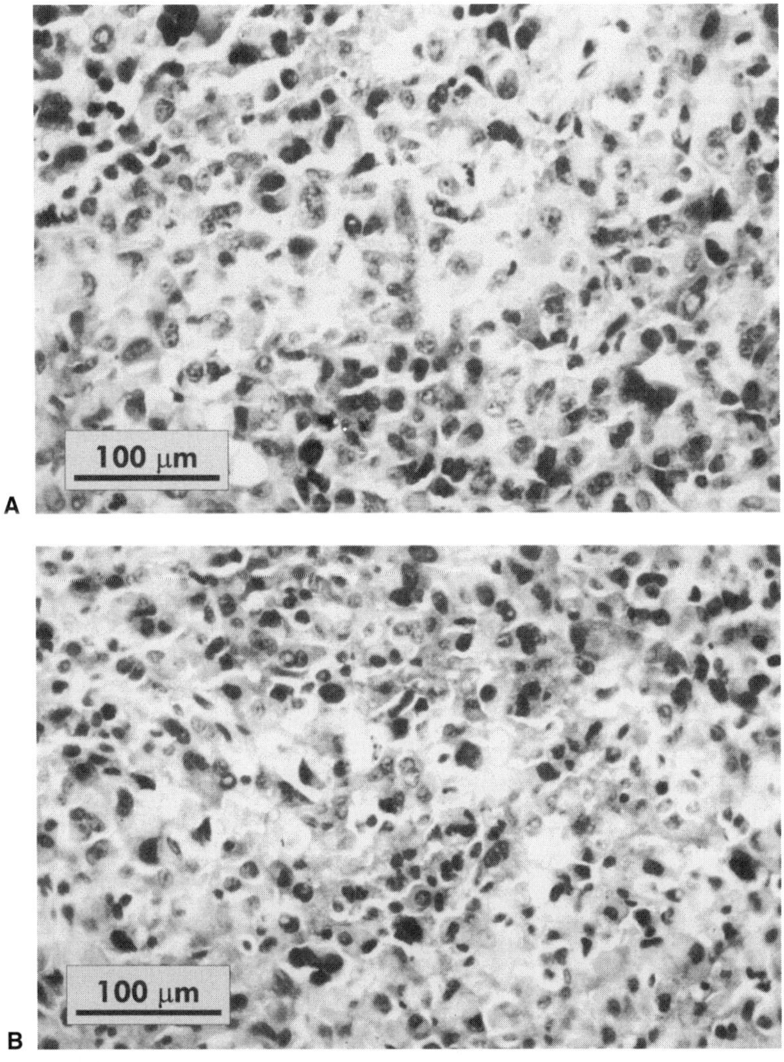

Figure 7. Histologic examination of malignant Nelson-adenoma before (**A**) and 4 months after (**B**) Gamma Knife treatment (reference dose, 50 Gy). H&E stain.

with malignant characteristics (Fig. 7). However, there was neither a difference in the morphology nor of the proliferation index (MIB-1 before 10.1% and 10.2% after the Gamma Knife treatment) that was significantly higher than in other pituitary adenomas.[1]

Nelson adenomas are notoriously aggressive tumors.[34,35] Endocrine cures are difficult to achieve and are only of relative importance (maintaining gonadal function), since a major deficit (total adrenal function loss, necessitating a permanent substitution with gluco- and mineralocorticoids) already exists. We therefore consider control of the tumor size and ACTH hypersecretion, analogous to the nonsecreting adenomas, a success.

Prolactinoma

The Gamma Knife treatment of prolactinomas has been less popular than the treatment of acromegaly because dopamine agonists offer an effective and cheap alternative that can be used for extended time periods. Table 5 summarizes our review of the literature with reports summarizing 73 patients.[13,16–18,20–25,36] The results are less favorable than in acromegaly. It is interesting to note that a measurement of the tumor shrinkage done by Martinez et al shows that prolactinomas decreased less than growth hormone-secreting adenomas.[16] Pan et al consider the results of prolactinoma treatment to be less satisfactory than treatment of acromegaly and Cushing's disease.[17]

We have treated 20 patients suffering from prolactinomas who were either unresponsive to dopamine agonists, or, doses large enough to normalize prolactin levels were not tolerated by the patients because of side effects. Five patients were treated successfully. Their prolactin values became normal (<20 ng/mL) 5 to 41 months after the treatment. Three started to menstruate normally and two became pregnant. One patient who suffered from primary amenorrhea uses contraceptive pills because no pregnancy is intended, and one is of postmenopausal age. She was treated because of symptomatic trigeminal neuralgia. The situation improved in 11 patients who achieved normal prolactin values, but continued to need medical treatment, or who had persisting hyperprolactinemia

Table 5
Gamma Knife Treatment of Prolactinomas: Review of the Literature

First Author (Year)	*Criteria for Cure*	*Margin Dose (Gy)*	*Maximal Dose (Gy)*	*Follow-up (years)*	*No. of Patients*	*Percent "Normal"*
Ganz (1993)[13]	<18 ng/mL	6–20	30–50	>1.5	3	0
Martinez (1998)[16]	<20 ng/mL	27–35	70–80	2.2–3.8	5	0
Pan (1998)[17]	?	9–35	17–70	2–3	23	17*
Lim (1998)[18]	<25 ng/mL	30–35	60–70	0.25–3	18	56
Morange-Ramos (1998)[20]	<25 ng/mL	25–30	?	1–3	4	0
Witt (1998)[21]	?	9.6–30	20–60	?	7	0
Hayashi (1999)[22]	?	23.9	?	>0.5	13	15.4
Kim (1999)[23,36]	?	18–40	35–80	?	31	19
Laws (1999)[24]	<20 ng/mL	>18	?	>0.5	13	7
Mokry (1999)[25]	?	7.5–25	16–50	0.25–5.5	21	21

*1 pregnancy, 15 (65%) normal menses.

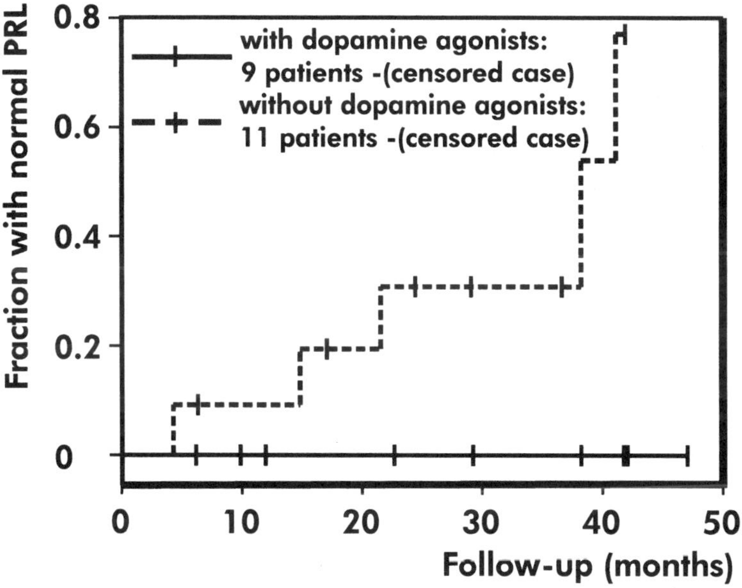

Figure 8. Cumulative distribution function (Kaplan-Meier estimate) showing successful results obtained in 20 prolactinomas, treated and not treated with dopamine agonists at the time of radiosurgery. Significance in log-rank test ($p=0.03$). Reprinted with permission from Landolt and Lomax.[9]

but needed less medication. Two of these patients became pregnant. One needed only a small dose of cabergoline. The second who had suffered from a large invasive adenoma and had microsurgical decompression needed cabergoline plus gonadotropin stimulation. Four patients showed no improvement after radiosurgery.

Retrospective analysis of our data showed again, similar to acromegaly, that the antisecretory dopamine agonists have a negative influence on prolactin normalization after radiosurgery (Fig. 8).[9] None of the patients treated with dopamine agonists at the time of the Gamma Knife application became normal. We have started, therefore, to use the Gamma Knife during a gap in the dopamine agonist treatment, similar to the octreotide gap in acromegalics.

Thyroid-Stimulating Adenomas

Thyroid-stimulating hormone-producing adenomas are rare. We are not aware of any patients reported in the literature. We have treated only one patient, a 43-year-old man who had undergone transsphenoidal microsurgery elsewhere and continued to suffer from hyperthyroidism despite octreotide therapy. This patient was lost to follow-up.

Nonsecreting Adenomas

Evaluation of the treatment result for patients with nonsecreting adenomas is usually based on a qualitative assessment of the volume changes shown on follow-up MRI studies. Only Martinez and collaborators have presented quantitative measurements of the adenoma volumes.[16] Tumor growth control signifies only that the tumor volume did not increase during the observation period. Control rates of 93 to 100% have been reported (Table 6).[12–16,21–23,25,37] It must be considered, however, that the follow-up time of most reported patients is short if the slow proliferation, particularly of nonsecreting adenomas, is taken into account.[1]

In our personal series of patients with 32 nonsecreting adenomas we found a control rate of 97% using a reference dose of 50 Gy and a prescription dose of 25 Gy. However, this standard dosage regime was violated in several cases because of the proximity of the optic nerve optic tract or chiasm. These cases demonstrated that lower doses are able to control the growth and even shrink nonsecreting pituitary adenomas (Fig. 9). The minimal dose required for achieving control of the adenoma's growth remains to be determined.

Radiosurgery failed to control further growth in only one patient. This was a 60-year-old man who complained about a right 3rd nerve weakness of recent onset. A pituitary adenoma invading the posterior parts of the right cavernous sinus was found on MRI examination and was decompressed using a transsphenoidal approach. The histologic examination showed a nonsecreting adenoma with an abnormally high proliferation index (Ki-67 expression 6.9%; usual average value in this group 0.61% with a maximum of 2.1%).[38] A rapid postoperative improvement of the 3rd nerve weakness was observed. The tumor, however, recurred 6 months later and was treated with the Gamma Knife (50 Gy to the maximum and 25 Gy to the margin). The MRI demonstrated a cystic lesion 1 year later and the oculomotor function was again normal. A second recurrence became evident, because a new partial 3rd nerve weakness had appeared 17 months after the first Gamma Knife treatment. This was treated a second time with the Gamma Knife (again, dose 50 Gy to the maximum and 25 Gy to the margin, because of the aggressive behavior of the tumor). There was a slow and incomplete recovery of the 3rd nerve palsy and appearance of a partial 6th nerve palsy on the right side. A new MRI demonstrated again a cyst. The cyst was reexplored 4 months later on a second transnasal intervention, because of the previous recurrence appearing after a transitory cyst formation. No remaining tumor could be found. The 6th nerve palsy has progressed and is now total; we consider this to be a radiation-related complication. The 6th nerve was irradiated in the region of Duello's canal with a dose of 23.7 Gy during the first treatment, and 24.0 Gy during the second. The dose used in this patient was therefore far above the dose of 20 Gy considered to be safe by Pan et al.[17]

Table 6
Gamma Knife Treatment on Nonsecreting Adenomas: Review of the Literature
(Including Growth Control of Secreting Adenomas)

First Author (Year)	Follow-up (yrs)	Dose (Gy)		Adenoma Size			No. of Patients	Control Rate (%)
		Margin	Max	Smaller	Equal	Larger		
Stephanien (1992)[12]	1	15–>25	?	9	5	0	14*	100
Ganz (1993)[13]	>1.5	10–25	28–60	8	9	1	18*	94
Pollock (1994)[14]	0.5–5	10–30	20–60	4	6	0	10**	100
Motti (1996)[15]	0.5	12–22	?	1	1	0	2**	50
Lim (1998)[18]	<4.5	15–36	?	37	3	0	40*	100
Martinez (1998)[16]	2.2–3.8	15–30	50–80	12	2	0	14**	100
Witt (1998)[21]	0.2–8.6	9.6–30	20–60	33	34	4	71*	94
Hayashi (1999)[22]	>0.5	19.5	?	3	15	0	18**	94
Inoue (1999)[37]	>2	9–42	?	18	15	2	35*	93
Kim (1999)[23]	2	18–40	35–80	19	19	0	28*	100
Mokry (1999)[25]	0.25–6	9–15	18–38	6	24	1	31**	97
Total				150	133	6	283	98

*Pooled secreting and nonsecreting adenomas.
**Only nonsecreting adenomas.

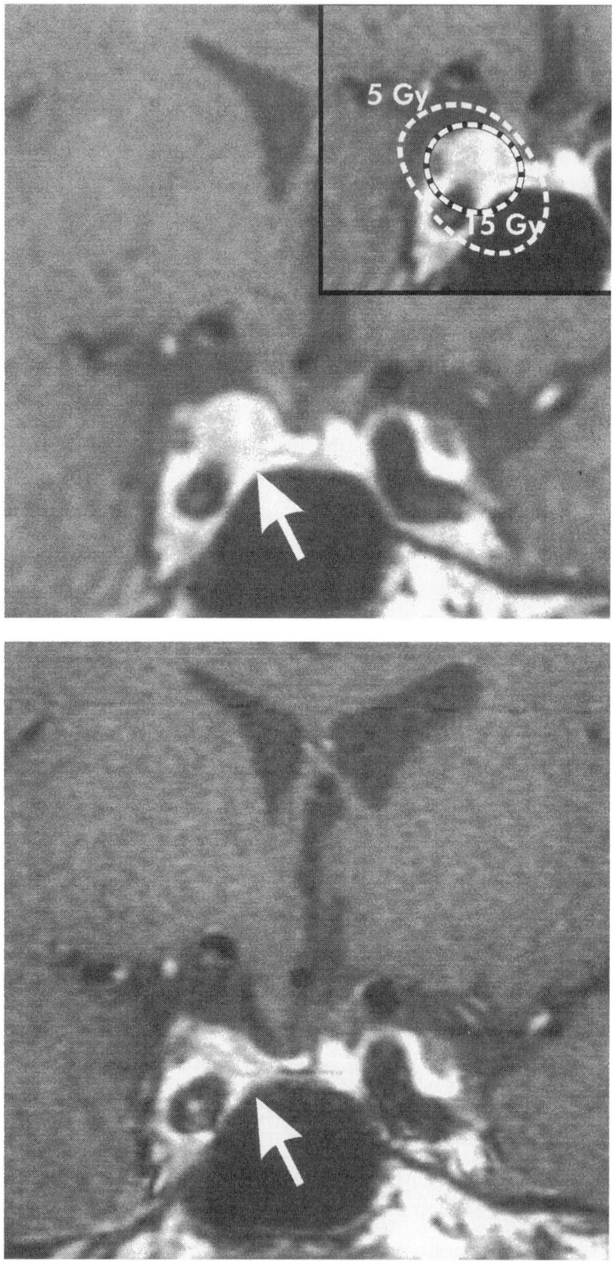

A

B

Figure 9. MRI of nonsecreting adenoma recurrence at the time of radiosurgery (**A**) (prescription dose 15 Gy to the 50% isodose) with treatment plan (inset). Note that the optic tract receives no more than 5 Gy. (**B**) Control MRI obtained 4 1/2 years after Gamma Knife treatment.

Complications

Three groups of possible complications will be discussed: cranial nerve injury (particularly the optic and occulomotor nerves), brain injury (injury of the pons and temporal lobe), and endocrine deficits (injury of the normal gland and median eminence). Their incidence is difficult to estimate. The reports summarized in Table 7 suggest that about 3.4% of the patients will suffer from endocrine deficits, 2.3% from optic nerve damage, and 1.6% from cavernous sinus nerve deficits. The final numbers, however, may be higher. It should be kept in mind that the time schedule of the appearance of the lesions may differ. The endocrine deficits after conventional radiotherapy develop only with latencies of up to 9 years and, therefore, appear later than neurological disorders.[40] Höybye et al[33] found new endocrine deficits more than 10 years after the application of very high doses (maximum total dose, 60–230 Gy). A final rate of 11 of 16 patients developed gradually pituitary insufficiency. The rare optic neuropathy appears after fractionated radiotherapy of pituitary adenomas typically after an interval of 4 to 18 months.[41] The low incidence of hypopituitarism in Table 10 therefore may be due to the short follow-up periods. No patients suffering from Gamma Knife-induced brain tumors have come to our attention yet. Brada et al, reexamining a cohort of 334 pituitary adenoma patients treated with fractionated radiotherapy (median dose, 45 Gy), reported an incidence of 1.9% with intervals of 6 to 21 years.[42]

Table 7

Complications of Gamma Knife Treatment of Pituitary Adenomas: Review of the Literature

Complication	*Latency (mos)*	*Reported*	*Total Cases**	*Percent***	*References*
Hypopituitarism	6–24	15	439	3.4	18–20, 25, 31
Vision	6–18	10	439	2.3	12, 17, 18, 20–22
Occulomotor	48 hrs–14	5	439	1.1	16, 17, 20, 21
Trigeminal	"Soon"–14	2			20, 21
Hypothalamic necrosis†	11	1			21
Temporal lobe necrosis	6	1			22
Carotid occlusion	4 yrs	1			39
Intratumoral hemorrhage	37	1			17
Central pontine myelinolysis†	13	1			21

*Total number of patients in reviewed reports.

**No percentages calculated if less than 5 patients.

†Fatal complication.

Visual disturbances observed after Gamma Knife treatment may be caused either by a radiation-induced swelling of the adenoma, or a radiation injury to the optic nerves and optic chiasma. The former condition can be treated either by prompt surgical decompression,[17] or with steroids.[16] Three of the four eye movement disorders observed by us corresponded to the direct actinic type of lesion, whereas the fourth one seemed to be pressure-related. The most severe, a total 3rd nerve palsy, was observed in a woman with acromegaly who had undergone fractionated radiotherapy (total dose, 50.4 Gy, fractions of 1.8 Gy) 10 years before the Gamma Knife treatment (dose to 3rd nerve $<$23.1 Gy). The 3rd nerve palsy appeared 8 months after the Gamma Knife treatment. An MRI examination showed an irregular contrast enhancement in the 3rd nerve (Fig. 10). Previous fractionated radiotherapy was frequently involved in this type of complication. Three of the 10 patients reported in the literature and two of our four patients with eye movement complications had undergone previous radiotherapy. The same is true in the only case with a temporal lobe necrosis reported after using the Gamma Knife.[22]

One patient in our series had a Gamma Knife-induced adenoma swelling. The patient experienced a 6th nerve palsy with abrupt onset 5 1/2 months after the treatment of a microprolactinoma remaining in the cavernous sinus. The area of Duello's canal was irradiated with 26.2 Gy. An MRI scan showed no contrast enhancement in the affected nerve. The early onset and the negative imaging study cast some doubt on the possibility of a radiation-related injury. A prompt improvement after intramuscular injection of 50-mg long-acting bromocriptine supports the in-

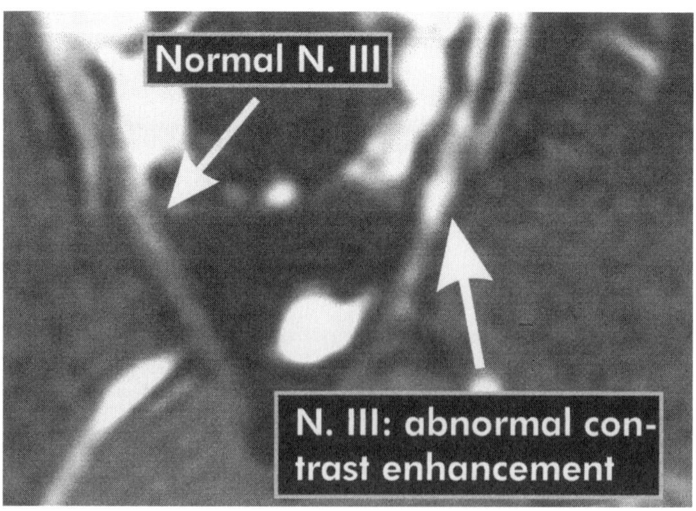

Figure 10. Axial MRI scan showing postactinic occulomotor palsy. The nerve shows an irregular contrast enhancement compared to the contralateral side.

Table 8
Endocrine Deficits After Gamma Knife Treatment of Nonsecreting Adenomas

	(Personal Series)				
Hormone	*Patients Examined*	*Normal Before GK*	*Deficient Before GK**	*New Deficiency After GK*	*Interval Since GK (mos)*
Growth hormone	8	1	7	1	17
Steroids	21	11	10	3	16, 19, 48
Thyroid	22	11	11	0	
Estrogens Testosterone	23	8	15**	0	
Adiuretin	23	23	0	0	
Follow-up: 12–60 months; average, 23.6 months.					

GK, Gamma Knife treatment.
*Caused by destruction of gland by neoplasm, surgery, and possible previous radiation.
**Includes patients after menopause and andropause.

terpretation of a swelling of the adenoma probably caused by the radiation, because we experienced a similar reaction in an estrogen-induced prolactinoma swelling.[43]

Table 8 shows the results of the endocrine findings in our group of nonsecreting macroadenomas followed for periods longer than 1 year. The table shows that endocrine failure is a minor issue. It should be kept in mind, however, that the follow-up is short in comparison to the cohorts treated with fractionated radiotherapy when the onset of radiation-induced pituitary deficits (GH, 100%; gonadotrophins, 96%; corticotrophin, 84%; thyrotrophin, 49%) is generally after 8 years.[40]

Stereotactic Linear Accelerator Radiosurgery and Radiotherapy

Linear accelerators are used in two possible ways: either as single-fraction stereotactic radiosurgery[44–47] or as multiple-fraction stereotactic radiotherapy.[44,48–50] A relocatable stereotactic frame should be used for multiple-fraction treatments. The number of isocenters is usually limited to one, or in rare instances, up to three. This results in a less than optimal target coverage and conformity unless a micromultileaf collimator is available. However, no published results obtained with this new device have come to our attention yet.

Single-Fraction Stereotactic Linear Accelerator Radiosurgery

Valentino reported 52 pituitary adenoma patients who were treated with a single dose of 10 to 20 Gy using one or two radiation isocenters.[46] Although 67% of patients with increased growth hormone and prolactin levels improved, no patient achieved hormonal normalization. No adverse effects were described. Rocher et al treated 42 patients with pituitary adenomas.[45] Using 15 to 20 Gy to the 70% isodose line, hormonal cures were reported for two of four patients with Cushing's disease, and one of six patients with acromegaly. Tumor regression was observed in nine adenomas. However, a high rate of visual complications was observed in this series: two patients became blind and six patients suffered a unilateral visual loss. Four additional patients had a chiasma syndrome and two developed a minor reduction in visual acuity and/or visual field. Based on this experience, the authors stopped using LINAC radiosurgery for treating pituitary adenomas. Voges et al presented their follow-up results obtained from 26 patients suffering from pituitary adenomas (12 acromegalics, 4 Cushing's, 3 Nelson's, 4 prolactinomas, and 3 nonsecreting adenomas).[47] Using three isocenters and radiation doses of 8 to 20 Gy, significant tumor volume reductions were obtained. Only one prolactinoma patient was cured. Complications included seizures (n=2), and one patient developed periodic somnolence, hyperphagia, and sexual hyperactivity (Kline-Levine syndrome).[51] Mitsumori and collaborators had similar experiences.[44] The authors reviewed 18 patients with pituitary adenomas in whom one or two isocenters were used. The 3-year tumor size control rate was 100%. Only two of five patients with Cushing's disease were cured. But three patients showed abnormal enhancements in the medial aspect of the ipsilateral temporal lobe consistent with radiation necrosis. Two of these three patients suffered from temporal lobe seizures. The authors therefore recommended stereotactic, fractionated radiotherapy and not radiosurgery as the primary method for treating pituitary adenomas. A single case of acute hyperthermia occurring 1 hour after radiosurgery (2 isocenters with 16 Gy to the 90% isodose) was described recently.[52] The hypothalamus was irradiated to a dose of approximately 16 Gy. A peak temperature of 105.1°F (40.6°C) was reached within 5 hours, the patient suffered from severe headaches and his speech was incoherent. He recovered completely but developed hypothyroidism and hypoadrenalism 2 years after radiosurgery.

Multiple-Fraction Stereotactic Linear Accelerator Radiotherapy

Multiple-fraction stereotactic radiotherapy represents a refinement of the classical, fractionated radiotherapy using three fields by improving the dose conformality to the target. This improved radiation delivery reduces the radiation exposure to the adjacent structures and thus is associated with fewer radiation-related complications. Coke et al obtained 100% control of tumor size in 19 patients with pituitary macroadenomas using a median dose of 46 Gy applied in daily 2-Gy fractions.[48] Mitsumori et al reported a tumor control rate of 85%.[44] Normal endocrine values were reached within the observation period of 3 years in one of five acromegalics, one of two Cushing patients, and five of eleven patients with prolactinomas. A total dose of 45 Gy at the 90 or 95% isodose line applied in 1.8-Gy fractions was used. Colin et al used one isocenter and daily fractions of 1.8 Gy (mean total dose, 50 Gy) to treat 42 patients.[49] No adenoma enlarged during follow-up of up to 5 years (100% control rate). Complete or partial tumor regression was seen in 79% of patients. Endocrine remissions were observed in two of six patients with Cushing's disease, seven of eighteen patients with acromegaly, and in four of seven patients with prolactinomas. No radiation-induced visual deficits were noted. However, radiation-induced pituitary insufficiency occurred in up to 20% of patients. Welsh et al treated six patients with Cushing's disease and three patients with prolactinomas (median dose, 33.3 Gy using fractions of 1.8 Gy).[50] Four patients had undergone previous conventional fractionated radiotherapy. This resulted in a median total dose of 47.7 Gy. Four of the six Cushing patients were normalized. The prolactin levels of the prolactinomas improved, but none became normal. One pregnancy was achieved, but no comment was made about the possible use of dopaminergic drugs in this case. The cited results show that stereotactic radiotherapy can achieve improvements of the endocrine disease but that they do not match those obtained with the Gamma Knife.

Conclusions

Stereotactic radiosurgery done with the Gamma Knife is characterized by a high precision and a sharp dose fall-off at the edge of the target, together with an excellent target coverage and dose conformity to the target volume. This allows an improved treatment of the slow-growing pituitary adenomas with application of the entire dose in one session leading to an improved biological activity. The tumor growth can be controlled in nearly all cases. Tumor growth control requires lower doses than hormonal normalization. Endocrine control is more difficult to achieve and depends on the endocrine type. The best results are obtained in acromegaly followed by Cushing's disease. Prolactinomas are more difficult to control. A control of Nelson's syndrome is almost impossible. Antisecretory drugs (dopamine agonists, somatostatin receptor ligands) should be discontinued before radiosurgery because they may increase the radioresistence of secreting adenomas. Few complications (cranial nerve damage, secondary hypopituitarism) are to be expected. Higher complication rates have been observed in patients who have been treated previously with conventional fractionated radiotherapy. Large adenomas must be decompressed surgically or, if not feasible, treated with stereotactic fractionated radiotherapy. Based on published reports, LINAC radiosurgery is characterized by a high rate of radiation-related complications, which are not typically seen after fractionated stereotactic LINAC radiotherapy or Gamma Knife radiosurgery.

References

1. Landolt AM: Growth of pituitary adenomas, malignant adenomas. In Landolt AM, Vance ML, Reilly PL (eds): Pituitary Adenomas. New York, Churchill Livingstone, 1996, pp 73–82.
2. Hall EJ, Brenner DJ: The radiobiology of radiosurgery: rationale for different treatment regimes for AVMs and malignancies. Int J Radiat Oncol Biol Phys 1993;25:381–385.
3. Frankel KA, Levy RP, Fabrikant JI, et al: Heavy-charged-particle radiosurgery: rationale and method. In Alexander E III, Loeffler JS, Lunsford LD (eds): Stereotactic Radiosurgery. New York, McGraw-Hill, 1993, pp 87–103.
4. Swearingen B, Thornton AF, Zervas NT: Proton radiosurgery for pituitary adenomas. In Landolt AM, Vance ML, Reilly PL (eds): Pituitary Adenomas. New York, Churchill Livingstone, 1996, pp 453–459.
5. Giovanelli M, Losa M, Mortini P: Acromegaly: surgical results and prognosis. In Landolt AM, Vance ML, Reilly PL (eds): Pituitary Adenomas. New York, Churchill Livingstone, 1996, pp 333–351.
6. Flickinger JC: Dosimetry and dose-volume relationships in radiosurgery. In Alexander E III, Loeffler JS, Lunsford LD (eds): Stereotactic Radiosurgery. New York, McGraw-Hill, 1993, pp 31–41.
7. Lam KSL, Wang C, Yeung RTT, et al: Hypothalamic hypopituitarism following cranial irradiation for nasopharyngeal carcinoma. Clin Endocrinol 1986; 24:643–651.
8. Samaan NA, Vieto R, Schultz PN, et al: Hypothalamic, pituitary and thyroid dysfunction after radiotherapy to the head and neck. Int J Radiat Oncol Biol Phys 1982;8:1857–1867.
9. Landolt AM, Lomax N: Gamma Knife treatment for prolactinomas. Neurosurgery 2000;93(suppl 3):14–28.
10. Kondziolka D, Atteberry DS, Lunsford LD: Gamma Knife radiosurgery for meningiomas, schwannomas, and pituitary tumors. In Germano IM (ed): LINAC and Gamma Knife Neurosurgery. Park Ridge, IL, American Association of Neurological Surgeons, 2000, pp 207–219.
11. Thorén M, Rähn T, Guo W-Y, et al: Stereotactic radiosurgery with the cobalt-60 gamma unit in the treatment of growth hormone-producing pituitary tumors. Neurosurgery 1991;29:663–668.
12. Stephanian E, Lunsford LD, Coffey RJ, et al: Gamma knife surgery for sellar and suprasellar tumors. Neurosurg Clin North Am 1992;3:207–218.
13. Ganz JC, Backlund E-O, Thorsen FA: The effect of gamma knife surgery of pituitary adenomas on tumor growth and endocrinopathies. Stereotact Funct Neurosurg 1993;61(suppl 1):30–37.
14. Pollock BE, Kondziolka D, Lunsford LD, et al: Stereotactic radiosurgery for pituitary adenomas: imaging, visual and endocrine results. Acta Neurochir 1994;62(suppl):33–38.

15. Motti EDF, Losa M, Pieralli S, et al: Stereotactic radiosurgery of pituitary adenomas. Metabolism 1996;45(suppl 1):111–114.
16. Martinez R, Bravo G, Burzaco J, et al: Pituitary tumors and Gamma Knife surgery: clinical experience with more than two years of follow-up. Stereotact Funct Neurosurg 1998;70(suppl 1):110–118.
17. Pan L, Zhang N, Wang E, et al: Pituitary adenomas: the effect of Gamma Knife radiosurgery on tumor growth and endocrinopathies. Stereotact Funct Neurosurg 1998;70(suppl 1):119–126.
18. Lim YJ, Leem W, Kim TS, et al: Four years' experience in the treatment of pituitary adenomas with Gamma Knife radiosurgery. Stereotact Funct Neurosurg 1998;70(suppl 1):95–109.
19. Ikeda H, Jokura H, Yoshimoto T: Gamma knife radiosurgery for pituitary adenomas: usefulness of combined transsphenoidal and gamma knife radiosurgery for adenomas invading the cavernous sinus. Radiat Oncol Invest 1998;6:26–34.
20. Morange-Ramos I, Régis J, Dufour H, et al: Gamma-Knife surgery for secreting pituitary adenomas. Acta Neurochir 1998;140:437–443.
21. Witt TC, Kondziolka D, Flickinger JC, et al: Gamma knife radiosurgery for pituitary tumors. In Lunsford DL, Kondziolka D, Flickinger JC (eds): Gamma Knife Brain Surgery: Progress in Neurological Surgery. Vol 14. Basel, S. Karger, 1998, pp 114–127.
22. Hayashi M, Izawa M, Hiyama H, et al: Gamma Knife radiosurgery for pituitary adenomas. Stereotact Funct Neurosurg 1999;72(suppl 1):111–118.
23. Kim SH, Huh R, Chang JW, et al: Gamma Knife radiosurgery for functioning pituitary adenomas. Stereotact Funct Neurosurg 1999;72(suppl 1):101–110.
24. Laws ER Jr, Vance ML: Radiosurgery for pituitary tumors and craniopharyngiomas. Neurosurg Clin North Am 1999;10:327–336.
25. Mokry M, Ramschak S, Simbrunner J, et al: A six year experience with the postoperative radiosurgical management of pituitary adenomas. Stereotact Funct Neurosurg 1999;13(suppl 1):88–100.
26. Landolt AM, Haller D, Lomax N, et al: Octreotide may act as a radioprotective agent in acromegaly. J Clin Endocrinol Metab 2000;85:1287–1289.
27. Landolt AM, Haller D, Lomax N, et al: Stereotactic radiosurgery for recurrent surgically treated acromegaly: comparison with fractionated radiotherapy. J Neurosurg 1998;88:1002–1008.
28. Lancranjan I, Bruns C, Grass PO, et al: Sandostatin LAR: a promising therapeutic tool in the management of acromegalic patients. Metabolism 1996; 45(suppl 1):67–71.
29. Oldfield EH, Friedman R, Kinsella T, et al: Reduction of radiation-induced brain injury by use of pentobarbital or lidocaine protection. J Neurosurg 1990; 72:737–744.
30. Copeland ES: Mechanisms of radioprotection: a review. Photochem Photobiol 1978;28:839–844.
31. Rähn T, Thorén M, Hall K, et al: Stereotactic radiosurgery in Cushing's syndrome: acute radiation effects. Surg Neurol 1980;14:85–92.
32. Seo Y, Fukuoka S, Takanashi M, et al: Gamma Knife surgery for Cushing's disease. Surg Neurol 1995;43:170–175.
33. Höybye Ch, Grenbäck E, Rähn T, et al: Adrenocorticotropic hormone-producing pituitary tumors: 12- to 22-year follow-up after treatment with stereotactic radiosurgery. Neurosurgery 2001;49:284–292.
34. Kovacs K, Horvath E: Tumors of the pituitary gland. In Hartmann WH (ed): Atlas of Tumor Pathology. Vol 21. Washington DC, Armed Forces Institute of Pathology, 1986, p 48.
35. Laws ER, Randall RV, Kern EB, et al: Management of Pituitary Adenomas

and Related Lesions with Emphasis on Transsphenoidal Microsurgery. New York, Appleton-Century-Croft, 1982, pp 288–291.
36. Kim MS, Lee SI, Sim JH: Gamma Knife radiosurgery for functioning pituitary microadenoma. Stereotact Funct Neurosurg 1999;72(suppl 1):119–124.
37. Inoue HK, Kohga H, Hirato M, et al: Pituitary adenomas treated with or without Gamma Knife surgery: experience in 122 cases. Stereotact Funct Neurosurg 1999;72(suppl 1):125–131.
38. Landolt AM, Shibata T: Growth, cell proliferation, and prognosis of pituitary adenomas. In Faglia G, Beck-Peccoz P, Ambrosi B, et al (eds): Pituitary Adenomas: New Trends in Basic and Clinical Research. International Congress Series. Vol 961. Amsterdam, Excerpta Medica, 1991, pp 169–178.
39. Lim YJ, Leem W, Park BJT, et al: Cerebral infarction with ICA occlusion after Gamma Knife radiosurgery for pituitary adenoma: a case report. Stereotact Funct Neurosurg 1999;72(suppl 1):132–139.
40. Littley MD, Shalet SM, Beardwell CG, et al: Hypopituitarism following external radiotherapy for pituitary tumours in adults. World J Med 1989; 262:145–160.
41. Sallet G, Kestelyn P: Radiation-induced optic neuropathy. Bull Soc Belge Ophthalmol 1992;243:99–107.
42. Brada M, Ford D, Ashley S, et al: Risk of secondary brain tumour after conservative surgery and radiotherapy for pituitary adenoma. BMJ 1992;304: 1343–1346.
43. Landolt AM, Del Pozo E, Hayek J: Injectable bromocriptine to treat acute, oestrogen-induced swelling of invasive prolactinoma. Lancet 1984;2:111.
44. Mitsumori M, Shrieve DC, Alexander E III, et al: Initial clinical results of Linac-based stereotactic radiosurgery and stereotactic radiotherapy for pituitary adenomas. Int J Radiat Oncol Biol Phys 1999;42:573–580.
45. Rocher FP, Sentenac I, Berger C, et al: Stereotactic radiosurgery: the Lyon experience. Acta Neurochir 1995;(suppl 63):109–114.
46. Valentino V: Postoperative radiosurgery of pituitary adenomas. J Neurosurg Sci 1991;35:207–211.
47. Voges J, Sturm V, Deuss U, et al: LINAC-radiosurgery in pituirary adenomas: preliminary results. Acta Neurochir 1996;65(suppl 1):41–43.
48. Coke C, Andrews DW, Corn BW, et al: Multiple fractionated stereotactic radiotherapy of residual pituitary macroadenomas: initial experience. Stereotact Funct Neurosurg 1997;69:183–190.
49. Colin P, Scavarda D, Delemer B, et al: Radiothérapie stéréotaxique fractionnée: résultats dans les adénomes hypophysaires, les neurinomes de l'acoustique et les méningiomes du sinus caverneux. Cancer Radiother 1998;2: 207–214.
50. Welsh JS, Wharam MD, Nauta H, et al: Stereotactic radiotherapy for Cushing's disease and prolactinoma. J Radiosurg 1999;2:23–29.
51. Martin JB, Reichlin S, Brown GM: Clinical Neuroendocrinology. Contemporary Neurology Series, Vol 14. Philadelphia, FA Davis, 1977, pp 268–269.
52. Kalapurakal JA, Silverman CL, Akhtar N, et al.: Acute hyperthermia following stereotactic radiosurgery for pituitary adenoma. Br J Radiol 1999;72: 1218–1221.

Comment
Chapter 10

Mary Lee Vance

Dr. Landolt and colleagues have summarized the experience with Gamma Knife radiosurgery for the treatment of patients with a pituitary adenoma, including secretory and nonsecretory adenomas. This review includes the personal experience of the authors and a discussion of the published studies.

Gamma Knife radiosurgery has been used to treat pituitary adenomas for over 30 years and with the refinement of dose planning using MRI, it is not appropriate to compare results of earlier series with more recent studies. This chapter includes primarily reviews of studies from the more modern era and is a comprehensive review of the subject. Inherent in such a review is the inclusion of studies of variable quality, thus rendering some of the information confusing and contradictory. Additionally, some authors use different and not always correct criteria to define "cure" of hormone-producing adenomas.

The proposed place of stereotactic radiosurgery in the treatment of pituitary adenomas is shown in Table 1, with treatments listed sequentially. In clinical practice, a combination of treatments is often given simultaneously. In the treatment of acromegaly, patients are usually given somatostatin analog treatment (octreotide, lanreotide) at the time of, or after, stereotactic radiosurgery, and it is discontinued at later intervals to assess the efficacy of radiation. In patients with a prolactinoma, a dopamine agonist is usually administered (if the patient is responsive) after radiosurgery and is also discontinued at later intervals. Regarding Cushing's disease, medical treatment of lower cortisol production *should* be given while awaiting the desired effect of radiosurgery since the drugs do not affect the pituitary gland but diminish adrenal steroid synthesis. At my institution, medications that inhibit hormone production are discontinued every 6 months and the appropriate hormone tests (acromegaly: serum IGF-I, growth hormone response to oral glucose; prolactinoma: serum prolactin; Cushing's disease: 24-hour urine free cortisol) are obtained to assess the effectiveness of Gamma Knife radiosurgery. Additionally other studies are conducted to determine if new pituitary hormone deficiencies have developed.

As shown in Table 3, the effectiveness of Gamma Knife radiosurgery in the treatment of acromegaly is variable and dependent upon the criteria for cure. Unfortunately, 6 of the 16 studies reported do not provide information on criteria for cure and thus should not be considered valid assessments. Additionally, the criteria for cure have changed over the years; thus a single growth hormone level of less than 5 ng/mL, less than 7 ng/mL, or less than 12 ng/mL cannot be considered a "cure." A recent consensus conference of experts in endocrinology, neurosurgery, and radiotherapy concluded that the criteria for cure of acromegaly include a serum growth hormone of less than 1 ng/mL after oral glucose ingestion and a normal age adjusted serum IGF-1 level.[1] A caveat about measuring these hormones when the patient is being treated with a long-acting somatostatin analog (Sandostatin LAR, lanreotide) is that there should be a sufficient amount of time since the last dose before obtaining the study (e.g., 8 weeks for Sandostatin LAR, 4–8 weeks for lanreotide depending on the formulation and dose).

Dr. Landolt et al present convincing information from their investigations about the potentially deleterious effect of administration of a somatostatin analog at the time of stereotactic radiosurgery. As shown in Figure 5, patients treated with octreotide at the time of radiosurgery had a substantially reduced cure rate compared with those who did not receive octreotide for the 2 weeks prior to radiosurgery. Thus, administration of octreotide at the time of radiosurgery is to be avoided.

Results of Gamma Knife radiosurgery for Cushing's disease are subject to the same criticism as for acromegaly. Review of the literature (Table 4) reveals that 6 of the 15 studies did not report a criterion or criteria for cure. Additionally, a "normal" ACTH or serum cortisol of less than 15.5 ug/100 mL are not valid criteria for cure. ACTH is secreted in bursts or pulses and levels vary considerably. The only acceptable definition of cure is a normal 24-hour urine-free cortisol which reflects overall ACTH activity. The normal 24-hour urine-free cortisol concentration may vary depending on the specific method of assay (e.g., HPLC, RIA).

Treatment of prolactinomas with stereotactic radiosurgery is less effective than is the treatment of growth hormone- and ACTH-producing adenomas. This appears to be a fairly uniform finding. Once again, in a review of ten studies, five authors did not report the criteria for cure (should be a normal serum prolactin off of medication), so interpretation of the results is problematic (Table 5). Dr. Landolt et al make the important observation that administration of a dopamine agonist at the time of radiosurgery likely interferes with the effectiveness of the treatment. As shown in Figure 8, no patients who received a dopamine agonist at the time of radiosurgery achieved a normal serum prolactin during the almost 50 months of follow-up. Approximately 80% of patients who received radiosurgery without concomitant dopamine agonist treatment achieved a normal serum prolactin within 50 months.

Since there is no biochemical tumor marker to measure in patients who have a nonsecretory adenoma, assessment of tumor size is the only method of determining efficacy. Definition of "control" poses the same problems in interpretation as occurs for the secretory tumors: different definitions among authors (Table 6). For example, some authors consider reduction in tumor size as control while others include patients with no increase in size as control. Of the 11 studies reported in Table 6, six of them included both secretory and nonsecretory tumors in the analysis. This is a definite shortcoming since the definition of "control" for a secretory tumor differs from that of a nonsecretory tumor.

Complications of stereotactic radiosurgery are extremely important to document. In Table 7 are listed biochemical, visual, and anatomical adverse consequences of Gamma Knife radiosurgery. Once again, the summarized data are dependent on the quality of the individual studies. For example, a 3.4% rate of new pituitary function loss is likely a drastic underestimation since it is dependent on both the duration of follow-up and the stringency of the investigations. We recently published our series of 43 patients with Cushing's disease treated with Gamma Knife radiosurgery. New pituitary hormone deficiency developed in 16% of patients.[2] In our patients with acromegaly, we have observed a 28% incidence of new pituitary hormone deficiency (unpublished observations). With longer follow-up and more precise evaluations (e.g., stimulation test to diagnose growth hormone deficiency), the incidence of new hypopituitarism will most likely be much higher than is currently reported. While development of new hormone deficiency is not desirable, this can be treated successfully with appropriate hormone replacement. The more serious matter is the adverse effects on vision, occulomotor function, and brain anatomy and function. Damage to vision and occulomotor function is certainly dependent upon several factors including prior effects on vision from a tumor compressing the optic apparatus (resected prior to stereotactic radiosurgery), prior conventional radiotherapy, tumor location (cavernous sinus invasion), and the radiation dose to the optic chiasm. The development of hypothalamic or temporal necrosis or central pontine myelinolysis is of great concern and raises questions regarding the dose administered and the accuracy of the treatment field. One complication, intratumoral hemorrhage 37 months after treatment, may not be related to radiosurgery since any pituitary tumor may undergo spontaneous hemorrhage.

From the available information it is evident that Gamma Knife radiosurgery is a very effective adjuvant treatment for patients with a pituitary adenoma. This is particularly obvious in patients with acromegaly. Results in Cushing's disease are perhaps better than those of conventional radiation while results in patients with a prolactinoma are not quite as encouraging. However, the important observations of Dr. Landolt and colleagues are that medical therapy for patients with acromegaly or a prolactinoma at the time of radiosurgery likely delays effectiveness. Thus, these patients should not receive medication at the time of Gamma Knife treatment. With larger numbers of patients treated, accurate assessment of hormone function, and longer follow-up, Gamma Knife radiosurgery will likely become a treatment of choice in patients with residual disease after surgical resection of the adenoma or failure of medical therapy.

References

1. Guistina A, Barkan A, Casanueva FF, et al: Criteria for cure of acromegaly: a consensus statement. J Clin Endocrinol Metab 2000;85:526–529.
2. Sheehan JM, Vance ML, Sheehan JP, et al: Radiosurgery for Cushing's disease after failed transsphenoidal surgery. J Neurosurg 2000;93:738–742.

Chapter 11

Stereotactic Radiosurgery for Brain Metastases

Bruce E. Pollock, Paul D. Brown

Introduction

Cancer is the second leading cause of death in developed nations. More than 1,000,000 people are diagnosed with cancer each year in the USA alone. Of these patients, it is estimated that 20 to 40% will have the disease spread to their brain, resulting in several hundred thousand people developing brain metastases annually.[1,2] Moreover, this figure appears to be increasing as patients live longer from their primary tumor and a greater percentage of patients undergo either computed tomography (CT) or magnetic resonance imaging (MRI) of their head as part of their original evaluation for disseminated disease. In comparison, it is estimated that approximately 30,000 people are discovered to have a primary tumor of the brain (gliomas) or its coverings (meningiomas, schwannomas). Thus, brain metastases are by far the most common brain tumor.

Despite significant advances in the detection and treatment of brain metastases, the prognosis for this patient group remains poor even in the modern era with median survival rates reported between 2.9 and 3.4 months.[3,4] However, within this patient population subgroups appear to exist that are associated with improved survival. Gaspar et al used recursive partitioning analysis (RPA) to evaluate patient survival from three consecutive Radiation Therapy Oncology Group (RTOG) trials involving more than 1200 patients.[5] The best median survival (7.1 months) was observed for patients less than 65-years old, a Karnofsky Performance Score (KPS) greater than or equal to 70, and a controlled primary tumor with the brain as the only site of metastases. Patients with a KPS less than 70 had a median survival of only 2.3 months. Unfortunately,

From Pollock BE (ed). *Contemporary Stereotactic Radiosurgery: Technique and Evaluation.* Armonk, NY, Futura Publishing Company, Inc. © 2002.

only 3 to 20% of patients with brain metastases are Class I by the RTOG RPA criteria.[4,5]

The majority of brain metastasis patients are treated with palliative whole brain radiation therapy (WBRT) alone. The average patient survival for patients managed in this fashion ranges from 3 to 6 months. However, several recent reports have demonstrated that the addition of either tumor resection or stereotactic radiosurgery to radiation therapy significantly improves survival for patients with a single brain metastasis.[6–9] Unfortunately, less than half of brain metastasis patients present with a single tumor, and few reports demonstrate any survival benefit after neurosurgical intervention (either resection or radiosurgery) for patients with multiple brain metastases.[10,11] Consequently, patients with multiple brain metastases are generally treated with WBRT alone and their prognosis remains poor. This chapter will present the results of radiosurgery for patients with brain metastases, and outline a management strategy that incorporates radiosurgery as part of a protocol that also includes surgical resection and WBRT to improve survival for selected patients with brain metastases.

Indications for Aggressive Intervention

It is critical to consider the characteristics of patients being reported when assessing the outcomes of any management option for brain metastasis patients. There are three major factors dictating whether or not an individual patient with brain metastases will benefit from either surgical resection or radiosurgery: systemic disease status, functional status, and number of brain metastases. First, and most important, is the extent of systemic disease dissemination. Smalley et al reviewed 229 consecutive patients with a single brain metastasis and found that the presence of systemic disease was significantly associated with inferior survival.[12] The significant negative influence that ongoing systemic disease has upon the survival of patients with brain metastases has been confirmed in virtually every study that has addressed this issue.[3,4,6,11,13–18] In fact, the primary criticism of a recent prospective, randomized, multicenter study evaluating the efficacy of tumor resection in addition to radiotherapy for patients with a single brain metastasis was that almost three-fourths of the patients entered into the trial had either extracranial metastases or uncontrolled primary disease.[19] In the study of Mintz et al,[19] no survival benefit was seen for patients who underwent surgery. Conversely, survival 2 or more years after surgery has been documented for patients with no evidence of systemic disease if tumor control can be achieved intracranially. Thus, the addition of tumor resection or radiosurgery has little effect on overall survival for patients with ongoing systemic disease.

Second, is the patient's functional status. Patients with a KPS greater than or equal to 70 (independent in their activities of daily living) survive longer than patients with a KPS less than 70 (require assistance to perform their activities of daily living).[3,6,15,17–20] A poor performance status typically reflects either widespread body disease or tumors in critical brain locations (brainstem, thalamus, sensorimotor cortex) that result in a significant neurological deficit. Third, the number of brain metastases inversely correlates with the chance of intracranial disease control. Theoretically, if one assumes an 80% chance of local tumor control (after either resection + WBRT or radiosurgery + WBRT) and a 20% incidence of developing new tumors, at 1 year the likelihood of intracranial progression-free survival is 64%, 51%, 41%, and 33%, for patients with one, two, three, and four brain tumors, respectively.[21] Patchell et al found an approximately 75% 1-year progression-free survival rate for patients having resection of a single metastasis and WBRT.[22] Alternatively, our group found a 43% 1-year progression-free survival rate for a group of 52 patients with multiple brain metastases (median number of tumors, three) managed by a either resection, radiosurgery, or both.[23] For this reason, the vast majority of patients with multiple brain metastases which have been analyzed to date after resection,[10] radiosurgery,[11] or both,[23] have had only two or three brain metastases. Other factors that correlate with improved patient survival include tumor histology,[1,3,7] a longer interval between primary diagnosis and the discovery of brain metastases,[12,24] and younger patient age.[3,13,15,18] Thus, a complete evaluation of each brain metastases patient is required prior to recommending either tumor resection or radiosurgery.

Patient Evaluation and Management

Patients with brain metastases should have undergone a recent work-up to evaluate the degree of primary tumor control, and to determine if the brain is the only site of tumor dissemination. This evaluation should include a CT of the chest, abdomen, and pelvis, as well as a radionuclide bone scan if the cancer has a tendency to produce osseous metastases or if the patient complains of a specific region of bone pain. If widespread systemic disease is discovered during this evaluation, we recommend that patients proceed to WBRT for symptom palliation (Fig. 1). The exception to this rule is for patients with symptomatic mass effect related to a large lesion which could be life threatening without immediate tumor resection. Although post-contrast CT of the head may be adequate as a screening examination, patients found to have brain metastases should then undergo MRI to accurately determine the number of brain tumors present. Recent work has shown that the addition of double or even triple dose gadolinium may enhance our ability to detect small lesions.

If a patient has good primary disease control and a KPS greater than 70, a decision is made whether to proceed with surgical resection, radio-

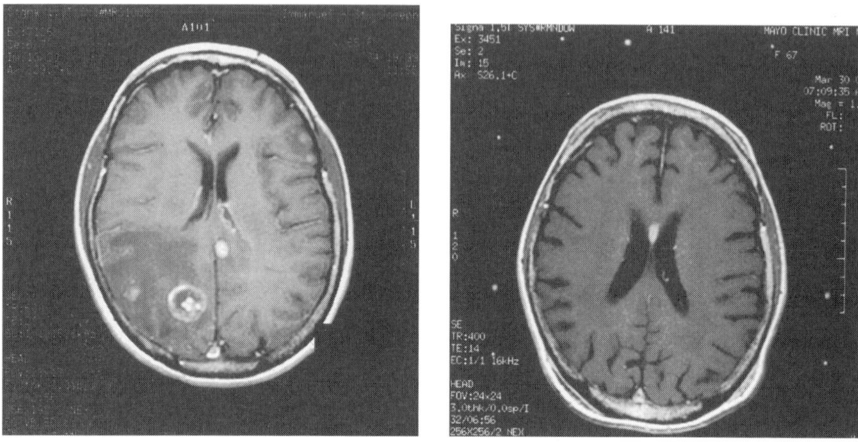

Figure 1. Axial T1-weighted postgadolinium MRIs of a 67-year-old woman with non-small cell lung cancer. (**Left**) MRI showing multiple brain metastases. Due to the patient's poor performance status, she was treated with fractionated radiation therapy (30 Gy). (**Right**) MRI 23 months later shows complete resolution of the previous brain tumors, but several new tumors involving the basal ganglia, corpus callosum, and fornices were discovered.

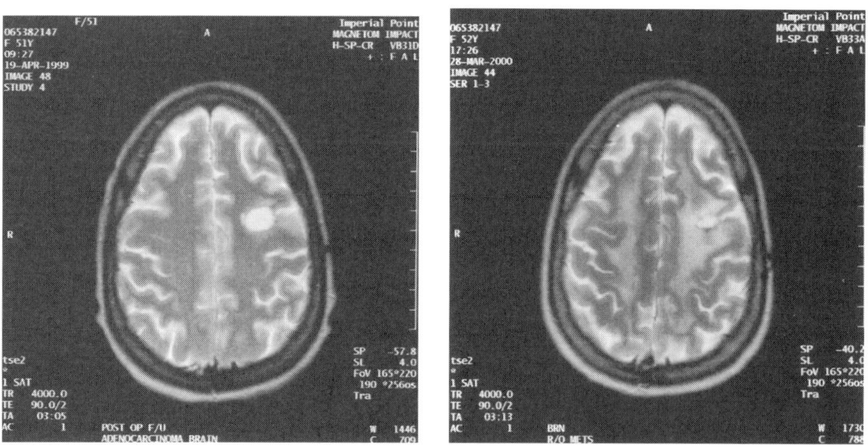

Figure 2. Axial T2-weighted MRIs of a 51-year-old woman with non-small cell lung cancer. (**Left**) MRI performed 2 months after the patient underwent tumor resection and fractionated radiation therapy (40 Gy). (**Right**) MRI 11 months later shows no evidence of residual tumor, only diffuse regions of increased signal throughout both cerebral hemispheres. The patient was suffering from generalized cognitive decline.

surgery, or both. Typically, resection is recommended for larger tumors causing symptomatic mass effect and radiosurgery is performed for smaller tumors. Diabetic patients are given special consideration for tumor resection in order to simplify their postoperative care by minimizing the need for corticosteroids. Occasionally, patients have several large tumors and simultaneous craniotomies are performed to resect separate metastases. This treatment algorithm is based on the fact that local tumor control is quite similar for tumors having resection and WBRT or radiosurgery and WBRT (approximately 85%).[6–9] If a patient undergoes tumor removal, we almost always follow this with WBRT to reduce the chance of local tumor recurrence.[22,23] For patients having radiosurgery, although some reports have found better tumor control when radiosurgery is combined with WBRT,[7,25] others have questioned the usefulness of WBRT for patients having radiosurgery.[26,27] It is argued that if patients develop additional brain tumors following radiosurgery, the procedure can be repeated thereby minimizing the chance of delayed cognitive decline frequently noted after WBRT (Fig. 2).[28]

Results of Brain Metastases Radiosurgery

Stereotactic radiosurgery is an attractive option for patients with brain metastases. Unlike gliomas where the tumor cells infiltrate the surrounding normal brain, metastases typically have discrete borders that are clearly visualized with modern neuro-imaging. Recent studies have shown that the local tumor control rate after radiosurgery ranges from 77 to 94%,[6,7,13,14,16–18,24,27,29] and several studies suggest that higher prescribed doses correlate with greater local tumor control.[14,16,29] Shiau et al reviewed 119 patients having radiosurgery between 1991 and 1994 at the University of California at San Francisco.[29] The actuarial local control was 93% and 90% at 6 and 12 months after radiosurgery for tumors receiving greater than or equal to 18 Gy, compared to 70% and 55% for tumors treated with 15 to 18 Gy, and 28% at 6 months for tumors receiving less than 15 Gy. Likewise, Matsuo et al in their study of 92 patients with 162 tumors found a 1-year local control rate of 93% for tumors receiving greater than or equal to 25 Gy at the tumor margin compared to 60% for tumors treated with lower doses.[14] Of course, the prescribed radiation dose must take into account the chance of a radiation-related complication for each patient. Shaw et al in the RTOG protocol 90-05 sought to better understand the maximum tolerable dose for radiosurgery based on acute complications (within 3 months of radiosurgery) for patients with recurrent previously irradiated primary brain tumors and metastases.[30] Overall, 6% of patients required reoperation for symptomatic radiation necrosis (Fig. 3). Multivariate analysis found that tumor volumes greater than or equal to 8.2 cm^3 and a ratio of maximum dose to prescribed dose

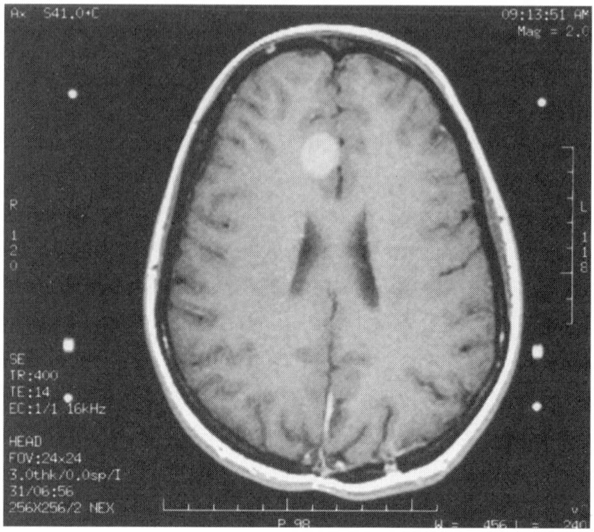

Figure 3. Axial MRIs of a 30-year-old woman with metastatic melanoma. She had previously undergone resection of a parasagittal tumor; no postoperative radiation was given. (**A**) T1-weighted postgadolinium MRI at the time of radiosurgery showing a right frontal tumor (volume, 3.3 cm^3; tumor margin/maximum dose, 15 Gy/30 Gy). Two additional tumors were treated in the right temporal region. *(Continued.)*

(MD/PD) greater than or equal to 2 were associated with unacceptable toxicity. Based on the results of this study, radiation doses were escalated to 24 Gy for tumors less than or equal to 20 mm in maximum diameter, 21 Gy for tumors 21 to 30 mm, and 18 Gy for tumors 31 to 40 mm. However, the final report on RTOG 90-05 found a greater incidence of radiation necrosis with 5%, 8%, 9%, and 11% of patients developing this complication at 6, 12, 18, and 24 months after radiosurgery, respectively.[31] Again, tumor size strongly correlated with an increased risk of neurotoxicity: patients with tumors from 21 to 40 mm were 7.3 to 16 times more likely to develop radiation necrosis compared to patients with tumors less than 20 mm. Of note, this study found that although patients having linear accelerator (LINAC) radiosurgery were 2.84 times more likely to have tumor progression compared to patients undergoing Gamma Knife radiosurgery, there was no difference in the rate of radiation necrosis. This underscores the important point that dose inhomogeneity by itself is not undesirable provided that treatment plan tightly conforms to the target volume, thereby minimizing the exposure of the surrounding normal brain to radiation "hot spots."

Radiosurgery also has several obvious advantages compared to surgical resection for patients with brain metastases: (1) Radiosurgery has almost zero immediate procedural risks (neurological deficit, infection)

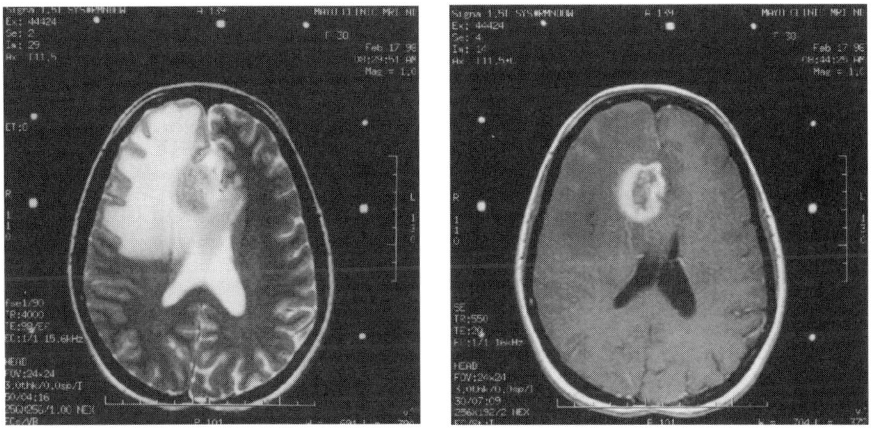

B C

Figure 3. (**B** and **C**) T2-weighted and T1-weighted postgadolinium MRIs performed 8 months after radiosurgery. The patient had developed increasing headaches that were not controlled with steroids. Note area of enhancement is larger and there is adjacent edema and mass effect. She underwent resection of this mass; no tumor was discovered only radiation necrosis.

and is performed under local anesthesia. As a result, patients have little or no recovery time and are able to resume their normal activities on the day of or following the procedure. This is vital for a patient group in which the typical several week convalescence after surgery often comprises a significant portion of their remaining survival. (2) Radiosurgery is not constrained by tumor location like surgical resection (Fig. 4). Thus, although advances in surgical technique and stereotactic guidance make many deep, subcortical tumors accessible for removal, tumors located within the basal ganglia, thalamus, or brainstem continue to be unresectable except in exceptional instances. (3) With radiosurgery, it is possible to treat patients with multiple tumors in a single setting. This is critical because more than 50% of patients with brain metastases will have two or more tumors. (4) Radiosurgery appears to be quite effective against tumor histologies that are traditionally considered radioresistant (melanoma, renal cell carcinoma, sarcoma).[25,32–34]

Radiosurgery was performed on 271 patients with brain metastases at the Mayo Clinic, Rochester, MN, between January 1990 and December 2000 (Table 1). As expected, the most common tumor treated was lung carcinoma (41%), followed by breast (18%), melanoma (11%), and renal (11%). Our crude local tumor rate is approximately 85%, and the incidence of symptomatic radiation-related complications is approximately 5 to 8%. We have recently reviewed in detail two subsets of this patient group: patients with radioresistant tumors and patients with multiple tumors. Brown et al examined 41 consecutive patients presenting with 83 brain metastases from radioresistant primaries.[25] Tumor histology in-

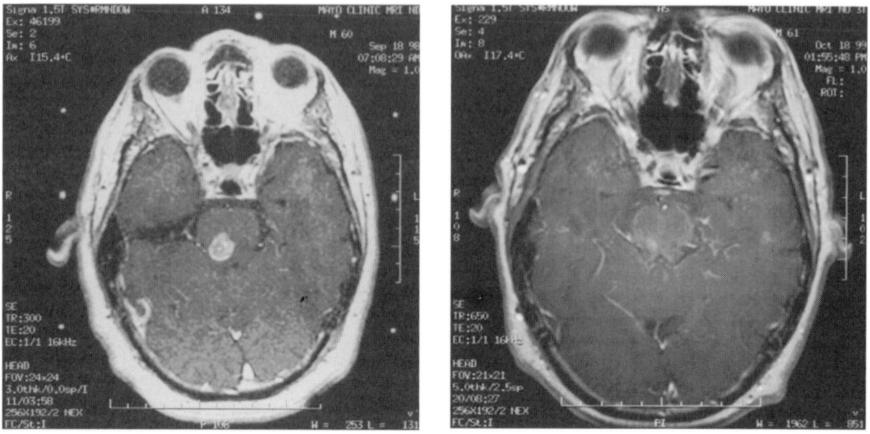

Figure 4. Axial T1-weighted postgadolinium MRIs of a 60-year-old man who developed left hand and face numbness. Work-up revealed a lung mass which was biopsied and found to be a non-small cell lung cancer. (**Left**) MRI at the time of radiosurgery (volume, 1.9 cm^3; tumor margin/maximum dose, 15 Gy/30 Gy). In addition, he was treated with fractioned radiation therapy (37.5 Gy). (**Right**) MRI 13 months after radiosurgery shows near complete resolution of the brainstem metastasis. The patient remains well 33 months after radiosurgery.

Table 1
Tumor Histology*

Tumor Type	*No. of Patients (%)*
Lung	112 (41)
Breast	48 (18)
Melanoma	31 (11)
Renal	30 (11)
Colorectal	12 (5)
Unknown	11 (4)
Other†	28 (10)

*Brain metastases patients represent 15% of the total number of radiosurgical procedures (n=1846) performed between 1990 and 2000.

†Tumor histology included endometrial (n=2), paraganglioma (n=2), cholangiocarcinoma (n=1), esophageal (n=1), germ cell (n=1), hurthle cell (n=2), insulinoma (n=2), adenoid cystic (n=3), lacrimal (n=1), leiomyosarcoma (n=3), ovarian (n=1), prostate (n=1), squamous cell (n=2), spindle cell (n=1), thyroid (n=3).

cluded renal cell carcinoma (n=16, 39%), melanoma (n=23, 56%), and sarcoma (n=2, 5%). Eighteen (44%) patients had solitary metastasis and 23 (56%) had multiple metastases. The median patient age at the time of radiosurgery was 58 years. Twenty-six patients (63%) had either no evidence or stable primary disease; 38 patients (93%) were RTOG RPA Class I (n=12, 29%) or Class II (n=26, 64%). Four patients (10%) had progressed after prior radiation therapy. The median Gamma Knife dose to the margin was 16 Gy with a median maximum dose of 32 Gy. Fourteen patients received adjuvant WBRT with the Gamma Knife procedure. The median overall survival was 18.9 months from the time of diagnosis of brain metastasis and 14.2 months from the time of radiosurgery. Univariate analysis found systemic disease status (p=0.006) and RPA Class (p=0.005) correlated with survival. The median survival was 23.5 months for RPA Class I compared to 10.5 months for RPA Class II–III. There was a trend (p=0.12) for improved survival for patients with a renal cell primary (17.8 months) versus melanoma primary (9.7 months). Multivariate analysis revealed RPA Class (p=0.0001) and primary histology (p=0.002) to be independent predictors for overall survival. Of the 35 patients with follow-up imaging, 9 of 73 tumors (12%) recurred locally and 54% developed distant brain failure (DBF). WBRT was found to improve local control and decrease DBF on univariate and multivariate analysis. Patients receiving adjuvant WBRT with Gamma Knife had a 6-month actuarial local control of 100% versus 85% for those not receiving WBRT (p=0.018). Those patients receiving adjuvant WBRT and Gamma Knife had a 6-month actuarial DBF of 15% compared to 64% for those patients undergoing Gamma Knife alone (p=0.0027). Thus, it appears that patients with brain metastases from radioresistant primaries undergoing radiosurgery have improved survival compared to historical controls. Although adjuvant WBRT improved local control and decreased DBF, it did not impact overall survival. Further studies are needed to determine which patients should receive WBRT.

The second group of patients that were reviewed are those with multiple brain metastases managed between April 1997 and March 2000.[23] Fifty-two consecutive patients with multiple brain metastases had initial treatments including multiple craniotomies and tumor resection (n=5, 10%), radiosurgery (n=31, 60%), or resection and radiosurgery (n=16, 30%) (Fig. 5). Twenty patients (39%) had progressed after prior radiation therapy. Tumor histology included lung (n=18, 35%), breast (n=11, 21%), renal (n=6, 12%), and melanoma (n=6, 12%). The median patient age was 58 years, median number of tumors was three, and median KPS was 90. Median survival was 15.5 months; the 1- and 2-year actuarial survivals were 63% and 27%, respectively. Multivariate analysis found RPA Class (I vs. II/III) correlated with improved survival. The median time to neurological progression was 8.0 months after neurosurgical intervention. Multivariate analysis found patients with radiosensitive tumors had

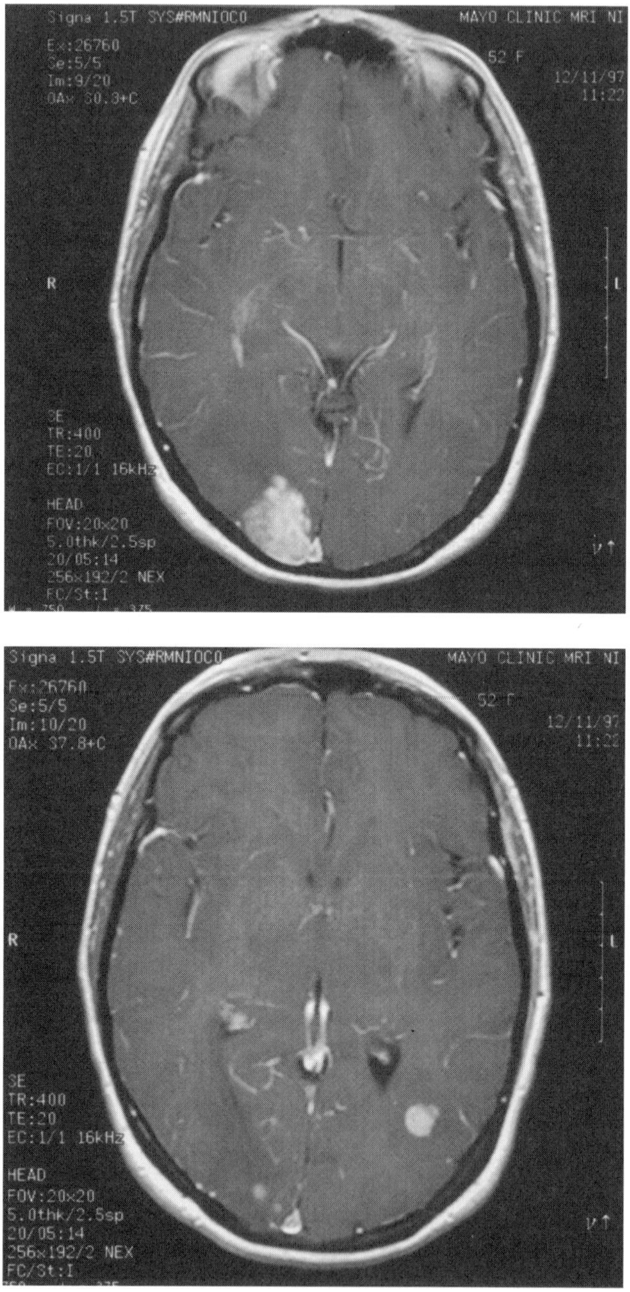

A

B

Figure 5. Axial T1-weigthed postgadolinium MRIs of a 52-year-old woman with breast cancer. (**A** and **B**) MRI showing two tumors involving the right occipital and left temporal regions. The patient underwent resection of the larger occipital tumor, radiosurgery to the smaller contralateral tumor (volume, 0.6 cm^3; tumor margin/maximum dose, 20 Gy/40 Gy), and fractionated radiation therapy (37.5 Gy). *(Continued.)*

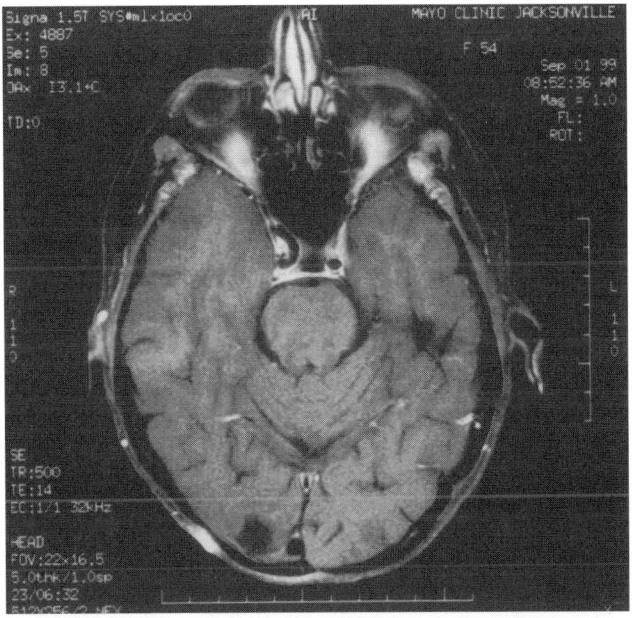

C

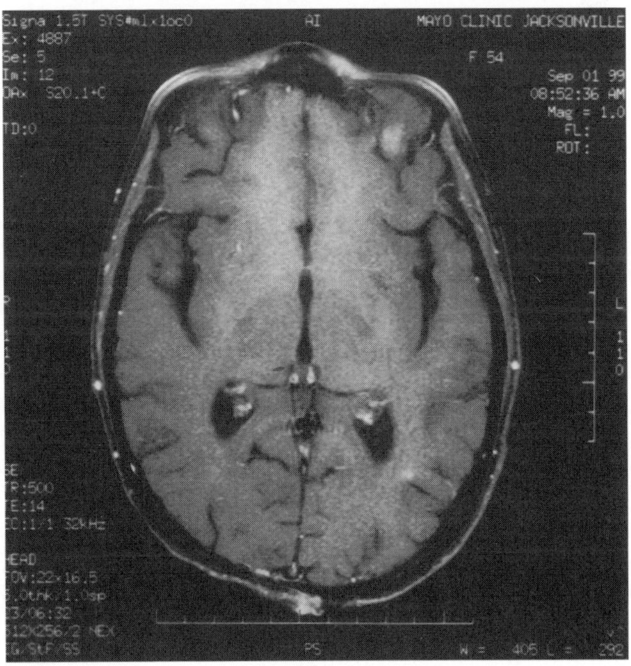

D

Figure 5. (**C and D**) MRI 21 months later showing good control of both the right and left tumors.

fewer intracranial recurrences compared to patients with radioresistant tumors. No difference in local tumor control was detected after resection and radiation therapy, radiosurgery alone, or radiosurgery and radiation therapy; only patients having resection alone had higher local tumor recurrence rates. As a result, aggressive intervention improves survival for good prognosis patients with multiple brain metastases compared to historical controls. In our patients, tumor histology correlated with intracranial disease progression although a patient's overall disease status as described by the RPA classification was a better predictor of survival. Thus, radiosurgery should be strongly considered for the majority of brain metastasis patients not suffering from symptomatic mass effect, who are performing well on a daily basis with limited or stable systemic disease.

Radiosurgery or Surgical Resection

The best management strategy for good prognosis brain metastases patients is controversial. Although prospective randomized trials have been performed comparing outcomes for patients with a single metastasis having resection with or without WBRT,[8,9,19,22] and for patients with two to four tumors having either radiosurgery or WBRT,[11] there is no study that has adequately compared surgical resection to radiosurgery. To date, there are two published papers that have retrospectively compared these two treatment options for patients with a single brain metastasis.[35,36] Bindal et al reviewed 31 patients having radiosurgery between 1991 and 1994 and compared this group to 62 patients undergoing surgical resection over the same time interval (out of more than 500 operated patients, or approximately 12%).[35] Patients were treated with LINAC radiosurgery: the median tumor size was 2 cm^3, and the median tumor margin dose was 18.7 Gy. These authors found that survival was longer in the patients having tumor removal (16.4 months vs. 7.5 months), and that the decreased survival related to neurological progression, not systemic disease progression. Moreover, the higher mortality rate in the radiosurgical group did not relate to the development of new brain metastases, but rather, it related to progression of the radiosurgically treated tumors. Based on these results, the authors concluded that surgical resection was superior to radiosurgery in the treatment of brain metastases patients. However, this study has been criticized on several points relating primarily to patient selection and the comparability of the treatment groups. For example, the median time to local progression in this study (6 months) is far less than other published reports on brain metastases radiosurgery.[6,7,11,13,14–18,23–25,27,29,32–34] Conversely, the median survival in the surgical resection arm (16.4 months) is far greater than other published reports on brain metastasis surgery that found survival times ranging from 5.6 to 11 months.[8,12,19,20,22] Moreover, the median survival of patients having surgical resection in this paper exceeds the results found by the same authors on brain metastasis surgery.[10,37] Thus, although this paper matched patients in regard to primary tumor type, age, and other variables, it is likely that patients having radiosurgery (approximately 6% of treated patients) were thought to be in relatively poor condition after their evaluation and were thus deemed "poor candidates" for surgical resection.

The second study that has compared surgical resection and radiosurgery for brain metastases patients was recently published by Muacevic et al.[36] Patients in this study had a single metastasis less than 3.5 cm in diameter; all patients having tumor removal received postoperative WBRT (median dose, 50 Gy). The pretreatment characteristics were similar, with the exception that patients with larger tumors more often had tumor resection. No difference was noted in the 1-year survival rates; 53% for patients having tumor resection compared to 43% in patients having radiosurgery. Likewise, 1-year local tumor control rates (75% for surgical resection vs. 83% for radiosurgery) and 1-year neurological death rates (37% for surgical resection vs. 39% for radiosurgery) were quite comparable between the two treatment groups. There was also no difference in the treatment-related morbidity and mortality. These authors concluded that radiosurgery provided local tumor control rates as good as resection and WBRT for selected patients.

We have recently compared patient survival and local tumor control rates for patients with a single brain metastasis having either surgical resection or radiosurgery at the Mayo Clinic between 1991 and 1999.[38] In a retrospective study of 97 patients, actuarial analysis showed no difference in patient survival (15.4 months for resection vs. 12.8 months for radiosurgery) or local tumor control (85% for resection vs. 100% for radiosurgery). Recursive partitioning analysis showed improved survival for patients with either nonevident or stable systemic disease compared to patients with progressive disease, and for patients less than 66.5 years old. Thus, we have interpreted our own experience combined with the available published data as showing little difference in regard to local tumor control after surgical resection and WBRT when compared to radiosurgery. Consequently, we approach good prognosis brain metastasis patients with the bias that the majority of tumors are not large and can be effectively managed with radiosurgery. Still diabetic patients frequently benefit from tumor removal to minimize the need for prolonged steroid usage; Shaw et al in the initial report on RTOG 90-05 found that over 40% of brain metastasis patients required corticosteroids 3 to 12 months after radiosurgery.[30] Last, it appears that radiosurgery is more cost effective compared to surgical resection and WBRT for patients with a single brain tumor based on data available from the Medicare Provider Analysis and Review database.[39] If, in fact, this is true, the cost savings to society would be measured in the millions of dollars if appropriate patients had radiosurgery rather than surgical resection.

Usefulness of Whole Brain Radiation Therapy

The use of WBRT in conjunction with radiosurgery is controversial.[11,26,27] Although it appears quite clear that patients having tumor resection have improved local control with addition of WBRT,[12,22,23] the role of WBRT is not as clear after radiosurgery. Several studies have found that the combination of radiosurgery and WBRT results in greater local control rates than radiosurgery alone[7,25,40]; other reports have not detected any difference in local control rates for patients having radiosurgery alone.[16,23,27,36] Moreover, the effect on patient survival is even less well established, especially since radiosurgery can be repeated for patients who remain in a good functional state but develop new distant brain tumors. Therefore, quality of life after WBRT is of great importance.

Neurocognitive function directly correlates with quality of life in brain tumor patients.[41] Neurocognitive deficits induced by WBRT have a negative impact on quality of life. A frequently quoted study by DeAngelis et al reported 12 patients who developed delayed complications of whole brain radiotherapy (8 also underwent surgical resection).[28] The incidence of WBRT-induced dementia was 1.9 to 5.1% in the two populations reviewed. Frequently, when this study is referenced, important considerations are omitted which are emphasized in the original paper. For example, the relevance of dose fraction is typically not discussed. Thus, although the total dose of WBRT was only 25 to 39 Gy, daily fractions of 3 to 6 Gy were used in these patients. The authors noted that these fractionation schedules predispose patients to delayed neurological toxicity. The authors recommended more protracted schedules to improve the safety and efficacy of WBRT for "good-risk" patients with brain metastases.

Several studies have not found the addition of radiotherapy to be a significant predictor of neurocognitive decline in brain tumor patients.[42,43] Murray et al analyzed the Mini-Mental State Examination (MMSE) scores (before and after WBRT) of brain metastasis patients randomized to the standard arm (30 Gy in 10 fractions) in a phase III RTOG trial.[44] Improvement in MMSE score over time was assessed for patients surviving long enough to undergo follow-up MMSE and in patients with a baseline score of less than 30 (30 was the maximum score). Overall, 55% of these patients showed improvement in their MMSE scores on follow-up visits. To better assess neurocognitive function after WBRT, the RTOG is piloting a feasibility study in patients treated with WBRT (37.5 Gy in 15 fractions) for brain metastases. Five neurocognitive measures and a quality of life instrument will be performed in patients with brain metastasis. Although a randomized trial of WBRT with serial neurocognitive function testing and a quality of life component would be preferred, the RTOG trial, when completed, should provide helpful information regarding the decision for WBRT in patients with brain metastases.

References

1. Nussbaum ES, Djalilian HR, Cho KH, et al: Brain metastases: histology, multiplicity, surgery and survival. Cancer 1996;78:1781–1788.
2. Posner J: Management of brain metastases. Rev Neurol 1992;148:477–487.
3. Lagerwaard FJ, Levendag PC, Nowak PJ, et al: Identification of prognostic factors in patients with brain metastases: a review of 1292 patients. Int J Radiat Oncol Biol Phys 1999;43:795–803.
4. Nieder C, Nestle U, Motaref B, et al: Prognostic factors in brain metastases: should patients be selected for aggressive treatment according to recursive partitioning analysis (RPA) classes? Int J Radiat Oncol Biol Phys 2000;46: 297–302.
5. Gaspar L, Scott C, Rotman M, et al: Recursive partitioning analysis (RPA) of prognostic factors in three Radiation Therapy Oncology Group (RTOG) brain metastases trials. Int J Radiat Oncol Biol Phys 1997;37:745–751.
6. Auchter RM, Lamond JP, Alexander E III, et al: A multiinstitutional outcome and prognostic factor analysis of radiosurgery for resectable single brain metastasis. Int J Radiat Oncol Biol Phys 1996;35:27–35.
7. Flickinger JC, Kondziolka D, Lunsford LD, et al: A multi-institutional experience with stereotactic radiosurgery for solitary brain metastasis. Int J Radiat Oncol Biol Phys 1994;28:797–802.
8. Patchell RA, Tibbs PA, Walsh JW, et al: A randomized trial of surgery in the treatment of single brain metastases to the brain. N Engl J Med 1990;322: 494–500.
9. Vecht CJ, Haaxma-Reiche H, Noordijk EM, et al: Treatment of single brain metastasis: radiotherapy alone or combined with neurosurgery. Ann Neurol 1993;33:583–590.
10. Bindal RK, Sawaya R, Leavens ME, et al: Surgical treatment of multiple brain metastases. J Neurosurg 1993;79:210–216.
11. Kondziolka D, Patel A, Lunsford LD, et al: Stereotactic radiosurgery plus whole brain radiotherapy versus radiotherapy alone for patients with multiple brain metastases. Int J Radiat Oncol Biol Phys 1999;45:427–434.
12. Smalley SR, Laws ER Jr, O'Fallon JR, et al: Resection for solitary brain metastasis: role of adjuvant radiation and prognostic variables in 229 patients. J Neurosurg 1992;77:531–540.
13. Alexander E III, Moriarty TM, Davis RB, et al: Stereotactic radiosurgery for the definitive, noninvasive treatment of brain metastases. J Natl Cancer Inst 1995;87:34–40.
14. Matsuo T, Shibata S, Yasunga A, et al: Dose optimization and indications of Linac radiosurgery for brain metastases. Int J Radiat Oncol Biol Phys 1999;45:931–939.
15. Joseph J, Adler JR, Cox RS, et al: Linear accelerator-based stereotactic radiosurgery for brain metastases: the influence of number of lesions on survival. J Clin Oncol 1996;14:1085–1092.
16. Pirzkall A, Debrus J, Lohr F, et al: Radiosurgery alone or in conjunction with whole-brain radiotherapy for brain metastases. J Clin Oncol 1998;16:3563–3569.
17. Schoeggl A, Kitz K, Ertel A, et al: Prognostic factor analysis for multiple brain metastases after gamma knife radiosurgery: results in 97 patients. J Neurooncol 1999;42:169–175.
18. Weltman E, Salvajoli JV, Brandt RA, et al: Radiosurgery for brain metastases: a score index for predicting prognosis. Int J Radiat Oncol Biol Phys 2000;46:1155–1161.

19. Mintz AH, Kestle J, Rathbone MP, et al: A randomized trial to assess the efficacy of surgery in addition to radiotherapy in patients with single cerebral metastasis. Cancer 1996;78:1470–1476.
20. Agboola O, Benoit B, Cross C, et al: Prognostic factors derived from recursive partitioning analysis (RPA) of Radiation Therapy Oncology Group (RTOG) brain metastases trials applied to surgically resected and irradiated cases. Int J Radiat Oncol Biol Phys 1998;42:155–159.
21. Pollock BE: Management of patients with multiple brain metastases. Cont Neurosurgery 1999;21:1–6.
22. Patchell RA, Tibbs PA, Regine WF, et al: Postoperative radiotherapy in the treatment of single metastasis to the brain: a randomized trial. JAMA 1998;280:1485–1489.
23. Pollock BE, Brown PD, Foote RL, et al: Properly selected patients with multiple brain metastases may benefit from aggressive treatment of their intracranial disease. J Neurooncol (submitted for publication).
24. Buatti JM, Friedman WA, Bova FJ, et al: Treatment selection factors for stereotactic radiosurgery of intracranial metastases. Int J Radiat Oncol Biol Phys 1995;32:1161–1166.
25. Brown PD, Brown CA, Pollock BE, et al: Stereotactic radiosurgery for patients with radioresistant brain metastases. Neurosurgery (in press).
26. Shaw EG: Radiotherapeutic management of multiple brain metastases: "3000 in 10" whole brain radiation radiation is no longer a "no brainer." Int J Radiat Oncol Biol Phys 1999;45:253–254.
27. Sneed PK, Lamborn KR, Forstner JM, et al: Radiosurgery for brain metastases: is whole brain radiotherapy necessary. Int J Radiat Oncol Biol Phys 1999;43:549–558.
28. DeAngelis LM, Delattre JY, Posner JB: Radiation-induced dementia in patients cured of brain metastases. Neurology 1989;39:789–796.
29. Shiau C, Sneed PK, Shu H, et al: Radiosurgery for brain metastases: relationship of dose and pattern of enhancement to local control. Int J Radiat Oncol Biol Phys 1997;37:375–383.
30. Shaw E, Scott C, Souhami L, et al: Radiosurgery for the treatment of previously irradiated recurrent primary brain tumors and brain metastases: initial report of Radiation Therapy Oncology Group protocol 90–05. Int J Radiat Oncol Biol Phys 1996;34:647–654.
31. Shaw E, Scott C, Souhami L, et al: Single dose radiosurgical treatment of recurrent previously irradiated primary brain tumors and brain metastases: final report of RTOG protocol 90–05. Int J Radiat Oncol Biol Phys 2000;47:291–298.
32. Lavine SD, Petrovich Z, Cohen-Gadol AA, et al: Gamma knife radiosurgery for metastatic melanoma: an analysis of survival, outcome, and complications. Neurosurgery 1999;44:59–66.
33. Mori Y, Kondziolka D, Lunsford LD, et al: Stereotactic radiosurgery for brain metastases from renal cell carcinoma. Cancer 1998;83:344–353.
34. Somoza S, Kondziolka D, Lunsford LD, et al: Stereotactic radiosurgery for cerebral metastatic melanoma. J Neurosurg 1993;79:661–666.
35. Bindal AK, Bindal RK, Hess KR, et al: Surgery versus radiosurgery in the treatment of brain metastasis. J Neurosurg 1996;84:748–754.
36. Muacevic A, Kreth FW, Horstmann GA, et al: Surgery and radiotherapy compared to gamma knife radiosurgery in the treatment of solitary cerebral metastases of small diameter. J Neurosurg 1999;91:35–43.
37. Bindal RK, Sawaya R, Leavens ME, et al: Reoperation for recurrent metastatic brain tumors. J Neurosurg 1995;83:600–604.

38. Dagam SA, Link MJ, O'Neill B, Pollock BE: Comparison of microneurosurgery with stereotactic radiosurgery in the treatment of solitary brain metastases. J Neurosurg 2001;94:387A. Abstract.
39. Rutigliano MJ, Lunsford LD, Kondziolka D, et al: The cost effectiveness of stereotactic radiosurgery versus surgical resection in the treatment of solitary metastatic brain tumors. Neurosurgery 1995;37:445–455.
40. Chidel MA, Suh JH, Reddy CA, et al: Application of recursive partitioning analysis and evaluation of the use of whole brain radiation among patients treated with stereotactic radiosurgery for newly diagnosed brain metastases. Int J Radiat Oncol Biol Phys 2000;47:993–999.
41. Weitzner MA: Psychosocial and neuropsychiatric aspects of patients with primary brain tumors. Cancer Invest 1999;17:285–291.
42. Taylor BV, Buckner JC, Cascino TL, et al: Effects of radiation and chemotherapy on cognitive function in patients with high-grade glioma. J Clin Oncol 1998;16:2195–2201.
43. Taphoorn MJB, Schiphorst AK, Snoek FJ, et al: Cognitive functions and quality of life in patients with low-grade gliomas: the impact of radiotherapy. Ann Neurol 1994;36:48–54.
44. Murray KJ, Scott C, Zachariah B, et al: Importance of the mini-mental status examination in the treatment of patients with brain metastases: a report from the Radiation Therapy Oncology Group protocol 91-04. Int J Radiat Oncol Biol Phys 2000;48:59–64.

Comment

Chapter 11

Edward G. Shaw

The incidence of metastatic brain disease, the most common neurological manifestation of cancer, is in excess of 200,000 cases per year, similar to or exceeding the incidence of newly diagnosed lung, breast, or prostate cancer.[1] The availability and efficacy of stereotactic radiosurgery (SRS) has completely changed the management of patients with metastatic brain disease, as outlined in the preceding chapter by Pollock and Brown. This commentary will highlight the advances made by SRS, and challenge the "conventional wisdom" regarding the routine use of WBRT in the treatment of patients with metastatic brain disease.

The radiosurgical treatment of brain metastases (with or without WBRT) results in a crude local control rate of approximately 75 to 95%,[2] even in radioresistant histologies like melanoma and renal cell carcinoma.[2] This compares with 0 to 50% when WBRT alone is used.[3,4] Radiosurgically treated patients with metastatic brain disease have a lower neurological death rate [3] and an enhanced quality of life.[5] With a median survival time of 6 to 12 months in most series, and a 2-year survival rate of 25% in selected patients, patients are living longer and manifesting an irreversible and often fatal late side effect of WBRT, radiation-induced dementia.[6] Is the routine use of WBRT appropriate for all patients with metastatic brain disease? The answer is no.[7]

Based on autopsy and imaging series, approximately 50% of cancer patients will have a solitary brain metastasis. Another 20% will have two metastases, and 30% will have three or more.[8,9] For the subset of patients with a favorable overall prognosis (good performance status, controlled or absent primary tumor, and stable or absent extracranial metastatic disease) with one to four metastases,[10,11] local treatment alone (i.e., surgical resection or SRS) with delayed WBRT should be an alternative strategy worth considering. The European Organization for the Research and Treatment of Cancer is testing this approach in two prospective randomized clinical trials. Patients with a solitary metastasis undergo surgical resection or SRS and are then randomized to either immediate WBRT or WBRT delayed to the time of recurrence in the brain. Those with two or three metastases undergo SRS and then the same randomization to immediate or delayed WBRT. The RTOG is about to initiate a similar trial for patients with two or three metastases. The RTOG trial for those with a solitary metastasis will be randomized to local treatment (SRS to the resection cavity) or WBRT.

The advances in the treatment of metastatic brain disease that have resulted from SRS have generated several challenges as well. Despite a crude local control rate of 85 ± 10%, the 2-year actuarial local rate falls to 65%.[2] Radiation sensitizers are needed to enhance efficacy. While the risks of SRS are modest, in one series that included patients with recurrent brain metastases, 68% of patients were steroid-dependent and 11% developed radionecrosis that required an operation following SRS.[12] Radiation protectors and more effective treatment for cerebral edema are needed to minimize toxicity. Last, there is room for technical improvement, including ways to more routinely achieve a consistently high degree of conformity using LINAC SRS, and greater geometric flexibility and collimator selection for Gamma Knife SRS.

References

1. Greenlee RT, Hill-Harmon MB, Murray T, Thun M: Cancer Statistics, 2001. CA Cancer J Clin 2001;51:15–36.
2. Flickinger JC, Kondziolka D, Lunsford LD, et al: A multi-institutional outcome and prognostic factor analysis in radiosurgery for solitary brain metastasis. Int J Radiat Oncol Biol Phys 1994;28:797–802.
3. Kondziolka D, Patel A, Lunsford LD, et al: Stereotactic radiosurgery plus whole brain radiotherapy versus radiotherapy alone for patients with multiple brain metastases. Int J Radiat Oncol Biol Phys 1999;45:427–434.
4. Shaw EG, Gaspar LE, Gibbs FA, et al: Multiple brain metastases. American College of Radiology. ACR Appropriateness Criteria. Radiology 2000;215 (suppl):1121–1128.
5. Sperduto PW, Scott C, Andrews D, et al: Preliminary report of RTOG 9508: a phase III trial comparing whole brain irradiation alone versus whole brain irradiation plus stereotactic radiosurgery for patients with two or three unresected brain metastases (abstract). Int J Radiat Oncol Biol Phys 2000;48 (suppl):113.
6. DeAngelis LM, Delattre JY, Posner JB: Radiation-induced dementia in patients cured of brain metastases. Neurology 1989;39:789–796.
7. Shaw EG: Radiotherapeutic management of multiple brain metastases: "3000 in 10" whole brain radiation is no longer a "no brainer." Int J Radiat Oncol Biol Phys 1999;45:253–254.
8. Posner JB, Chernik NL: Intracranial metastases from systemic cancer. Adv Neurol 1978;45:741–744.
9. Delattre JY, Krol G, Thaler HT, Posner JB: Distribution of brain metastases. Arch Neurol 1988;45:741–744.
10. Gaspar L, Scott C, Rotman M, et al: Recursive partitioning analysis (RPA) of prognostic factors in three radiation therapy oncology (RTOG) brain metastases trials. Int J Radiat Oncol Biol Phys 1997;37:745–751.
11. Swift PS, Phillips T, Martz K, et al: CT characteristics of patients with brain metastases treated in RTOG study 79–16. Int J Radiat Oncol Biol Phys 1993; 25:209–214.
12. Shaw E, Scott C, Souhami L, et al: Single dose radiosurgical treatment of recurrent previously irradiated primary brain tumors and brain metastases: final report of RTOG protocol 90-05. Int J Radiat Oncol Biol Phys 2000;47:291–298.

Chapter 12

Stereotactic Radiosurgery for Glial Tumors

Gene H. Barnett, John H. Suh

Introduction

While metastases are often cited as being ideally suited for radiosurgical treatment (i.e., typically small at presentation, spherical in shape, and both radiographically and histologically well demarcated from surrounding brain), gliomas often possess none of these properties.[1–4] This notwithstanding, they constitute the vast majority of primary brain tumors in adults and exist along a continuum of greater or lesser histologic malignancy. Depending upon subtype, traditional treatments include surgery, chemotherapy, and/or radiotherapy. Unfortunately, with few exceptions (notably anaplastic oligodendrogliomas), the prognosis for these tumors has not materially improved in the last 30 years.[5–7]

Although it was observed for years that some of these tumors were responsive to radiotherapy, the clinical response of high-grade gliomas was scientifically established by the Brain Tumor Study Group (BTSG). BTSG 6901 was a randomized trial that showed that survival from malignant glioma was 14 weeks with supportive care alone, but 36 weeks with radiotherapy.[6] The benefit of radiotherapy over chemotherapy was demonstrated by the same investigators in Brain Tumor Cooperative Group (BTCG) 7201 where survival after radiation (with or without chemotherapy) was superior to chemotherapy alone.[7]

Buoyed by the results of focal reirradiation for recurrent disease, the notion that more is better, and considering that initial dosage of conventional radiotherapy may be limited by toxicity to normal brain, more regional approaches of radiation "boosts" have been applied to newly diagnosed tumors. These were initially delivered by brachytherapy boosts

From Pollock BE (ed). *Contemporary Stereotactic Radiosurgery: Technique and Evaluation.* Armonk, NY, Futura Publishing Company, Inc. © 2002.

using temporary or permanent radioactive sources.[8–11] Although survival appeared to increase in phase II trials, toxicity was high. However, no survival advantage was found in two subsequent North American phase III trials of brachytherapy boosts, suggesting that much of the apparent benefit seen in the phase II trials was due to the effects of selection bias that led to more favorable patients in the brachytherapy group.[8,10,12]

Currently, based on anecdote and some phase II data, certain investigators have great enthusiasm for radiosurgery as an up-front radiation boost for malignant gliomas. Will radiosurgery prove to be more effective than brachytherapy? In this chapter, we will attempt to provide a rational perspective for the role of radiosurgery in glioma, not only for malignant glioma, but also for lower grade astrocytoma and World Health Organization (WHO) Grade I pilocytic astrocytomas.

Radiosurgery for Pilocytic and Optic Nerve Tumors

Pilocytic astrocytoma tends to be an exceptional, yet not inconsequential, member of the astrocytoma family. These tumors of childhood and adolescence usually have the capacity for surgical cure, assuming the anatomical location is favorable, such as in the cerebellar hemispheres. Unfortunately, they often occur in surgically untreatable areas such as the optic nerves and chiasm, or in regions where only incomplete surgery is feasible. Also, these tumors may behave more aggressively and defy surgery by early recurrence or metastasis in the central nervous system.

Radiosurgery is an appealing option for treatment of some of these lesions as it may be applicable to surgically inaccessible lesions, allow for "mopping up" of surgically incomplete resection, potentially minimize long-term radiation toxicity in children, and be applied to recurrence without the need for surgery. Nonetheless, focused reports of the successful use of radiosurgery to treat these lesions are few.

Proust et al reported a case of a deep hemispheric pilocytic astrocytoma that was treated with 21 Gy to the 70% isodose line using single-fraction radiosurgery.[13] Subsequent enlargement of the cystic component was addressed with intracavitary rhenium. Three years later there was no evidence of metabolic activity of the tumor by positron-emission tomography (PET) and the tumor and cyst remained stable.

Somaza et al presented their experience with radiosurgery for growing pilocytic astrocytomas in children.[14] This group of nine children represent an assortment of newly treated versus failed treatment, incompletely resected,[7] and failed radiotherapy[2] patients. All had growing lesions in regions barring definitive surgical cure and all had growth arrest, with five clear-cut regressions. They reported no toxicity, but long-term results (both favorable and unfavorable) were not addressed.

Lim and Leem reported one case of juvenile optic nerve gliomas treated with single-fraction stereotactic radiosurgery (SRS) delivering 12

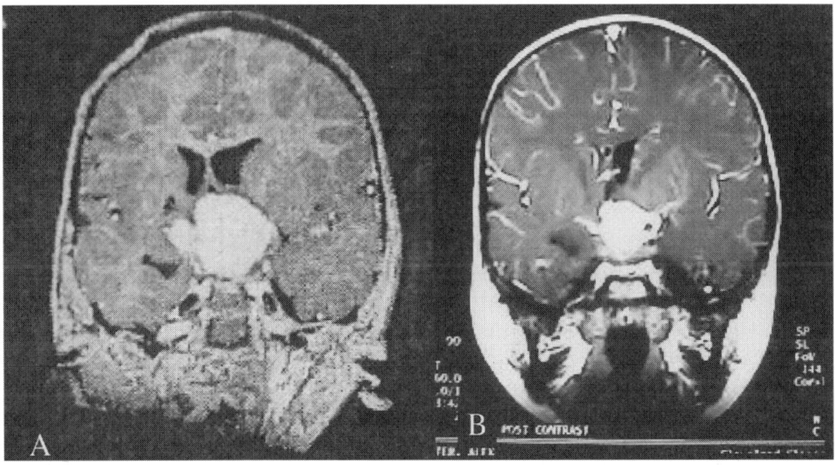

Figure 1. (**A**) A 41-month-old boy with biopsy-proven pilocytic astrocytoma of the optic nerve and chiasm. The child was blind preoperatively, and the tumor was treated with 12 Gy to the 48% isodose line with initial shrinkage. (**B**) Eight months later there was substantial reduction in the size of the tumor. Unfortunately, the child had no return of vision and suffered from leptomeningeal dissemination of the tumor. He remained alive 4 1/2 years later.

Gy to the 40% isodose line with the Gamma Knife.[15] Follow-up was 24 months with tumor shrinkage and visual improvement. Figure 1A shows a similar case treated at our institution of a 41-month-old boy with biopsy-proven pilocytic astrocytoma of the optic nerve and chiasm. The child was blind preoperatively, and the tumor treated with 12 Gy to the 48% isodose line with initial shrinkage. Unfortunately, he had no return of vision and suffered from leptomeningeal dissemination of the tumor 4 1/2 years later.

Clearly, single-fraction radiosurgery of gliomas of the optic apparatus risks worsening of vision from the treatment itself, particularly when the nerve receives more than 8 Gy in a single fraction. In an effort to reduce this risk, Debus et al treated 10 patients with optic nerve glioma using fractionated radiosurgery delivering 1.8 Gy daily for a total of 54 Gy.[16] Nine of 10 tumors responded with three complete remissions associated with improvement of vision.

These reports *suggest* that radiosurgery (single or multiple fraction) may be an effective treatment for inoperable or recurrent pilocytic tumors, even those situated in functionally critical areas. Surgical resection probably remains the treatment of choice, when feasible.

Radiosurgery for Low-Grade Glioma

Fibrillary low-grade astrocytomas tend to be genetically unstable tumors that frequently evolve into more malignant forms. Extent of resection of these lesions has often been cited as a favorable survival factor, although this assertion remains controversial because tumor cells may exist well beyond the radiographic boundaries of these lesions. Despite impressive improvements in the results of surgery due to surgical navigation,[17] awake craniotomy,[18] and resection control using intraoperative magnetic resonance imaging (MRI),[19] a complete resection of these lesions may be limited by poor surgical access or by its location in a functionally critical area of the brain.

Some inoperable lesions may lend themselves to radiosurgical treatment. Plowman reported radiographic control at 2 and 5 years in two cases of low-grade tumor treated with radiosurgery.[20] Barcia et al presented 16 cases of deeply seated low-grade glioma treated with radiosurgery.[21] A mean dose of 22 Gy was delivered and 13 lesions shrunk, of which eight had a complete response. Six cases had previously been treated with conventional radiotherapy. Three cases of brainstem glioma did not respond and the patients succumbed to their disease.

Tectal brainstem lesions were, however, successfully treated with Gamma Knife radiosurgery in a report by Kihlstrom et al.[22] Six of the seven tumors responded to doses of 14 to 35 Gy at the treatment isodose line. However, two cases treated with greater than or equal to 30 Gy developed radiation necrosis with permanent deficits. The authors concluded that this was an effective treatment and safe if the treatment dose did not exceed 14 Gy.

We have seen three cases of low-grade, nonenhancing tumors developing contrast enhancement several months after treatment. Figure 2 il-

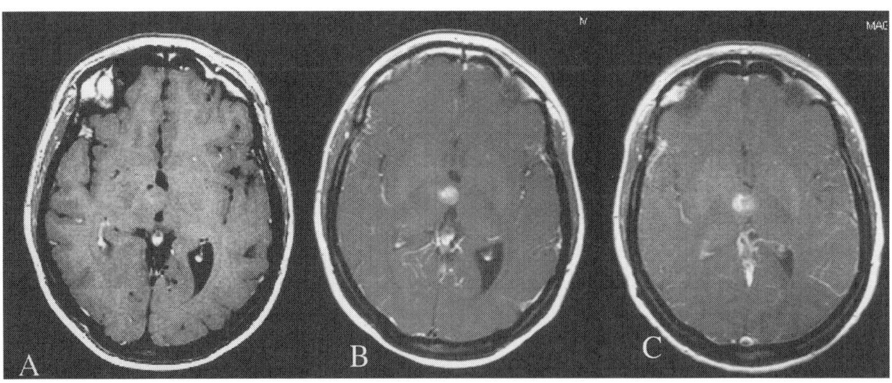

Figure 2. (**A**) A 34-year-old female had a biopsy-proven WHO Grade II astrocytoma of the right thalamus. This 6-mm lesion was treated with radiosurgery using 18 Gy to the 77% isodose line. (**B**) Six months later, the patient developed headaches, the tumor avidly enhanced, and she required steroids for peritumoral edema. A fluorodeoxyglucose PET scan demonstrated hypometabolism, but she required a cerebrospinal fluid diversion procedure for hydrocephalus. (**C**) Four years after treatment, the tumor remains stable in size and the patient is asymptomatic, but ongoing enhancement is found.

lustrates such a case where a 34-year-old woman had a biopsy-proven WHO Grade II astrocytoma of the right thalamus. This 6-mm lesion was treated with radiosurgery using 18 Gy to the 77% isodose line. Six months later, she developed headaches, the tumor had avidly enhanced, and she required steroids for peritumoral edema. A fluorodeoxyglucose PET scan demonstrated hypometabolism, but she required a cerebrospinal fluid diversion procedure for hydrocephalus. Four years after treatment the tumor has remained stable and she is asymptomatic, but ongoing enhancement has been found.

The role of radiosurgery in low-grade infiltrating astrocytoma remains controversial. The natural history of these tumors is such that years, and even decades, may elapse before observing tumor progression. Convincing evidence that radiosurgery extends survival in these lesions is lacking, although its use in small, surgically inaccessible tumors is seductive. However, some lesions may respond adversely, even when treated with nominal doses of radiosurgery. The use of SRS in small, inoperable tumors or residual tumors after best surgical resection is reasonable, but should be balanced with the knowledge that adverse reactions can occur and that improved survival has not been proven.

Radiosurgery for High-Grade Glioma

Collectively, high-grade (WHO Grades III and IV) astrocytomas represent the most common primary brain tumors in adults. As mentioned earlier, the value of radiotherapy as part of the management of these lesions was established in the late 1970s. Efforts to enhance control and minimize radiation-induced toxicity by delivering a boost to the tumor and its immediate surroundings rest on the observation that tumor recurrence or failure is usually local–with 80% recurring within 2 cm of the primary tumor and half recurring within 1 cm.[23,24] Indeed, whole brain radiation therapy does not provide superior survival or local control over partial field treatment of these lesions.

Thus, standard radiotherapy of these tumors, as defined by the Radiation Therapy Oncology Group (RTOG), uses the "shrinking field" method of treating the region of edema (defined on T2-weighted MRI) plus 2 cm with 4600 cGy in 23 fractions of 200 cGy each, and a conedown field, determined by the region of enhancement (or resection bed) on T1-weighted MRI plus 2.5 cm, treated with an additional 1400 cGy in 7 fractions of 200 cGy each.

Building on these observations and practices, the notion that even higher "boosts" of radiation limited to the tumor and its immediate surroundings evolved. The development of image-guided stereotactic techniques allowed for precise targeting of structures that could be visualized on neuroimaging studies such as CT, MRI, and PET. Stereotactic brachytherapy (temporary or permanent)[8–12] and radiosurgery allowed for focal escalation of radiation dose with sharp dose fall-off that spared normal brain tissue.

At present, encouraging reports of the results of radiosurgery for malignant glioma abound and are presented here. However, these data are limited to case reports, clinical series and phase I or II trials. Until phase III trials data becomes available, it is *essential* to interpret these studies in the context of the pattern of observations and results that derived from brachytherapy for such tumors a decade ago. These issues will be discussed following a review of reports of radiosurgery for malignant glioma.

Radiosurgery for Recurrent Malignant Glioma

Much of the initial enthusiasm for the use of radiosurgery for these tumors stems from reports on its impact on recurrent tumor that failed conventional treatment.

In 1995, Hall et al reported on the results of SRS in 35 patients with malignant glioma (75% glioblastoma multiforme [GBM]) that had failed conventional treatment.[25] The actuarial survival was 8 months from radiosurgery with the vast majority (85%) dying of local failure. Nearly a third of the patients required reoperation after radiosurgery although the rate of radionecrosis was only 14%. They concluded that SRS was a useful treatment, with lower morbidity than brachytherapy, for recurrent malignant glioma. Similarly, median survival was 9 months after SRS in a group of 62 patients with recurrent GBM treated by van Kampen et al with half the patients showing improved quality of life (neurological findings, frequency of seizure, and steroid dose) at 4.5 months after treatment.[26] We found a median progression-free survival of 4.7 months in 22 patients with recurrent GBMs (median volume, 9.9 cm^3) when treated with 15 Gy delivered to the 60% isodose line (median).[27]

Early reports of SRS for glioma suggested a rather high toxicity. For example, Chamberlain et al treated 20 patients with various recurrent gliomas with SRS.[28] Of these, seven had early radiation complications, including one death. Efficacy of this treatment was regarded as "modest." In an effort to define acceptable treatment doses for these treatments, the RTOG conducted a phase I/II dose-escalation trial of SRS (RTOG 9005) in patients with recurrent malignant gliomas and metastases.[4] They derived maximum treatment doses based on acceptable levels of toxicity (Table 1). Higher toxicity was found in maximum tumor diameters greater than or equal to 21 mm and those treated with linear accelerators (LINACs) compared with the Gamma Knife. Also, treatment using the LINAC versus Gamma Knife had 2.84 times greater risk for local progression.

Shrieve et al more formally compared the efficacy and toxicity of radiosurgery to brachytherapy for treatment of recurrent malignant

Table 1
Maximum Radiosurgical Treatment Dose for Acceptable Toxicity in Recurrent Malignant Tumor: Results of RTOG 9005[46]

Maximum dimension	≤20 mm	21–30 mm	31–40 mm
Treatment dose	2400 cGy	1800 cGy	1500 cGy

RTOG, Radiation Therapy Oncology Group.

gliomas.[29] While survival after SRS was nearly as good as for I-125 brachytherapy, the rate of reoperation was substantially less. Comparative results for brachytherapy and SRS from the Brigham and Women's Hospital (Joint Center for Radiation Therapy), University of California San Francisco, and the Cleveland Clinic Foundation are shown in Table 2.

As fractionation of a radiosurgical treatment may reduce normal tissue toxicity, Cho et al compared the results of single-fraction radiosurgery (median, 17 Gy to the 50% isodose line) to fractionated radiosurgery (median, 37.5 Gy in 15 fractions to the 85% isodose line) in a group of 71 patients with recurrent malignant glioma.[30] Although prognostic factors (age, performance status, tumor size) were more favorable in the SRS group, survival was longer in the fractionated SRS (FSRS) patients (11 months vs. 12 months, respectively) and complications were lower (30% vs. 8%, respectively). These results suggested that FSRS may be a more appropriate choice in this setting, especially for large tumors or those in critical areas. In another report, median survival of 7 months was achieved in 88 patients with recurrent GBM when Taxol (120 mg/m^2) was used as a radiation sensitizer for FSRS (mean, 24 Gy in 4 fractions).[31,32] Patients with tumor volume less than 30 cm^3 survived significantly longer than those with larger tumors.

Table 2
Selected Results for Recurrent Glioblastoma Treated with Brachytherapy or Stereotactic Radiosurgery

Center	*Technique*	*Dose (Gy)*	*Survival*	*Reop Rate*
JCRT[48]	I-125	50.0	11.5 m	44%
UCSF[19]	I-125	64.4	12.0 m	38%
JCRT[48]	SRS	13.0	10.0 m	22%
CCF[37]	SRS	15.0	10.3 m	18%

Reop, reoperation; JCRT, Joint Center for Radiation Therapy; UCSF, University of California San Francisco; CCF, Cleveland Clinic Foundation; SRS, stereotactic radiosurgery.

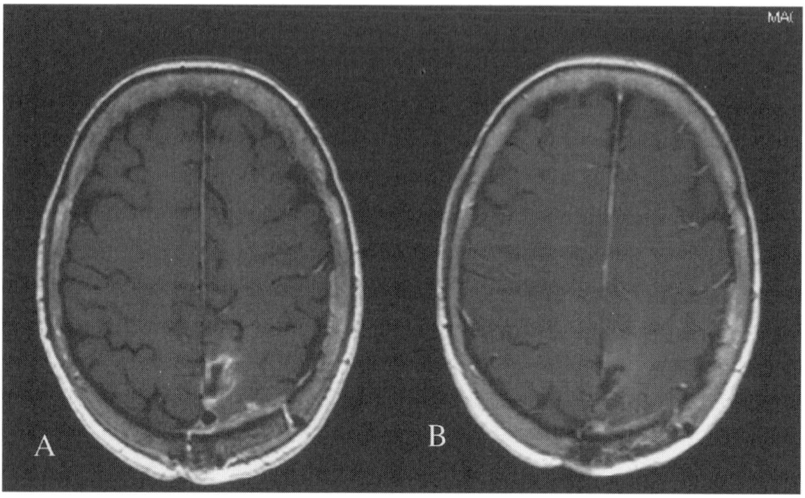

Figure 3. (**A**) A 63-year-old female with recurrent glioblastoma, which was treated with Gamma Knife radiosurgery using 18 Gy to the 50% isodose line. (**B**) Tumor regression is shown 9 months later. The patient survived 23 months after treatment.

Clearly, there are objective responses to SRS in the setting of recurrent malignant glioma. Figure 3, shows a 63-year-old female with recurrent glioblastoma. She was treated with Gamma Knife radiosurgery using 18 Gy to the 50% isodose line. Tumor regression is shown and the patient survived 23 months after treatment. The literature suggests that these treatments are, however, only palliative as local failure from SRS is the norm.

It remains unclear if SRS is the best treatment for recurrent malignant glioma, especially at doses that have limited toxicity. Nonetheless, SRS should be considered in cases of focal recurrence, particularly if other treatment options have been exhausted.

Radiosurgery for Newly Diagnosed Malignant Glioma

It is generally held that cancer treatments that show benefit at tumor recurrence are likely to yield even greater benefit when delivered as part of initial management. As such, SRS has been aggressively applied at some centers as a regional "boost" delivered to the tumor along with conventional radiotherapy.

Among the earliest reports of radiosurgery as a boost for malignant gliomas was one from the Joint Center by Loeffler et al.[33] Twenty-three

GBM and 14 anaplastic astrocytoma patients underwent radiosurgery of enhancing tissue 2 to 4 weeks after completion of conventional radiotherapy (max, 5940 cGy). Median radiosurgical minimum dose was 12 Gy (range, 10 to 20 Gy) and maximum dose was 15 Gy (range, 12.5 to 25 Gy). Tumor size range from 1.2 to 72 cm^3. Only 24% of patients died at 19-month median follow-up. This, as well as many subsequent studies, concluded that SRS was a useful adjunct in the management of these lesions.[34–37] The Joint Center for Radiation Therapy, University of Wisconsin, and University of Florida pooled their data and found that median survival was 24 months among 115 GBM patients treated with radiosurgery as part of initial management.[38] Alexander et al found results similar to those of brachytherapy, both in terms of benefit and toxicity.[39] Results using FSRS have been reported to be even more favorable.[40,41]

The importance of selection to the success of the procedure (potentially introducing bias in analysis of the results) was recognized early.[42] Mehta et al, and Sarkaria et al, attempted to minimize the influence on outcome analysis by interpreting their results according to several classifications of outcome as derived by the RTOG (see next section).[38,43] Although the smaller, single institution study found the median survival difficult to assess and 2-year survival for GBM patients significantly better than predicted,[43] the larger, multi-institutional report showed significant improvement over expected outcome in both categories.[38]

While equivocal reports of the benefit of early SRS for malignant glioma are not uncommon,[44] exceptions to the use of early, adjuvant radiosurgery are few. Among these, Masciopinto et al found that median survival was 9.5 months–with no significant difference from standard therapy.[45,46] Interpretation of their data is hampered, however, by nonstandard reporting of treatment dosing. All 11 patients treated with LINAC radiosurgery to the enhancing lesion with malignant glioma progressed within 1 year in a report from Buatti et al.[47] Shenouda et al found limited benefit when SRS was combined with accelerated radiotherapy.[48]

Although the impact of SRS on the typical patient with malignant glioma remains obscure, some patients with malignant glioma treated with SRS have prolonged survival.[49] Figure 4 shows a 36-year-old female with a biopsy-proven glioblastoma of the right temporal stem. It was treated with LINAC radiosurgery using 25 Gy to the 80% isodose line and 59.4 Gy in 33 fractions of radiotherapy. She remains alive today 110 months after SRS, with no evidence of tumor recurrence or progression. Despite these anecdotal cases, it is clear that the procedure may be associated with toxicity, especially for high doses or when large lesions are treated. Distinguishing recurrent tumor from radiation necrosis may require special imaging studies such as PET, SPECT, or even biopsy.[50–54]

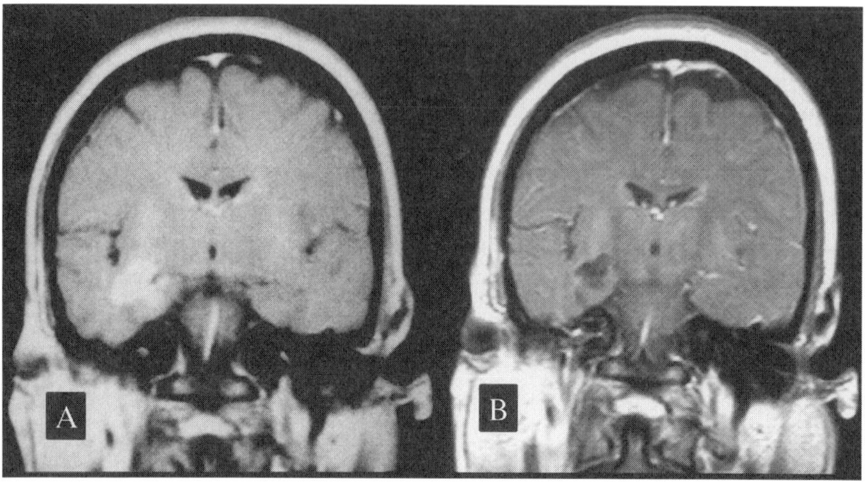

Figure 4. (**A**) A 36-year-old female with a biopsy-proven glioblastoma of the right temporal stem. It was treated with LINAC radiosurgery using 25 Gy to the 80% idodose line and 59.4 Gy in 33 fractions of radiotherapy. (**B**) The patient remained alive 110 months after SRS, with no evidence of tumor recurrence or progression.

Radiosurgery and Brachytherapy for Malignant Glioma–Déjà Vu?

These collective results of SRS for newly diagnosed malignant glioma are eerily similar to those obtained from brachytherapy when applied in this setting. In the early 1990s there was much enthusiasm for brachytherapy boosts in the initial management of these tumors with survivals that bordered on spectacular. Patients with anaplastic astrocytomas and glioblastomas had median survivals of 38 and 20 months, respectively, when so treated.[9,11] It was recognized that these were high morbidity procedures that often required operation to treat radionecrosis–so much so that operability became a criteria for its use in many centers. Nonetheless, the extended survival was felt to make these risks worthwhile.

However, skeptics cautioned that these survivals could not be taken at face value due to selection bias.[8,55] Limitations on tumor size, patient performance status, operability, number of lesions, unilaterality, and lack of subependymal involvement clearly selected a group of patients with a better prognosis than the average patient with a newly diagnosed glioblastoma. Brachytherapy boost was eventually subjected to phase III randomized trials. Two such trials were conducted in North America. One by Bernstein in Canada, the other by BTCG 87-01[10,12] (Selker R, personal communication). Both trials found that brachytherapy provided *no benefit* over radiotherapy and carmustine (BCNU) alone.

When determining the efficacy and risk of a treatment, such as brachytherapy or SRS, for a given disorder, such as malignant glioma, it is imperative to consider the strength of the evidence that supports its use.[56] Criteria for evidence-based medicine recommendations are accepted and range from Class C (case report, series with historical controls) to Class A (phase III randomized trial) as shown in Table 3. When only Class C evidence existed, brachytherapy appeared to be a breakthrough in the management of these tumors. Discredited by Class A evidence, brachytherapy has largely fallen into disuse (although enjoying something of a resurgence of interest–and no proof of benefit—with "liquid" brachytherapy).[57]

Studies of treatment benefit on malignant glioma are particularly susceptible to the outcomes that are perturbed by selection bias because of the short life expectancy and powerful impact of several factors on survival. The RTOG analyzed several of these factors by recursive partitioning analysis and was able to define several clear classes of survival (Table 4).[55] Of note is that expected median survival for anaplastic tumors ranges from 17.9 to 58.6 months, while for glioblastoma it is 4.6 to 17.9 months. When other biases such as small lesion size, unifocality, unilaterality, lack of subependymal spread, and use of toxic doses (in some studies) are considered, much, if not all, of the potential benefit of this treatment may be negated.[42]

As of November 2001 (the time at which this chapter was written), despite many vocal advocates and substantial evidence limited to Class C recommendations, the efficacy and role of radiosurgery, if any, in the initial management of malignant glioma remained unproven. There is, however, hope that the first Class A or B recommendation is near at hand. RTOG 9305 was a phase III trial comparing SRS followed by daily radiotherapy with BCNU to radiotherapy and BCNU, alone. The trial is currently closed to accrual. Candidates included patients with a supratentorial tumor of less than 4 cm in maximum dimension. Radiosurgical dosing was based on the doses established from RTOG 9005 (Table 1), with radiotherapy using 6000 cGy delivered in 30 fractions and dosage of BCNU at 80 mg/m^2 on days 1 to 3 of radiotherapy, and then every 8 weeks for 6 cycles.

Table 3

Categories of Evidence-Based Medicine*

Level I: Grade A recommendations from a single significant randomized clinical trial (RCT) or meta-analysis of randomized clinical trials with consistent positive results.
Level II: Grade B recommendations coming from a single RCT or meta-analysis of RCT where the treatment effects overlap the clinically important benefit or disparate results of RCTs.
Level III: Grade C recommendations where results come from nonrandomized concurrent cohort studies.
Level IV: Grade C recommendations where results come from nonrandomized historical cohort studies.
Level V: Grade C recommendations where results come from case series.

*Adapted from Guyatt et al.[56]

Table 4
Classification of Malignant Gliomas by RTOG Recursive Partitioning Analysis[11]

Definitions Class	*Clinical Criteria*	*Survival Class*	*Median Survival (mos)*	*2-Year Survival (mos)*
1	AA, age <50, normal mental status	1	58.6	76
2	AA, age <50, KPS ≥70, duration >3 mos	2	37.4	68
3	AA, age <50, abnormal mental status	3	17.9	35
3	GBM, age <50, KPS ≥90			
4	AA, age ≥50, KPS ≥70, duration ≤3 mos, STR or GTR, working	4	11.1	15
4	GBM, age <50, KPS <90, STR or GTR, working			
4	GBM, age >50, KPS ≥70, STR or GTR, working			
5	GBM, age ≥50, KPS ≥70, STR or GTR, not working	5	8.9	6
5	GBM, age ≥50, KPS ≥70, Bx			
5	AA or GBM, age ≥50, KPS <70, normal mental status			
6	GBM or AA, age ≥50, KPS <70, abnormal mental status	6	4.6	4

RTOG, Radiation Therapy Oncology Group; AA, anaplastic astrocytoma; KPS, Karnofsky performance score; GBM, glioblastoma multiforme; STR, subtotal resection; GTR, gross total resection; Bx, biopsy.

Only when these results are presented will we have our first and best evidence that SRS belongs in the initial management of these tumors. It is irresponsible to state that SRS *should* be part of the initial management of these tumors, particularly when its use often excludes patients from subsequent investigational trials. Until then, we will need to rely on the best Class C and potentially biased information on which to make these decisions, and consider SRS in the initial management of some malignant gliomas.

References

1. Buatti JM, Friedman WA, Bova FJ, et al: Treatment selection factors for stereotactic radiosurgery of intracranial metastases. Int J Radiat Oncol Biol Phys 1995;32:1161–1166.

2. Coffey RJ, Flickinger JC, Bissonette DJ, et al: Radiosurgery for solitary brain metastases using the cobalt-60 gamma unit: methods and results in 24 patients. Int J Radiat Oncol Biol Phys 1991;20:1287–1295.
3. Kondziolka D, Patel A, Lunsford LD, et al: Stereotactic radiosurgery plus whole brain radiotherapy versus radiotherapy alone for patients with multiple brain metastases. Int J Radiat Oncol Biol Phys 1999;45:427–434.
4. Shaw E, Scott C, Souhami L, et al: Single dose radiosurgical treatment of recurrent previously irradiated primary brain tumors and brain metastases: final report of RTOG 90-05. Int J Radiat Oncol Biol Phys 2000;47:291–293.
5. Cairncross JG, Ueki K, Zlatescu MC, et al: Specific genetic predictors of chemotherapeutic response and survival in patients with anaplastic oligodendrogliomas. J Natl Cancer Inst 1998;90:1473–1479.
6. Walker MD, Alexander E, Hunt WE, et al: Evaluation of BCNU and/or radiotherapy in the treatment of anaplastic gliomas: a cooperative clinical trial. J Neurosurg 1978;49:333–343.
7. Walker MD, Green SB, Byar DP, et al: Randomized comparisons of radiotherapy and nitrosoureas for the treatment of malignant glioma after surgery. N Engl J Med 1980;303:1323–1329.
8. Florell RC, Macdonald DR, Irish WD, et al: Selection bias, survival, and brachytherapy for glioma. J Neurosurg 1992;76:179–183.
9. Gutin P, Wara W, Larson D, et al: Stereotaxic interstitial iodine-125 'boost' in the initial management of malignant gliomas. Int J Radiat Oncol Biol Phys 1990;19(suppl 1):204.
10. Laperriere NJ, Leung PMK, McKenzie S, et al: Randomized study of brachytherapy in the initial management of patients with malignant astrocytoma. Int J Radiat Oncol Biol Phys 1998;41:1005–1011.
11. Prados MD, Gutin PH, Phillips TL, et al: Highly anaplastic astrocytoma: a review of 357 patients treated between 1977 and 1989. Int J Radiat Oncol Biol Phys 1992;23:3–8.
12. Green SB, Shapiro WR, Burger PC, et al: A randomized trial of interstitial radiotherapy (RT) boost for newly diagnosed malignant glioma: Brain Tumor Cooperative Group (BTCG) trial 8701. Proc Ann Meet Am Soc Clin Oncol 1994;13:174.
13. Proust F, Coche-Dequeant B, Carpentier P, et al: Traitement combine d'un astrocytome pilocytique: radiochirurgie stereotaxique et radiotherapie endocavitaire. Neurochirurgie 1998;44:50–54.
14. Somaza SC, Kondziolka D, Lunsford LD, et al: Early outcomes after stereotactic radiosurgery for growing pilocytic astrocytomas in children. Pediatr Neurosurg 1996;25:109–115.
15. Lim YJ, Leem W: Two cases of Gamma Knife radiosurgery for low-grade optic chiasm glioma. Stereotact Funct Neurosurg 1996;66(suppl 1):174–183.
16. Debus J, Kocagoncu KO, Hoss A, et al: Fractionated stereotactic radiotherapy (FSRT) for optic glioma. Int J Radiat Oncol Biol Phys 1999;44:243–248.
17. Barnett GH, Kormos DW, Steiner CP, et al: Use of a frameless, armless stereotactic wand for brain tumor localization with two-dimensional and three-dimensional neuroimaging. Neurosurgery 1993;33:674–678.
18. Taylor MD, Bernstein M: Awake craniotomy with brain mapping as the routine surgical approach to treating patients with supratentorial intraaxial tumors: a prospective trial of 200 cases. J Neurosurg 1999;90:35–41.
19. Black PM, Alexander E 3rd, Martin C, et al: Craniotomy for tumor treatment in an intraoperative magnetic resonance imaging unit. Neurosurgery 1999;45:423–431.
20. Plowman PN: Stereotactic multiple arc radiotherapy. V: Primary treatment of discrete low grade glioma. Br J Neurosurg 1997;11:331–334.

21. Barcia JA, Barcia-Salorio JL, Ferrer C, et al: Stereotactic radiosurgery of deeply seated low grade gliomas. Acta Neurochir Suppl (Wien) 1994;62:58–61.
22. Kihlstrom L, Lindquist C, Lindquist M, et al: Stereotactic radiosurgery for tectal low-grade gliomas. Acta Neurochir Suppl (Wien) 1994;62:55–57.
23. Hochberg FH, Pruitt A: Assumptions in the radiotherapy of glioblastoma. Neurology 1980;30:907–911.
24. Wallner KE, Galicich JH, Krol G, et al: Patterns of failure following treatment for glioblastoma multiforme and anaplastic astrocytoma. Int J Radiat Oncol Biol Phys 1989;16:1405–1409.
25. Hall WA, Djalilian HR, Sperduto PW, et al: Stereotactic radiosurgery for recurrent malignant gliomas. J Clin Oncol 1995;13:1642–1648.
26. van Kampen M, Engenhart-Cabillic R, Debus J, et al: Radiochirurgie des Glioblastoma multiforme in der Rezidivsituation. Heidelberger Erfahrungen im Literaturvergleich. Strahlenther Onkol 1998;174:19–24.
27. Park JL, Suh JH, Barnett GH, et al: Survival after stereotactic radiosurgery for recurrent glioblastoma multiforme. J Radiosurgery 2000;3:169–175.
28. Chamberlain MC, Barba D, Kormanik P, et al: Stereotactic radiosurgery for recurrent gliomas. Cancer 1994;74:1342–1347.
29. Shrieve DC, Alexander E, Wen PY, et al: Comparison of stereotactic radiosurgery and brachytherapy in the treatment of recurrent glioblastoma multiforme. Neurosurgery 1995;36:275–282.
30. Cho KH, Hall WA, Gerbi BJ, et al: Single dose versus fractionated stereotactic radiotherapy for recurrent high-grade gliomas. Int J Radiat Oncol Biol Phys 1999;45:1133–1141.
31. Lederman G, Arbit E, Odaimi M, et al: Fractionated stereotactic radiosurgery and concurrent taxol in recurrent glioblastoma multiforme: a preliminary report. Int J Radiat Oncol Biol Phys 1998;40:661–666.
32. Lederman G, Arbit E, Odaimi M, et al: Recurrent glioblastoma multiforme: potential benefits using fractionated stereotactic radiotherapy and concurrent taxol. Stereotact Funct Neurosurg 1997:69(1–4 Pt 2):162–174.
33. Loeffler JS, Alexander E III, Shea WM, et al: Radiosurgery as part of the initial management of patients with malignant gliomas. J Clin Oncol 1992; 10:1379–1385.
34. Addesa A, Shrieve D, Alexander E, et al: Stereotactic radiosurgery as primary adjuvant treatment for glioblastoma multiforme: the JCRT update (meeting abstract). Proc Annu Meet Am Soc Clin Oncol 1995;14:A274.
35. Gannett D, Stea B, Lulu B, et al: Stereotactic radiosurgery as an adjunct to surgery and external beam radiotherapy in the treatment of patients with malignant gliomas. Int J Radiat Oncol Biol Phys 1995;33:461–468.
36. Kondziolka D, Flickinger JC, Bissonette DJ, et al: Survival benefit of stereotactic radiosurgery for patients with malignant glial neoplasms. Neurosurgery 1997;41:776–783.
37. Shrieve DC, Alexander E, Black PM, et al: Treatment of patients with primary glioblastoma multiforme with standard postoperative radiotherapy and radiosurgical boost: prognostic factors and long-term outcome. J Neurosurg 1999;90:72–77.
38. Sarkaria JN, Mehta MP, Loeffler JS, et al: Radiosurgery in the initial management of malignant gliomas: survival comparison with the RTOG recursive partitioning analysis. Radiation Therapy Oncology Group. Int J Radiat Oncol Biol Phys 1995;32:931–941.
39. Alexander E, Loeffler JS, Alexander E 3rd: Radiosurgery for primary malignant brain tumors. Semin Surg Oncol 1998;14:43–52.
40. Regine WF, Patchell RA, Strottmann JM, et al: Preliminary report of a phase I study of combined fractionated stereotactic radiosurgery and conventional

external beam radiation therapy for unfavorable gliomas. Int J Radiat Oncol Biol Phys 2000;48:421–426.
41. Regine WF, Patchell RA, Strottmann JM, et al: Combined stereotactic split-course fractionated gamma knife radiosurgery and conventional radiation therapy for unfavorable gliomas: a phase I study. J Neurosurg 2000;93(suppl 3):37–41.
42. Loeffler JS, Shrieve DC, Alexander E, et al: Radiosurgery for glioblastoma multiforme: the importance of selection criteria. Int J Radiat Oncol Biol Phys 1994;30:731–733.
43. Mehta MP, Masciopinto J, Rozental J, et al: Stereotactic radiosurgery for glioblastoma multiforme: report of a prospective study evaluating prognostic factors and analyzing long-term survival advantage. Int J Radiat Oncol Biol Phys 1994;30:541–549.
44. van Kampen M, Engenhart-Cabillic R, Debus J, et al: Stellenwert der Radiochirurgie in der Primartherapie des Glioblastoma multiforme. Heidelberger Erfahrungen im Literaturvergleich. Strahlenther Onkol 1998; 174:187–192.
45. Masciopinto JE, Levin AB, Mehta MP, et al: Stereotactic radiosurgery for glioblastoma multiforme. Stereotact Funct Neurosurg 1994;63:233–240.
46. Masciopinto JE, Levin AB, Mehta MP, et al: Stereotactic radiosurgery for glioblastoma: a final report of 31 patients. J Neurosurg 1995;82:530–535.
47. Buatti JM, Friedman WA, Bova FJ, et al: Linac radiosurgery for high-grade gliomas: the University of Florida experience. Int J Radiat Oncol Biol Phys 1995;32:205–210.
48. Shenouda G, Souhami L, Podgorsak EB, et al: Radiosurgery and accelerated radiotherapy for patients with glioblastoma. Can J Neurol Sci 1997;24: 110–115.
49. Suh JH, Barnett GH, Sohn JW, et al: LINAC-based stereotactic radiosurgery as primary adjuvant treatment for newly diagnosed malignant gliomas (meeting abstract). Proc Annu Meet Am Soc Clin Oncol 1996;15:A299.
50. Chao ST, Suh JH, Raja S: The sensitivity and specificity of FDG PET in distinguishing recurrent brain tumor from radionecrosis in patients treated with stereotactic radiosurgery. J Cancer 2001;96:191–197.
51. Graves EE, Nelson SJ, Vigneron DB, et al: A preliminary study of the prognostic value of proton magnetic resonance spectroscopic imaging in gamma knife radiosurgery of recurrent malignant gliomas. Neurosurgery 2000;46:319–326.
52. Kline JL, Noto RB, Glantz M: Single-photon emission CT in the evaluation of recurrent brain tumor in patients treated with gamma knife radiosurgery or conventional radiation therapy. Am J Neuroradiol 1996;17:1681–1686.
53. Schlemmer HP, Bachert P, Herfarth KK, et al: Proton MR spectroscopic evaluation of suspicious brain lesions after stereotactic radiotherapy. Am J Neuroradiol 2001;22:1316–1324.
54. Schwartz RB, Hsu L, Kacher DF, et al: Intraoperative dynamic MRI: localization of sites of brain tumor recurrence after high-dose radiotherapy. J Magn Reson Imaging 1998;8:1085–1089.
55. Curran WJ, Scott CB, Horton J, et al: Recursive partitioning analysis of prognostic factors in three Radiation Therapy Oncology Group malignant glioma trials. J Natl Cancer Inst 1993;85:704–710.
56. Guyatt GH, Sackett DL, Sinclair J, et al: Users' guides to the medical literature: a method for grading health care recommendations. JAMA 1995; 274:1800–1804.
57. Monroe JI, Dempsey JF, Dorton JA, et al: Experimental validation of dose calculation algorithms for the GliaSite RTS, a novel 125I liquid-filled balloon brachytherapy applicator. Med Phys 2001;28:73–85.

Comment
Chapter 12

Philip H. Gutin

Focal radiation dose escalation done in selected patients as part of their initial treatment for glioblastoma can approximately double survival (over external radiation alone). This increased survival frequently comes at the expense of brain injury and reoperation for radiation necrosis. Various stereotactic radiation technologies can be used to accomplish a focal dose boost. Brachytherapy, radiosurgery, and charged particle irradiation all seem to increase survival to approximately the same extent in selected patients.[1–3] It is disappointing that the eventual tumor regrowth, even after very large focal doses, is within the high-dose volume.[4] Higher doses to attempt to effect complete control are out of the question, because the rate of symptomatic radiation necrosis, which is already high, would be unacceptable.

The authors of this chapter have no difficulty with the prospect of using radiosurgery for palliation of recurrent malignant tumors, and, indeed, it can be a very useful modality for small tumors. Shrieve et al write that radiosurgery is equal to brachytherapy for recurrent glioblastomas in their experience, but their data show that they treated far smaller volumes with radiosurgery than with brachytherapy.[5] The low dose rate irradiation of brachytherapy would allow larger volumes to be treated than the unfavorable (to normal tissue) rapid, single high-dose fraction of radiosurgery. Tumor volumes treated with brachytherapy in this series would currently receive fractionated stereotactic or other types of conformal radiotherapy.

The authors balk at the idea of embracing radiosurgery for adjuvant radiation boosts for newly diagnosed tumors, preferring to await Class A evidence, which can only be gained through randomized trials that eliminate selection bias. Brachytherapy boosts fell into disuse, they say, after Class A evidence was available from the BTCG trial, and a similar fate may await radiosurgery. Speaking for myself, as one of the principal brachytherapy advocates of earlier decades, I did not stop using brachytherapy because of the BTCG trial, which still is not published and which contains design flaws and technical difficulties inherent to a study including 14 centers of widely differing expertise in selection, technique, and physics. I stopped doing brachytherapy because it was clear that when radiosurgery techniques and conformal radiotherapy techniques became widely available, they were far safer and easier to use in tumors of all shapes, sizes, and locations. We acknowledged early on that some of the improved survivals seen with brachytherapy boosts were due to selection bias, but patients eligible for focal stereotactic boosts of all sorts *must* be carefully selected if there is to be any sort of success.[6] The authors are anxiously awaiting an RTOG multicenter randomized trial of radiosurgery boost that could be as flawed as the BTCG brachytherapy trial.

Until we have better treatments for glioblastoma, it is completely reasonable to continue to treat selected newly diagnosed younger patients with focal radiation boosts. In certain cases, particularly in younger patients, long-term survival can be achieved.[7]

References

1. Gutin PH, Prados MD, Phillips TL, et al: External irradiation followed by an interstitial high activity iodine-125 implant "boost" in the initial treatment of malignant gliomas: NCOG study 6G-82-2. Int J Radiat Oncol Biol Phys 1991;21:601–606.
2. Shrieve DC, Alexander E III, Black PM, et al: Treatment of patients with primary glioblastoma multiforme with standard postoperative radiotherapy and radiosurgical boost: prognostic factors and long-term outcome. J Neurosurg 1999;90:72–77.
3. Fitzek MM, Thornton AF, Rabinov JD, et al: Accelerated fractionated proton/photon irradiation to 90 colbalt gray equivalent for glioblastoma multiforme: results of a phase II prospective trail. J Neurosurg 1999;91:251–260.
4. Sneed PK, Gutin PH, Larson DA, et al: Patterns of recurrence of glioblastoma multiforme after external irradiation followed by implant boost. Int J Radiat Oncol Biol Phys 1994;29:719–727.
5. Shrieve DC, Alexander E, Wen PY, et al: Comparison of stereotactic radiosurgery and brachytherapy in the treatment of recurrent glioblastoma multiforme. Neurosurgery 1995;36:275–282.
6. Florell RC, Macdonald DR, Irish WD, et al: Selection bias, survival, and brachytherapy for glioma. J Neurosurg 1992;76:179–183.
7. Sneed PK, Prados MD, McDermott MW, et al: Large effect of age on the survival of patients with glioblastoma treated with radiotherapy and brachytherapy boost. Neurosurgery 1995;36:898–904.

Chapter 13

Stereotactic Radiosurgery of Chordomas, Glomus Tumors, and Malignant Skull Base Tumors

Robert L. Foote, Bruce E. Pollock

Introduction

Chordomas, glomus tumors, and malignant skull base tumors are a rare group of tumors that share numerous common features. They arise in similar locations along the skull base and are challenging tumors to treat with acceptable morbidity because they often infiltrate surrounding bone extensively. In addition, they are adjacent to vital structures such as the carotid artery, jugular vein, and cranial nerves. Recent advances in managing these patients have included improved skull base surgical techniques and the development of charged particle therapy, stereotactic radiation therapy, and stereotactic radiosurgery. These developments have improved tumor control rates and patient survival, and have also decreased the morbidity associated with treatment.

Chordomas

Chordomas may arise from the sacrum, spine, or skull base. Skull base chordomas comprise about 40% of all chordomas, and represent 0.1 to 0.7% of all intracranial tumors.[1–4] Skull base chordomas frequently extend to involve the cavernous sinus, petrous apex, cerebellopontine angle, sphenoethmoidal area, parasellar region, and clivus. Lower clival lesions can extend to involve the nasopharynx. With invasion through the dura,

From Pollock BE (ed). *Contemporary Stereotactic Radiosurgery: Technique and Evaluation.* Armonk, NY, Futura Publishing Company, Inc. © 2002.

chordomas can encase intracerebral vessels and invade or compress the brainstem. Skull base chordomas occur in all ages, but have a peak age of presentation between 38 to 50 years. There may be a slight male preponderance.

Chordomas arise from remnants of the notochord. Hence, in the skull base they tend to arise from the clivus and dorsum sellae. There are three histologic subtypes: conventional, dedifferentiated, and chondroid. Conventional chordomas make up the majority (70–90%) of all skull base chordomas. The dedifferentiated chordomas are aggressive tumors accounting for 2 to 10% of all chordomas. They tend to recur quickly following treatment and can metastasize in 10–20% of cases. Survival can be short, with death occurring within 6 to 12 months. They commonly present as recurrences of previously treated conventional chordomas. Chondroid chordomas make up 5–15% of all chordomas. They tend to occur in a slightly younger age group and appear to have a better survival.[1,5–7] Conversely, some have reported similar or worse survival for patients with chondroid chordomas.[8,9]

The natural history of untreated chordoma has been reported as an average patient survival of approximately 2 years.[1,4] Chordomas are typically slow-growing tumors that can present with a large tumor size and minimal symptoms. The most common presenting symptoms include headache and/or diplopia as a result of abducens nerve involvement.[1,5] Less commonly affected cranial nerves include the oculomotor, trigeminal, facial, and lower cranial nerves. Visual loss is uncommon. When there is tumor extension into the lower clivus and nasopharynx, patients can present with nasal obstruction or bleeding. Useful imaging studies include computed tomography (CT) to define the extent of bony destruction, and magnetic resonance imaging (MRI), which is helpful in visualizing the tumor margins and the location of adjacent structures. Extension into the nasopharynx and cavernous sinus are also well visualized with MRI.

The primary treatment modality for skull base chordomas is surgical resection. The goal of surgery is gross total resection whenever this is technically possible. However, diffuse bone invasion and involvement of neurovascular structures precludes this degree of tumor removal and patients are frequently left with residual tumor in 25 to 100% of reported cases.[6,10–13] Three published series using surgery alone for treatment are summarized in Table 1. Five-year relapse-free survival is low (17%) as is long-term survival (5 years, 35%; 10 years, 28%).[10–12] Because incomplete tumor resection is frequent, chordoma patients are often referred for radiation therapy either postoperatively or at the time of imaging or symptomatic tumor progression. As summarized in Table 2, the addition of external beam radiation therapy (EBRT) to surgery improves disease-free and overall survival.[11,12,14–16] Traditionally, chordomas have been felt to be relatively radioresistant, and conventionally fractionated doses

Table 1
Results of Surgery Alone for Skull Base Chordomas

Institution	No. Pts.	No. Pts. GTR/ <GTR	Local Control (GTR: <GTR)	5-yr RFS	Survival Median (yr)	Survival 5 yr	Survival 10 yr
CUSM[10]	12	8/4	8/8:2/4	—	—	—	—
ABMC[11]	32	—	—	—	0.25	35%	28%
Mayo Clinic[12*]	12	0/12	—	17%	—	—	—

GTR, gross total resection; RFS, relapse-free survival; CUSM, Catholic University School of Medicine, Rome, Italy; ABMC, Allan Blair Memorial Clinic, Regina, Saskatchewan, Canada.
*0% 10-yr relapse-free survival.

of 70 to 80 Gy have been recommended for optimal tumor control. Unfortunately, such doses exceed the tolerance of the surrounding brain and cranial nerves.[7,14]

Specialized radiation delivery systems have been developed to allow the delivery of higher doses to the tumor while lowering the dose to the surrounding sensitive normal tissues. These techniques have included charged particle beams, stereotactic radiation therapy, and stereotactic radiosurgery. Table 3 summarizes the results from series using these specialized techniques either alone or combined with EBRT. Additional improvements in local tumor control, disease-free survival, and overall survival are encouraging.[17–20] Using charged particle beams, a total fractionated dose of 50 to 75 cobalt Gy can be delivered to skull base chordomas. A 63% recurrence-free survival has been reported for postoperative

Table 2
Results of Combined Surgery and Conventionally Fractionated External Beam Radiation Therapy for Skull Base Chordomas

Institution	No. Pts.	Relapse-Free Survival 5 yr	Relapse-Free Survival 10 yr	Overall Survival Median	Overall Survival 5 yr	Overall Survival 10 yr
ABMC[11]	84	—	—	NR	65%	55%
Mayo Clinic[12]	39	39%	31%	—	—	—
PMH[15]	13	—	—	5.4 yr	50%	—
FRD[16]	12	—	8%	—	58%	35%

ABMC, Allan Blair Memorial Clinic, Regina, Saskatchewan, Canada; PMH, Princess Margaret Hospital, Toronto, Ontario, Canada; FRD, Florence Radiotherapy Department, Florence, Italy; NR, not reached, >7.5 yr.

Table 3
Results of Charged Particle Beam, Stereotactic Radiation Therapy, and Stereotactic Radiosurgery for Skull Base Chordoma

Institution	Treatment	No. Pts.	Follow-up (mos)	Tumor Volume (cc)	5-yr Local Control	Overall Survival		
						Median	*5 yr*	*10 yr*
UCLBL[17]	CPB	53	51 (4–191)	—	63%	—	—	—
MGH[18*]	CPB	115	41 (5–174)	46	59%	—	80%	—
UH GCRC[19]	SRT	37	27	—	50%	—	82%	—
UPSM[20]	SRS	9	40 (6–84)	3.3 (0.98–16.3)	56%	—	—	—
Mayo Clinic	SRS	20	43.5 (13.4–116)	18.5 (2.9–65.1)	72%	—	100%	—

CPB, charged particle beam; SRT, stereotactic radiation therapy; SRS, stereotactic radiosurgery; UCLBL, University of California Lawrence Berkeley Laboratory; MGH, Massachusetts General Hospital, Harvard Medical School; UH GCRC, University of Heidelberg, German Cancer Research Center; UPSM, University of Pittsburgh School of Medicine.

*44% 10-yr local control, 80% 5-yr disease-specific survival.

residual tumors or recurrent tumors.[17] Unfortunately, radiation-related complication rates of 13 to 26% have been associated with this technique.[13,21–26] To maximize the narrow therapeutic window between tumor control and toxicity for skull base chordomas, stereotactic radiosurgery has been evaluated. The aim of radiosurgery is to provide control of tumor growth while maintaining the normal function of surrounding brain and cranial nerves. Our initial experience has been encouraging.

Between September 1990 and May 1999, 20 patients were treated with stereotactic radiosurgery using the Leksell Gamma Unit. Median patient age was 43 years with a range of 10 to 81 years. Thirteen patients were female and seven were male. Sixteen patients had undergone prior treatment, including gross total resection in two and one or more attempts at subtotal resection in 14 patients. Two patients had biopsy only and two diagnoses were based on clinical and imaging evaluation alone without histologic confirmation. All patients had clinical signs or symptoms and/or imaging studies documenting tumor progression. In general, patients with smaller tumors were selected for radiosurgery. The median largest tumor diameter was 3.9 cm (range, 1.9–6.7 cm); the median tumor volume was 18.5 cm^3 (range, 2.9–65.1 cm^3). Thus, our patients had larger tumors than the patients reported in the University of Pittsburgh radiosurgical series but were smaller than those reported in the Massachusetts General Hospital charged particle beam series.[18,20] The median tumor margin dose was 15 Gy (range, 10–20 Gy), typically prescribed to the 50% isodose line (Fig. 1).

Patients have been followed for a median of 43.5 months after radiosurgery (range, 13–116 months). Serial MRI revealed a complete tumor response in 2 patients, a partial response in 9 patients, stabilization of the tumor with no further growth in 6 patients, and progressive enlargement of the tumor in 3 patients. The 5-year local tumor control rate was 72%. Overall survival was 100% at 5 years, and 73% at 8 years. Local control was 5 of 5 patients treated with radiosurgery alone, and 12 of 15 in patients treated with EBRT followed by a radiosurgery boost. The median external beam dose delivered was 50.4 Gy. All three patients having tumor progression had undergone prior surgery (two subtotal resections, one gross total resection). The volume of these tumors were 15.6, 52.1, and 65.1 cm^3, respectively. The tumor margin doses were 12 Gy (n=2) and 13 Gy (n=1). Two of the patients died of progressive chordoma at 63 and 67 months after radiosurgery. One patient is clinically stable 21 months following radiosurgery. We analyzed patient and treatment-based factors to identify predictors of local tumor control. Factors used in the model included patient age, tumor volume, tumor diameter, dose, and gender. On univariate analysis, tumor diameter less than or equal to 5 cm and dose greater than 12 Gy were associated with improved local tumor control. However, on multivariate analysis, none of the factors analyzed were predictive for local tumor control.

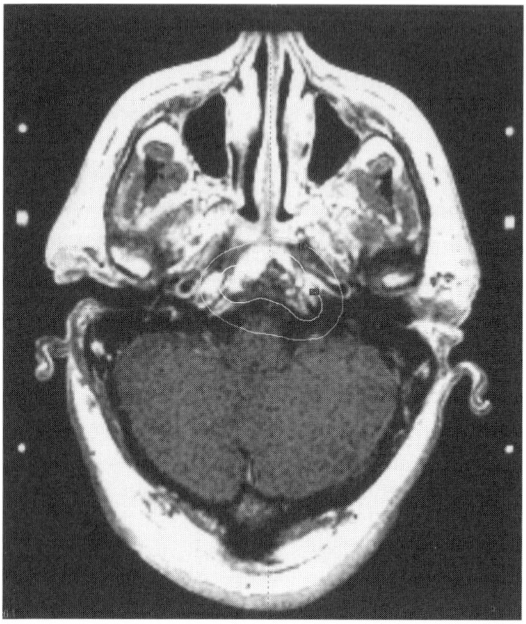

Figure 1. Dose plan for a skull base chordoma encompassed by the 50% isodose line. The minimum tumor dose (15 Gy) was prescribed to this isodose line.

Eleven of 20 patients (55%) experienced no complications from radiosurgery. Complications included a cranial nerve VI palsy (n=1, corrected with surgery), anterior pituitary dysfunction (n=2), decreased taste (n=1), and partial visual field deficit (n=1). However, the most frequent complication was radiation necrosis of the medial temporal lobe (n=4). One patient required a temporal lobectomy to relieve symptoms from mass effect. One patient with temporal lobe necrosis also developed decreased hearing and disequilibrium felt to be due to cranial nerve VIII dysfunction. All four patients developing temporal lobe necrosis also received EBRT as part of their treatment. Thus, it would appear that the combination of EBRT at 45–50.4 Gy with radiosurgical boost is associated with a significant risk of temporal lobe necrosis and pituitary dysfunction. Since all five patients treated with radiosurgery alone have experienced local tumor control, we would advise treating with radiosurgery alone without the addition of EBRT whenever possible.

While longer follow-up is needed to assess the long-term tumor control and complication rates associated with radiosurgery for skull base chordomas, our initial experience would suggest that, for tumors less than 6 cm in largest diameter, stereotactic radiosurgery is effective in preventing tumor growth in the majority of patients (72%). A minimum tumor dose of 15 Gy seems to be effective. The addition of conventionally fractionated EBRT does not seem to improve tumor control but is associated with a higher risk for temporal lobe necrosis and pituitary dysfunction. Complications may be reduced without compromising tumor control by eliminating EBRT. Physical and anatomical constraints (patient head size, extreme lateral location, inferior tumor extension below C1/C2) may limit application of this technique to all patients. Larger tumors can undergo partial tumor resection prior to radiosurgery as part of a planned staged approach for these difficult tumors.

Glomus Tumors

Glomus tumors make up a family of neoplasms that develop from the paraganglia, which are chemoreceptor organs of neural crest origin distributed throughout the body. The chief cell is probably the principal cell of origin in glomus tumors. The chief cells migrate with autonomic ganglion cells and are in close association with sympathetic ganglia, the aorta, and its main branches. Head and neck paraganglia, and their associated neoplasms, are distributed in relation to the vessels and cranial nerves of the primitive branchial arches. For this reason they are referred to as branchiomeric paraganglia. The jugulotympanic paragangliomas (glomus jugulare tumors) are related to the third gill arch and are the topic of this section. Glomus jugulare tumors arise from chief cells within the paraganglia located on the jugular bulb associated with the auricular branch of the vagus nerve. The cells of origin may function and serve as chemoreceptors which respond to changes in blood pH, oxygen, and carbon dioxide tensions, and can affect systemic blood pressure with the release of various neurotransmitters such as norepinephrine, dopamine, somatostatin, vasoactive intestinal polypeptide, and calcitonin.

Glomus jugulare tumors are the most common neoplasms in the middle ear and are second only to acoustic neuromas as the most common tumors involving the temporal bone.[27,28] The incidence has been estimated as 1 per 1.3 million people.[29] There is generally a very strong female predominance of 4:1 to 6:1.[27,30–32] Most patients present between the fifth and sixth decades of life, but patients as young as 6 months and as old as 88 years have been reported.[27,30,32,33] Bilateral glomus jugulare tumors are very rare. Glomus jugulare and carotid body tumors may occur synchronously in 7% of cases, and overall, multicentricity of paragangliomas has been reported in up to 10% of all cases.[27,34,35] Multicentric paragangliomas may be ipsilateral, contralateral, or bilateral and may arise from the glomus jugulare, glomus tympanicum, glomus vagale, or carotid body. Bilateral or multiple tumors are significantly more frequent in familial disease (31.8% of cases).[36,37] In general, glomus tumors grow slowly and metastasize very rarely.[38]

Presenting signs and symptoms depend on the size and anatomical extent of the tumor. Tumor within the middle ear often results in conductive hearing loss. Blood-tinged otorrhea, otalgia, and pulsatile tinnitus are also frequent symptoms. Auscultation may demonstrate a high pitched bruit over the mastoid. The tympanic membrane may be hypervascular, or a dark red mass may be seen in the hypotympanum. Visible margins 360° around the tumor permit the diagnosis of a glomus tympanicum tumor. Without circumferential visualization, the differentiation of tympanic from jugulare lesion is not possible on examination alone and a jugulare lesion should be expected. Cranial neuropathies involving primarily nerves VII, VIII, IX, X, XI, and XII may also be present in initial evaluation. The facial nerve is usually affected in the vertical mastoid segment rather than from intracranial extension of the tumor or brainstem compression. Hearing loss is usually conductive but can be sensorineural if there is labyrinth involvement, which can also result in vertigo. Hoarseness, dysphagia, aspiration, and/or shoulder weakness suggest lower cranial nerve involvement. A partial Horner's syndrome without facial anhydrosis is also sometimes seen with extensive tumors. Rarely, increased intracranial pressure or papilledema can result from tumor occluding a dominant sigmoid sinus. In general, there is a long duration of symptoms prior to the diagnosis being made. On average, there may be a 3.3- to 6-year interval between onset of symptoms and diagnosis with a range of 2 weeks to 42 years.[39] A history of palpitations, labile blood pressure, flushing, explosive diarrhea, headache, or excessive perspiration would indicate the possibility of a secretory tumor. This can be confirmed by measuring serum catecholamines, 24-hour urine catecholamines, vanillylmandelic acid, and metanephrines. The incidence of clinically functioning tumors is 1 to 3%.[40]

Imaging evaluation includes CT and MRI to determine the extent of bony destruction or remodeling, define the extent of the tumor, visualize nearby neural and vascular structures, and to look for other associated tumors. Glomus jugulare tumors are often intermediate signal intensity on T1-weighted MRI and are relatively bright on T2-weighted images. The tumors enhance following the administration of gadolinium. Small signal voids scattered throughout the tumor are characteristic but may not be present in small tumors. Transfemoral cerebral angiography is an integral part of the preoperative planning and assessment of glomus jugulare tumors. The uniform hypervascularity, combined with the MRI findings, make the diagnosis almost certain.

The management of glomus jugulare tumors is controversial. Observation, surgery, radiotherapy, and radiosurgery may alone or in combination be appropriate depending on the size and extent of the tumor, prior treatment, patient age, general health, and neurological condition. Yet, the uncertain natural history of untreated tumors combined with differences in patient selection and the lack of long-term follow-up of any large number of patients treated uniformly, make recommendations for the optimal treatment elusive. In our experience, surgical resection of glomus jugulare tumors has been associated with a high incidence of new postoperative cranial nerve deficits and a high rate of tumor persistence or recurrence. Between 1976 and 1998, 48 patients with 49 glomus jugulare tumors were operated at the Mayo Clinic using a combined intracranial-extracranial tumor resection. There was no operative mortality. Mean follow-up was 77.1 months with a range of 6 months to 20.5 years. New postoperative cranial nerve deficits were noted in 36 patients (74%). Cranial nerve VII was affected in 31 patients, VIII in 8 patients, IX in 3 patients, X in 17 patients, XI in 5 patients, and XII in 6 patients. Eleven patients developed tumor recurrence despite apparent gross total resection, for a local control rate of 77%.

We have had a favorable, although limited, experience using EBRT to manage patients with glomus tumors.[41] Between 1974 and 1988, 10 patients with unresectable, locally recurrent, or partially resected paragangliomas of the head and neck region underwent conventional radiation therapy at the Mayo Clinic. The median dose delivered was 46 Gy using conventional fractionation. The response to treatment could not be assessed in one patient because he died of renal failure 4 months following treatment. Follow-up among the remaining nine patients ranged from 3.5 to 16 years with a median of 7.5 years. All nine assessable patients had decreased symptoms and tumor control on follow-up imaging. Four patients had a complete response, one had a partial response, and four tumors remained stable in size. A review of all published reports of local control of paragangliomas of the head and neck region following EBRT revealed 367 of 401 patients (92%) with local tumor control. Serious complications following EBRT have included bone necrosis (1.7%), brain necrosis (0.84%), and secondary malignancy (0.28%) usually associated with using higher doses of radiation therapy.[42,43] Delayed hypopituitarism and dural necrosis with subsequent cerebral spinal fluid leak has also been reported.[44] As few patients die of residual or recurrent tumor unless there is intracranial extension,[45] the primary goal of glomus jugulare treatment should focus on reducing morbidity rather than trying to improve survival.

In discussing treatment options with patients, the risks of morbidity and mortality associated with each treatment should be discussed. The acute toxicity and chronic morbidity associated with treatment can have a significant impact on the patient's quality of life. Surgical resection can result in significant, permanent morbidity related to transection of the lower cranial nerves in as many as 50% of operated patients.[46,47] Rehabilitation often requires additional surgical procedures such as vocal cord medialization and palatal adhesion. Some young, healthy patients eventually resume adequate oral intake, but a few never attain the goal of normal swallowing. Few elderly patients resume normal oral intake.[47,48] Moreover, mortality rates up to 4% have been reported.[46,49–55] Thus, surgical resection is perhaps best indicated in patients with small tumors and functioning nerves, or larger tumors which have already caused cranial nerve deficits. Conversely, EBRT often results in acute dermatitis, alopecia, mucositis, external otitis, serous otitis media, altered taste, and xerostomia. Chronic toxicity may include brain necrosis, osteoradionecrosis of the temporal bone, mastoid sinusitis, and radiation-induced malignant disease. However, the incidence of these complications is low.[41,49,56–59] Conventionally fractionated radiation therapy has typically been reserved for symptomatic patients who are too old or too ill to undergo surgical resection, for patients whose tumors were deemed to be unresectable, and for patients with recurrent tumors following prior surgical resection. When discussing treatment options with symptomatic young patients, one needs to balance a long life of possible cranial nerve dysfunction and low risk of surgical mortality against a potential, but extremely low risk, of radiation-induced malignancy. Still, EBRT appears to offer patients long-term tumor control with little risk of cranial nerve morbidity.

Based on the results of EBRT for glomus tumors, we proposed that stereotactic radiosurgery could achieve local tumor control rates and symptom response similar to that noted with fractionated radiation therapy. Stereotactic radiosurgery would offer the advantage of a single, 1-day outpatient procedure with minimal exposure of normal tissues to radiation. As a result, the incidence of acute and chronic complications might be expected to be lower with radiosurgery compared to EBRT. Based on this rationale, we developed a prospective, institutional review board approved, clinical trial to evaluate the efficacy and toxicity of stereotactic radiosurgery in the treatment of patients with glomus jugulare tumors. Between March 1990 and December 1998, 25 consecutive patients with glomus jugulare tumors underwent stereotactic radiosurgery with a Leksell Gamma Knife Unit. Eligible patients had measurable residual, recurrent, or unresectable tumor with a maximum tumor diameter in any dimension less than or equal to 40 mm, Eastern Cooperative Oncology Group performance status (ECOG) of 0 to 2, neurological function status score of 0 to 3, and age greater than or equal to 12 years. Post-treatment evaluation included reexamination and serial scanning every 6 months for the first year, yearly for the next 2 years, and every other year thereafter.

The study group included 17 female and 8 male patients. Their ages ranged from 30 to 88 years with a median age of 62.5 years. Ten patients were 30 to 50 years old. Thirteen patients had undergone prior treatment including embolization and subtotal surgical resection in 1, subtotal surgical resection in 7, gross total surgical resection in 4, and an incomplete course of conventionally fractionated radiation therapy in 1. All patients were symptomatic or had documented tumor growth by serial imaging studies.

The treatment goal was to encompass the tumor without a normal tissue margin within the 50% or higher isodose line as imaged by stereo-

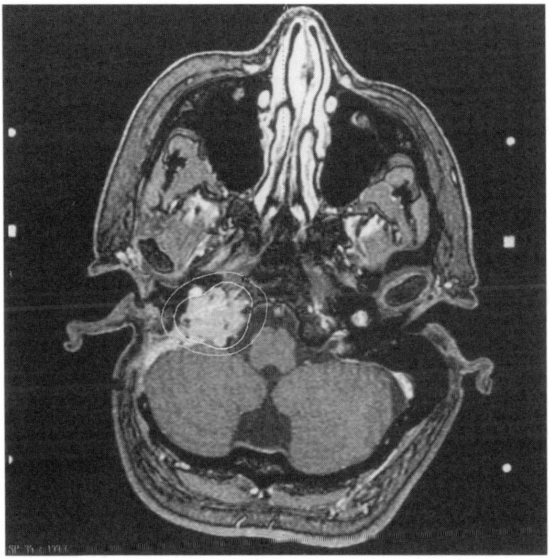

Figure 2. Dose plan for a glomus jugulare tumor encompassed by the 50% isodose line. The minimum tumor dose (15 Gy) was prescribed to this isodose line.

tactic multiplaner contrast-enhanced MRI scan (Fig. 2). The median largest tumor diameter was 3.3 cm (range, 1.7–4.7 cm). Median tumor volume was 10.4 cm^3 (range, 1.2–29.9 cm^3). The median dose delivered to the prescription isodose line was 15 Gy (range, 12–18 Gy). The median time from the date of radiosurgery to the most recent imaging follow-up was 24 months (range, 8–101 months). The median time from the date of radiosurgery to the most recent clinical follow-up was 35 months (range, 11–118 months). The first nine patients treated have a median imaging follow-up of 57 months (range, 24–101 months), and a median clinical follow-up of 67 months (range, 35–118 months).

No acute neurological toxicity was identified in this patient series. One patient who received 15 Gy to a tumor volume of 12.1 cm^3 developed significant disequilibrium 8.5 months after treatment which improved with vestibular training. This was the only neurological deficit that developed. With a median clinical follow-up of 35 months, 15 patients (60%) have reported a subjective improvement in their presenting symptoms. Eight of the first nine patients (89%) noted symptom improvement at a median follow-up of 67 months. After radiosurgery, 18 tumors have remained stable, 6 are smaller, and 1 completely resolved (Fig. 3). In the original group of 9 patients treated who have a median imaging follow-up of 57 months, 6 tumors remain stable in size, 2 are smaller, and 1 completely resolved. Three patients have died of causes unrelated to the glomus tumor: 1 of small cell lung cancer, 1 of an acute myocardial infarction, and 1 of gastrointestinal disease. The overall

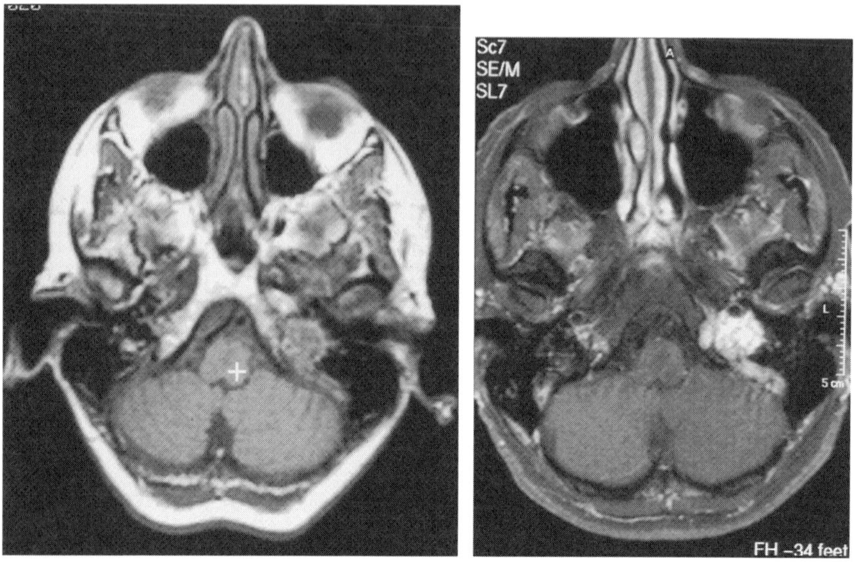

Figure 3. Axial T1-weighted MRI of a patient with a glomus jugulare tumor. (**Left**) MRI at the time of radiosurgery. (**Right**) Follow-up MRI scan 8.5 years later showing a stable tumor without growth.

5-year survival calculated using the Kaplan-Meier product limit method is 76% (±13%).

We have been able to achieve a rate of local tumor control using stereotactic radiosurgery comparable to the best surgical and conventional radiation therapy series. Table 4 outlines the published results of radiosurgery for glomus tumors.[60–63] Although it could be argued that our results merely reflect the slow growth of these tumors, we believe that radiosurgery does have an impact on the natural history of glomus jugulare tumors. In our series, all patients were symptomatic with serial imaging studies documenting progressive tumor enlargement. No patient experienced tumor growth after radiosurgery and most patients had an improvement in their symptoms. On the other hand, the majority (55%) of untreated jugulotympanic tumors will enlarge more than 20% within 4 years.[64] The median annual growth rate has been estimated at 0.8 mm, with tumor volume doubling time for untreated tumors of 13.8 years. Overall, radiosurgery is a promising new modality in the management of patients with glomus jugulare tumors and should be included in the discussion of treatment options. The early experience suggests that excellent tumor control with a low risk for cranial nerve deficits is possible. Longer follow-up will be needed to solidify radiosurgery within the treatment armamentarium for glomus jugulare tumors.

Table 4
Summary of Published Data Using Gamma Knife Radiosurgery for Glomus Tumors

Institution	No. Pts.	Follow-up (mos)	Tumor Response				Complications
			Regression	*Stable*	*Progression*	*Unknown*	
KFMS[60]	13	37.6* (5–68)	4	6	0	3	0
HNH[61]	66	24* (4–70)	19	28	0	19	3§
UTSMC[63]	8	27†(7–102)	4	3	0	1	1§
HNH[62]	14	20.5† (6–42)	4	7	0	3	3§
Mayo Clinic	25	35* (11–118)	7	18	0	0	1§

KFMS, Karl-Franzens Medical School, Graz, Austria; HNH, Hospital Na Homolce, Prague, Czech Republic; UTSMC, University of Texas Southwestern Medical Center, Dallas, TX.

*Median.

†Mean.

§Transient tinnitus, House-Brackmann Grade II facial neuropathy and deafness, House-Brackmann Grade IV facial neuropathy and vertigo; transient vertigo; decreased hearing in 3; transient vertigo.

Malignant Skull Base Tumors

The management of malignant tumors of the skull base presents a difficult challenge to physicians because many are advanced at the time of diagnosis. In addition, most persist or recur after conventional multimodality treatment including combinations of surgery, EBRT, and chemotherapy. Malignant tumors of the skull base that will be addressed in this section include malignant tumors arising from the major or minor salivary glands, advanced primary or recurrent nasopharyngeal carcinoma, advanced or recurrent squamous cell carcinoma of head and neck sites including nasal cavity and paranasal sinuses, sarcomas, and advanced or recurrent esthesioneuroblastoma.

Carcinomas of the nasal cavity, paranasal sinuses, and esthesioneuroblastomas can involve the anterior cranial base, the olfactory nerves, and frontal lobes. Vision can be affected by extension into the orbit, and nasal discharge and bleeding can occur from obstruction. Sphenoid sinus cancers, nasopharyngeal carcinoma, and adenoid cystic carcinoma can arise from the middle cranial base and extend to involve the pituitary, hypothalamus, optic nerve and chiasm, trigeminal nerve, lateral orbit, and infratemporal fossa. Chondrosarcomas can arise from and involve the posterior cranial base with involvement of the carotid and/or basilar artery, cranial nerves III through X, pons, and cerebellum. Cranial nerve involvement and bony destruction can result in craniofacial pain that can be debilitating to patients.

The optimal management of malignant skull base tumors should provide long-term tumor growth control, have minimal treatment-associated morbidity, and allow patients to return to their normal activities. Advances in neuroimaging, anesthesia, and microsurgical techniques have permitted many tumors in this region to be resected with acceptable morbidity. However, many tumors can be quite advanced and are frequently inoperable with acceptable risk. Modern skull base surgery can be performed, but because these approaches typically require extensive bone removal and often necessitate entrance into or transgression of potentially contaminated spaces, there is potential risk for complications such as cerebral spinal fluid leakage, infection, cosmetic defects, and cranial vertebral instability.[65] The exposure or manipulation of neurovascular structures also carries risks for stroke or cranial neuropathies. Cerebral spinal fluid leakage complicates cranial-based surgery in 5 to 30% of cases, whereas major neurological complications have occurred in 4 to 10% of cases.[65–67] In such cases, subtotal resection may be preferable, but tumor recurrence and progression with associated morbidity can be substantial.

Patients with large symptomatic tumors frequently undergo partial tumor resection to alleviate mass effect. This is typically followed by postoperative EBRT with or without chemotherapy depending upon the histology. Primary treatment and retreatment of malignant skull base tumors using EBRT is frequently constrained by the numerous dose-limiting structures. Treatment techniques that allow administration of higher doses of radiation are needed to optimize tumor control and survival. Stereotactic radiosurgery is one of several techniques available to accurately and precisely give additional dose, usually as a boost dose, in the advanced primary tumor setting, or as salvage treatment or palliation in the patient with recurrence following prior multimodality treatment. In the absence of distant metastatic disease, patients with recurrent or advanced malignant skull base tumors can live for extended periods, emphasizing the need for effective palliative treatments.

We have found stereotactic radiosurgery to be a valuable component of treatment for the patient with advanced, previously untreated, unresectable or subtotally resected or recurrent malignant skull base tumors.[68] Appropriate candidates for treatment should have a tumor less than or equal to 40 mm in maximum diameter and be in general good health with an ECOG performance status of 0 to 2. Between January 1990 and December 1995, we treated 24 consecutive patients with 27 tumors. There were 16 male and 8 female patients with a mean age of 56.5 years. Fifteen patients had received prior EBRT. Seven patients received EBRT following radiosurgery. One patient received EBRT both before and after radiosurgery. Tumor histology included adenoid cystic carcinoma, basal cell carcinoma, chondrosarcoma, nasopharyngeal carcinoma, osteogenic sarcoma, and squamous cell carcinoma. Tumor locations included cavernous sinus, clivus, petrous bone or apex, hypoglossal canal, and foramen rotundum.

Clinical follow-up has been available for all patients with a median of 2.3 years (range, 0.2–6.1 years). At the time of analysis, 16 of 24 patients (67%) remained alive. Follow-up imaging for these 24 patients revealed stable tumors in 12 (50%), partial regression in 3 (12.5%), complete resolution in 6 (25%), and progression in 3 (12.5%). Thus, local tumor control was 87.5%. Equally important, 16 of 18 patients (89%) with symptomatic tumors reported either a complete or partial response. All patient deaths were related to progression of their malignancies: 4 from regional progression outside of the radiosurgical treatment volume and 5 from distant metastases. No patient died from progression at the site of the radiosurgically treated lesion. Twelve patients with adenoid cystic carcinoma had 100% local tumor control at 2 years, 30% local-regional control at 2 years, and 81% 2-year survival. Eleven patients with nasopharyngeal carcinoma or squamous cell carcinoma of the head and neck region experienced an 80% 2-year local control, 30% 2-year local regional control, and 55% 2-year survival.

Table 5 summarizes the published experience of radiosurgery for skull base malignancies by tumor type and treatment technique.[69–85] These techniques can potentially deliver a high dose of radiation to a

Table 5

Local Control and Survival of Malignant Skull Base Tumors by Histology and Treatment Technique

Institution	Histology	Treatment	No. Pts.	Follow-up (mos)	Local Control Primary	Local Control Recurrent	Survival Primary	Survival Recurrent	Severe Complications
UCLBL[17*]	Nasopharynx	CPB	31	51 (4–191)	83%	45%	40%	—	15%
SUMC[69]	Nasopharynx	SRS	23	17 (1–60)	11/11	7/12	—	—	1/23
SUMC[70]	Nasopharynx	SRS	23	21 (2–64)	100%	—	—	—	0
TU[71†]	Nasopharynx	SRT	13	34 (24–65)	—	8/13	—	31%	0
UHK[72]	Nasopharynx	SRS	10	10.5 (8–27)	—	9/10	—	—	1/10
GUSM[73]	Nasopharynx	SRT	5	34 (4–61)	—	3/5	—	—	1/5
SMC[74]	Nasopharynx	SRT	3	9 (7–9)	—	3/3	—	—	0/3
UF[75]	Nasopharynx	SRS	3	9 (8–12)	—	1/3	—	—	1/3
UPSM[76]	Nasopharynx	SRS	1	7	—	0/1	—	—	0/1
MGH[77–79*]	Chondrosarcoma	CPB	200	63 (2–222)	99%		95%		8%
UCLBL[17,22,80*]	Chondrosarcoma	CPB	27	53 (4–201)	78%		83%		20–41%
UH GRC[19]	Chondrosarcoma	SRT	8	19 (up to 59)	8/8		8/8		1/8
Mayo	Chondrosarcoma	SRS	4	29 (20–85)	4/4		4/4		3/4
UCLBL[17,22,80*]	Sarcoma	CPB	19	53 (4–201)	58%		71%		20–41%
MGH[77–79*]	Sarcoma	CPB	15	40 (2–211)	59%		44%		8%
UCLBL[17*]	Salivary gland	CPB	44	51 (4–191)	58–68%		0–50%		15%
UCLBL[17*]	Paranasal sinus	CPB	22	51 (4–191)	60%		38%		15%
UG[81]	Esthesioneuroblastoma	SRS	3	50 (39–71)	3/3		—		0/3
NCCH[82]	Mixed	SRT	8	14 (6–59)	8/8		2/8		—
SUMC[69]	Mixed	SRS	29	9 (1–60)	53%		—		8.4%
UH[83]	Mixed	SRT	19	22	—		12/19		—
UPSM[84]	Mixed	SRS	12	4–17	8/8		7/12		0/12
UC[85]	Mixed	SRS	13	—	—		4/13		—

UCLBL, University of California Lawrence Berkeley Laboratory; SUMC, Stanford University Medical Center; TU, Turin University;UHK, University of Hong Kong; GUSM, Gunma University School of Medicine; SMC, Samsung Medical Center; UF, University of Florida; UPSM, University of Pittsburgh School of Medicine; MGH, Massachusetts General Hospital; UH GRC, University of Heidelberg, German Cancer Research Center; UG, University of Graz; NCCH, The National Cancer Center Hospital, Tokyo, Japan; UH, University of Heidelberg; UC, University of Cologne.

CPB, charged particle beam; SRS, stereotactic radiosurgery; SRT, stereotactic radiation therapy; Mixed, squamous cell carcinoma, rhabdomyosarcoma, adenoid cystic carcinoma, adenocarcinoma, malignant melanoma, mucoepidermoid carcinoma, sarcoma, nasopharyngeal carcinoma, salivary gland cancer, paranasal sinus cancer, chondrosarcoma.

*5-yr local control and survival.

†3-yr survival.

sharply delineated tumor volume without causing injury to normal neural structures in the region, especially when near-tolerance doses of EBRT already have been administered or are planned to be administered. This multi-institutional experience suggests that radiosurgery, when combined with surgery, EBRT and/or chemotherapy, can provide local tumor control with acceptable acute and chronic morbidity in the majority of patients with advanced or recurrent malignant skull base tumors. Local control at the skull base was excellent, and relief of symptoms occurred in the majority of patients. Continued follow-up of larger numbers of patients will be needed to draw definitive conclusions regarding long-term efficacy and toxicity.

Regional failure remains problematic in the setting of recurrent nasopharyngeal, squamous cell, and adenoid cystic carcinomas, as evidenced by the high failure rates outside the radiosurgically treated volumes for these patients. When feasible, EBRT was delivered after radiosurgery to attempt to control regional progression. However, in our experience, the goal of treatment in these patients was palliation of symptoms, and that goal was accomplished in the majority of cases.

References

1. Heffelfinger MJ, Dahlin DC, MacCarty CS, Beaubout JW: Chordomas and cartilaginous tumors of the skull base. Cancer 1973;32:410–420.
2. O'Neill P, Bell BA, Miller JD, et al: Fifty years of experience with chordomas in Southeast Scotland. Neurosurgery 1985;16:166–170.
3. Volpe R, Mazabraud A: A clinicopathologic review of 25 cases of chordoma. Am J Surg Path 1983;7:161–170.
4. Eriksson B, Gunterberg B, Kindblom LG: Chordoma: a clinicopathological and prognostic study of a Swedish National Series. ACTA Orthopedia Paedica Scandinavica 1981;52:49–58.
5. Raffel C, Wright DC, Gutin PH, Wilson CV: Cranial chordomas: clinical presentation and results of operative and radiation therapy in 26 patients. Neurosurgery 1985;17:703–710.
6. Rupa V, Rajshekhar V, Bhanu TS, Chandi SM: Primary chondroid chordoma of the skull base at the petrous temporal bone. J Laryngol Otol 1989; 103:771–773.
7. Cummings BJ, Hodgson DI, Bush RS: Chordoma: the results of megavoltage radiation therapy. Int J Radiat Oncol Biol Phys 1983;9:633–642.
8. Wold LE, Laws ER Jr: Cranial chordoma in children and young adults. J Neurosurg 1983;59:1043–1047.
9. Harbour JW, Lawton NT, Criscuolo GR, et al: Clivus chordoma: report of 12 cases and review of the literature. Skull Base Surg 1990;1:200–207.
10. Maira G, Pallini R, Anile C, et al: Surgical treatment of clival chordomas: transphenoidal approach revisited. J Neurosurg 1996;85:784–792.
11. Tai PTH, Craighead P, Bagdon F: Optimization of radiotherapy for patients with cranial chordoma: a review of dose-response ratios for photon techniques. Cancer 1995;75:749–756.
12. Forsyth PA, Cascino TL, Shaw EG, et al: Intracranial chordomas: a clinicopathological and prognostic study of 51 cases. J Neurosurg 1993;78:741–747.

13. Al-Mefty O, Borba LAB: Skull base chordomas: a management challenge. J Neurosurg 1997;86:182–189.
14. Amendola BE, Amendola AM, Oliver E, McClatchey KD: Chordoma: role of radiation therapy. Radiology 1986;158:839–843.
15. Catton C, O'Sullivan B, Bell R, et al: Chordoma: long-term follow-up after radical photon irradiation. Radiother Oncol 1996;41:67–70.
16. Magrini SM, Papi MG, Marletta F, et al: Chordoma: natural history, treatment and prognosis: the Florence Radiotherapy Department Experience (1956–1990) and a critical review of the literature. ACTA Oncologica 1992;31:847–851.
17. Castro JR, Linstadt DE, Bahary JP, et al: Experience in charged particle irradiation of tumors in the skull base: 1977–1992. Int J Radiat Oncol Biol Phys 1994;29:647–655.
18. Terahara A, Niemierko A, Goitein M, et al: Analysis of the relationship between tumor dose inhomogeneity and local control in patients with skull base chordoma. Int J Radiat Oncol Biol Phys 1999;45:351–358.
19. Debus J, Schulz-Ertner D, Schad L, et al: Stereotactic fractionated radiotherapy for chordomas and chondrosarcomas of the skull base. Int J Radiat Oncol Biol Phys 2000;47:591–596.
20. Muthukumar N, Kondziolka D, Lunsford LD, Flickinger JC: Stereotactic radiosurgery for chordoma and chondrosarcoma: further experiences. Int J Radiat Oncol Biol Phys 1998;41:387–392.
21. Castro JR, Collier M, Petti PL, et al: Charged particle radiotherapy for lesions encircling the brainstem or spinal cord. Int J Radiat Oncol Biol Phys 1989;17:477–484.
22. Berson AM, Castro JR, Petti P, et al: Charged particle irradiation of chordoma and chondrosarcoma of the base of skull and cervical spine: the Lawrence Berkeley experience. Int J Radiat Oncol Biol Phys 1988;15:559–565.
23. Habrand JL, Austin-Seymour M, Birbaum S, et al: Neurovisual outcome following proton radiation injury. Int J Radiat Oncol Biol Phys 1989;16:1601–1606.
24. Slater JD, Austin-Seymour M, Munzenrider J, et al: Endocrine function following high dose proton therapy for tumors of the upper clivus. Int J Radiat Oncol Biol Phys 1988;15:607–611.
25. Slater JM, Slater JD, Archambeau JO: Proton therapy for cranial base tumors. J Craniofacial Surg 1995;6:24–26.
26. Benk V, Liebsch NJ, Munzenrider JE, et al: Base of the skull and cervical spine chordomas in children treated by high-dose irradiation. Int J Radiat Oncol Biol Phys 1995;31:577–581.
27. Spector GJ, Gado M, Ciralsky R, et al: Neurologic implications of glomus tumors in the head and neck. Laryngoscope 1975;85:1387–1395.
28. Spector GJ, Sobol S, Thawley SE et al: Glomus jugulare tumors of the temporal bone: patterns of invasion in the temporal bone. Laryngoscope 1979; 89:1628–1639.
29. Moffat DA, Hardy DG: Surgical management of large glomus jugulare tumours: infra- and trans-temporal approach. J Laryngol Otol 1989;103: 1167–1180.
30. Alford BR, Guilford FR: A comprehensive study of tumors of the glomus jugulare. Laryngoscope 1962;72:765–87.
31. Woods CI, Strasnick B, Jackson CG: Surgery for glomus tumors: the Otology Group experience. Laryngoscope 1993;103:65–70.
32. Brown JS: Glomus jugulare tumors revisited: a ten-year statistical follow-up of 231 cases. Laryngoscope 1985;95:284–288.
33. Parkin JL: Familial multiple glomus tumors and pheochromocytomas. Ann Otol Rhinol Laryngol 1981;90:60–63.

34. Jackson CG, Glasscock ME, Harris PF: Glomus tumors: diagnosis, classification, and management of large lesions. Arch Otol 1982;108:401–406.
35. Olsen KD: Tumors and surgery of parapharyngeal space. Laryngoscope 1994;104:1–28.
36. Grufferman S, Gillman MW, Paternak LR, et al: Familial carotid body tumors: case report and epidemiologic review. Cancer 1980;46:2116–2122.
37. van Baars F, van den Broek P, Cremers C, et al: Familial non-chromaffinic paragangliomas (glomus tumors): clinical aspects. Laryngoscope 1981;91: 988–996.
38. Brown JS: Glomus jugulare tumors: methods and difficulties of diagnosis and surgical treatment. Laryngoscope 1967;77:26–67.
39. Gulya AJ, Glasscock ME, Jackson CG, et al: Skull base surgery; operative refinements. Otolaryngol Head Neck Surg 1986;94:315–321.
40. Schwaber MK, Glasscock ME, Jackson CG, et al: Diagnosis and management of catecholamine secreting glomus tumors. Laryngoscope 1984;94:1008–1015.
41. Schild SE, Foote RL, Buskirk SJ, et al: Results of radiotherapy for chemodectomas. Mayo Clin Proc 1992;67:537–540.
42. Leach W: Irradiation of the ear. J Laryngol Otol 1965;79:870–880.
43. Springate SC, Weichselbaum RR: Radiation or surgery for chemodectoma of the temporal bone: a review of local control and complications. Head Neck 1990;12:303–307.
44. Pluta RM, Ram Z, Patronas NJ, et al: Long-term effects of radiation therapy for a catecholamine-producing glomus juglare tumor. J Neurosurg 1994;80: 1091–1094.
45. van der Mey AGL, Fruns JHM, Cornelisse CJ, et al: Does intervention improve the natural course of glomus tumors? A series of 108 patients seen in a 32–year period. Ann Otol Rhinol Laryngol 1992;101:635–642.
46. Anand VK, Leonetti JP, Al-Mefty O: Neurovascular considerations in surgery of glomus tumors with intracranial extensions. Laryngoscope 1993;103:722–728.
47. Ojemann R: Skull base surgery: a perspective. J Neurosurg 1992;76:569–570.
48. Netterville JL, Civantos FJ: Rehabilitation of cranial nerve deficits after neurotologic skull base surgery. Laryngoscope 1993;103:45–54.
49. Springate SC, Haraf D, Weichselbaum RR: Temporal bone chemodectomas: comparing surgery and radiation therapy. Oncology (Huntington) 1991; 5: 131–137.
50. Watkins LD, Mendoza N, Cheesman AD, Symon L: Glomus jugulare tumours: a review of 61 cases. Acta Neurochir (Wien) 1994;130:66–70.
51. Green JD Jr, Brackmann DE, Nguyen CD, et al: Surgical management of previously untreated glomus jugulare tumors. Laryngoscope 1994;104:917–921.
52. Lenarz T, Plinkert PK: Glomustumoren des felsenbeines: operative konzept und ergebnisse. Laryngorhino-otologie 1992;71:149–157.
53. Patel SJ, Sekhar LN, Cass SP, Hirsch BE: Combined approaches for resection of extensive glomus jugulare tumors: a review of 12 cases. J Neurosurg 1994;80:1026–1038.
54. Spector GJ, Sobol S: Surgery for glomus tumors at the skull base. Otolaryngol Head Neck Surg 1980;88:524–530.
55. Gardner G, Cocke EW Jr., Robertson JH, et al: Skull base surgery for glomus jugulare tumors. Am J Otol 1985(suppl):126–134.
56. Powell S, Peters N, Harmer C: Chemodectoma of the head and neck: results of treatment in 84 patients. Int J Radiat Oncol Biol Phys 1992;22:919–924.
57. Cole JM, Beiler D: Long-term results of treatment for glomus jugulare and glomus vagale tumors with radiotherapy. Laryngoscope 1994;104:1461–1465.
58. Larner JM, Hahn SS, Spaulding CA, Constable WC: Glomus jugulare tumors: long-term control by radiation therapy. Cancer 1992;69:1813–1817.

59. Skolyszewski J, Korzeniowski S, Pszon J: Results of radiotherapy in chemodectoma of the temporal bone. Acta Oncol 1991;30:847–849.
60. Eustacchio S, Leber K, Trummer M, et al: Gamma knife radiosurgery for glomus jugulare tumours. Acta Neurochir 1999;141:811–818.
61. Liscak R, Vladyka V, Wowra B, et al: Gamma knife radiosurgery of the glomus jugulare tumour: early multicentre experience. Acta Neurochir (Wien) 1999;141:1141–1146.
62. Liscak R, Vladyka V, Simonova G, et al: Leksell Gamma Knife radiosurgery of the tumor glomus jugulare and tympanicum. Stereotact Funct Neurosurg 1998;70(suppl 1):152–160.
63. Jordan JA, Roland PS, McManus C, et al: Stereotactic radiosurgery for glomus jgulare tumors. Laryngoscope 2000;110:35–38.
64. Jansen JC, van den Berg R, Kuiper A, et al: Estimation of growth rate in patients with head and neck paragangliomas influences the treatment proposal. Cancer 2000;88:2811–2816.
65. Sen CN, Synderman CH, Sekhar LN: Complications of skull base operations. In Sekhar LN, Janecka IP (eds): Surgery of Cranial Base Tumors. New York, Raven Press, 1993, pp 831–839.
66. Gay E, Sekhar LN, Rubinstein E, et al: Chordomas and chondrosarcomas of the cranial base: results and follow-up of 60 patients. Neurosurgery 1995;36: 887–896.
67. Dolenc VV, Kregar T, Ferluga M, et al: Treatment of tumors invading the cavernous sinus. In Dolenc VV (ed): The Cavernous Sinus: A Multidisciplinary Approach to Vascular and Tumorous Lesions. New York, Springer-Verlag, 1987, pp 377–391.
68. Miller RC, Foote RL, Coffey RJ, et al: The role of stereotactic radiosurgery in the treatment of malignant skull base tumors. Int J Radiat Oncol Biol Phys 1997;39:977–981.
69. Cmelak AJ, Cox RS, Adler JR, et al: Radiosurgery for skull base malignancies and nasopharyngeal carcinoma. Int J Radiat Oncol Biol Phys 1997;37: 997–1003.
70. Tate DJ, Adler JR, Chang SD, et al: Stereotactic radiosurgical boost following radiotherapy in primary nasopharyngeal carcinoma: impact on local control. Int J Radiat Oncol Biol Phys 1999;45:915–921.
71. Orecchia R, Redda MGR, Ragona R, et al: Results of hypofractionated stereotactic re-irradiation on 13 locally recurrent nasopharyngeal carcinomas. Radiother Oncol 1999;53:23–28.
72. Chua DTT, Sham JST, Hung KN, et al: Stereotactic radiosurgery as a salvage treatment for locally persistent and recurrent nasopharyngeal carcinoma. Head Neck 1999;21:620–626.
73. Mitsuhashi N, Sakurai H, Katano S, et al: Stereotactic radiotherapy for locally recurrent nasopharyngeal carcinoma. Laryngoscope 1999;109:805–809.
74. Ahn YC, Kim DY, Huh SJ, et al: Fractionated stereotactic radiation therapy for locally recurrent nasopharynx cancer: report of three cases. Head Neck 1999;21:338–345.
75. Buatti JM, Friedman WA, Bova FJ, Mendenhall WM: Linac radiosurgery for locally recurrent nasopharyngeal carcinoma: rationale and technique. Head Neck 1995;17:14–19.
76. Kondziolka D, Lunsford D: Stereotactic radiosurgery for squamous cell carcinoma of the nasopharynx. Laryngoscope 1991;101:519–522.
77. Munzenrider JE, Liebsch NJ, Dubois W, et al: High dose fractionated combined proton and photon radiation therapy of chordoma and low-grade chondrosarcoma of the skull base and cervical spine. I. Results in adult patients. Int J Radiat Oncol Biol Phys 1991;21(suppl 1):166.

78. Munzenrider JE, Liebsch NJ, Efird JT: Chordoma and chondrosarcoma of the skull base: treatment with fractionated x-ray and proton radiotherapy. In Johnson JT, Didolkar MS (eds): Head and Neck Cancer 1993.Vol III. Amsterdam, Elsevier Science Publishers, 1993, pp 649–655.
79. Rosenberg AE, Nielsen GP, Keel SB, et al: Chondrosarcoma of the base of skull: a clinicopathologic study of 200 cases with emphasis on its distinction from chordoma. Am J Surg Path 1999;23:1370–1378.
80. Lillis-Hearne PK, Castro JR: Indications for heavy ions: lessons from Berkeley. In Linz U (ed): Ion Beams in Tumor Therapy. New York, Chapman & Hall, 1995, p 133.
81. Walch C, Stammberger H, Anderhuber W, et al: The minimally invasive approach to olfactory neuroblastoma: combined endoscopic and stereotactic treatment. Laryngoscope 2000;110:635–640.
82. Tokuuye K, Akine Y, Sumi M, et al: Reirradiation of brain and skull base tumors with fractionated stereotactic radiotherapy. Int J Radiat Oncol Biol Phys 1998;40:1151–1155.
83. Gademann G, Schlegel W, Debus J, et al: Fractionated stereotactically guided radiotherapy of head and neck tumors: a report on clinical use of a new system in 195 cases. Radiother Oncol 1993;29:205–213.
84. Firlik KS, Kondziolka D, Lunsford LD, et al: Radiosurgery for recurrent cranial base cancer arising from the head and neck. Head Neck 1996;18:160–166.
85. Kocher M, Voges J, Staar S, et al: Linear accelerator radiosurgery for recurrent malignant tumors of the skull base. Am J Clin Oncol 1998;21:18–22.

Comment

Chapter 13

Mark E. Linskey

There is a paucity of data regarding the efficacy of SRS for these types of skull base tumors. As such, this chapter by Foote et al is a welcome contribution to the growing radiosurgery literature. Paragangliomas are benign tumors that are locally aggressive and technically challenging to resect. Chordomas, on the other hand, are malignant skull base mesenchymal tumors. Chordomas are often lumped together with chondrosarcomas in order to swell patient numbers for series of rare mesenchymal skull base tumors. Despite their occurrence in similar locations, their similar neuroimaging appearance, and the possibility for both to demonstrate chondroid matrix on tissue histology, these are truly two separate disease entities with markedly different prognoses. Patients with chondrosarcoma fare much better than patients with chordoma.[1–3]

Glomus Tumors

It is rare for patients with glomus tumors to be referred for SRS. Reasons for this rarity include the fact that some glomus tumors are too large, and that some have soft tissue extensions that extend too far inferiorly into the neck at the time of diagnosis for safe and accurate SRS. However, the major reasons appear to be lack of familiarity with SRS as a therapeutic option for patients with this type of tumor, or reluctance on the part of many otolaryngologists to make the referral. One potential reason for this reluctance to recommend SRS for these patients is confusion of SRS with past experiences with fractionated radiation therapy for glomus tumors. At one time, fractionated radiation therapy was experimented with, and even advocated for, glomus tumors. Despite reports to the contrary,[4,5] the results of fractionated radiation therapy were considered to be disappointing. Tumor control was perceived to be permanent only rarely, and the resulting reactive fibrosis surrounding the extracranial cervical portion of the tumor rendered cranial nerve preservation at subsequent surgery, when tumor growth resumed, even more problematic. As a primary treatment modality, fractionated radiotherapy fell from favor for all but patients who were too ill or elderly to safely undergo microsurgical resection. Fractionated radiation therapy was also tried as a preoperative adjunctive therapy to attempt to reduce bleeding at subsequent surgery. The development of intravascular preoperative embolization techniques, as well as improvements in skull base microsurgical techniques, made this practice obsolete.

As neoplastic targets for SRS, glomus tumors would seem to be ideal. They are well circumscribed and make fine neuroimaging targets with clear, well-defined margins. Glomus tumors are benign, with low proliferative indices, and likely to behave as late-responding tissue to the effects of radiation. As such, we would expect high-dose single-fraction radiation to have a marked biological advantage with a corresponding greater therapeutic effect than fractionated approaches. Finally, these are highly vascular tumors, and would presumably be very susceptible to additional secondary therapeutic benefits from radiosurgery-induced vascular obliteration. The results from the Mayo Clinic presented in this chapter are extremely encouraging and support continued investigation of SRS for this tumor type.

Chordomas

Chordomas are malignant mesenchymal tumors. Local control measures such as microsurgery or SRS are not likely to be sufficient to maximize long-term tumor control. As "low-grade" malignancies, they have intermediate proliferative indices and presumably have intermediate alpha/beta ratios. Thus, fractionated radiation therapy is likely to provide a biological advantage to supplement either resection or SRS.

To date, proton beam treatment has been the most popular form of fractionated radiotherapy for patients with chordoma.[3,6] There are two potential reasons for preferring proton beam over photon irradiation. The first is the ability of the Bragg-peak effect to allow more conformal dose planning, thereby better limiting dose to adjacent structures. The second is a purported biological advantage of protons over photons for improved biological effect on tumor tissue for any given dose of radiation. This relative biological effect in favor of proton irradiation is solely based upon in vitro cell culture studies and in vivo animal studies, and has been approximated to be 1.1 for protons versus photons.[7] As a result, proton doses are reported in terms of "cobalt gray equivalents." However, we must keep in mind that, to date, there has been no clinical study in humans to confirm the laboratory findings of a greater relative biological effect of protons over photons, or to demonstrate improved tumor control for protons over photons once radiation dose is taken into account.

The argument over which local control measure should predominate–microsurgery or SRS–prior to fractionated radiotherapy is highly controversial. For tumors that are too large for primary SRS, we recommend a microsurgical approach. In this setting, SRS is reserved for any residual tumor identified on postoperative imaging (present in 33–56% of patients, even in the best microsurgical hands[1,2]). For smaller recurrent tumors with previously established histology, mounting data (including this chapter) suggest that SRS may provide an attractive, effective, and lower morbidity alternative to open microsurgery for providing local control.[8,9] Without tissue histology, it is almost impossible to distinguish skull base chordomas from skull base chondrosarcomas by neuroimaging criteria alone. In clinical situations where this distinction will alter the choice of future treatment, skull base microsurgery remains preferred.

The advent of SRS has certainly impacted intraoperative skull base microsurgical strategy. If only 80 to 90% of a tumor can be removed at surgery, it becomes far more important to remove 100% of the tumor from 80 to 90% of the original tumor volume, than to remove 80 to 90% from all involved regions. Second stage SRS can handle the remaining 10 to 20% of the original volume, but cannot treat the whole resection bed if the original volume is too large. Recurrence outside the SRS target volume but within the original microsurgical bed remains a serious concern. The issue of optimal targeting remains problematic (especially after prior microsurgery), and I strongly recommend relying on information from both CT and MRI for optimal targeting.

The authors present a series of 20 patients treated with SRS with a 5-year local control rate of 72%, and survival rates of 10% and 73% at 5 and 8 years, respectively. While these results are both impressive and encouraging, I disagree with the authors that one should consider eliminating adjunctive fractionated radiotherapy in these patients with malignant mesenchymal tumors. This is particularly true for patients treated with SRS after prior microsurgical subtotal resection since the whole resection bed (even without neuroimaging tumor mass) may be contaminated with microscopic disease. I do agree that conventional fractionated radiation therapy with traditional ports and wedges should be eliminated as a treatment modality for this disease.

Other Malignant Skull Base Tumors

In the last section of the chapter, the authors discuss a very heterogeneous group of "other" skull base malignancies with numbers for each histology too small for meaningful subset analysis. I would have preferred keeping basal cell carcinoma, chondrosarcoma, and even adenoid cystic carcinoma as a separate group. Each of these three tumor types are locally aggressive "low-grade" malignancies, where long-term control and survival are now possible with appropriately aggressive skull base microsurgical resection. They are quite different from squamous cell carcinoma and nasopharyngeal carcinoma where a beneficial survival role for aggressive cranial base microsurgery has yet to be proven, and where subtotal "debulking" has little, if any, role.

For "low-grade" skull base malignancies and anterior cranial base "high-grade" skull base malignancies, in our practice, SRS is used as an alternative to microsurgery in patients who are too ill or elderly to safely undergo microsurgical resection and for patients who refuse open microsurgery despite their candidacy. We also use SRS in conjunction with open microsurgery if we are not successful at achieving gross total imaging resection with the microsurgical attempt. For "high-grade" skull base malignancies involving deeper and more dangerous skull base regions, SRS has all but replaced open microsurgery as the treatment of choice for obtaining immediate local tumor control in our practice. Others are now reporting encouraging results using SRS as an alternative to skull base microsurgery in this clinical setting.[10,11] For those lesions that are too large for SRS alone, we now routinely resect the extradural tumor volume and treat the higher morbidity intradural and/or skull base component with SR. The SRS stage is performed first, in order to ensure tumor control short of the brainstem, prior to exposing the patient to the potentially higher risks of open skull base microsurgery of the extradural component. The results are often dramatic (particularly for sinonasal or mucinous carcinoma), with significant tumor shrinkage usually visible by neuroimaging within 2 months of treatment. Unfortunately, this response is not sustained, as the authors have shown, with loss of local control in 70% of patients by 2 years after SRS. For these patients, SRS is an effective but temporary palliative procedure with a lower morbidity than open microsurgical resection.

Another issue is how to treat patients with squamous cell carcinoma, nasopharyngeal carcinoma, or adenoid cystic carcinoma, who have no imaging evidence of cavernous sinus disease–but on histology after extradural orbital exenteration or infratemporal fossa resection are found to have perineural involvement or even positive microscopic trigeminal nerve margins. In these patients, we have begun prospectively targeting the trigeminal nerve from the pons, though the ganglia and the intracavernous course of all three divisions of the trigeminal nerve with SRS, and limiting fractionated radiation therapy fields to the extradural resection bed. Whether or not this approach will be effective remains to be seen.

References

1. Al-Mefty O, Borba LAB: Skull base chordomas: a management challenge. J Neurosurg 1997;86:182–189.
2. Gay E, Sekhar LN, Rubinstein E, et al: Chordomas and chondrosarcomas of the cranial base: results and follow-up of 60 patients. Neurosurgery 1995; 36:887–896.
3. Hug EB, Loredo LN, Slater JD, et al: Proton radiation therapy for chordomas and chondrosarcomas of the skull base. J Neurosurg 1999;91:432–439.
4. Cole JM, Beiler D: Long-term results of treatment for glomus jugulare and glomus vagale tumors with radiotherapy. Laryngoscope 1994;104:1461–1465.
5. Evenson LJ, Mendenhall WM, Parsons JT, et al: Radiotherapy in the management of chemodectomas of the carotid body and glomus vagale. Head Neck 1998;20:609–613.

6. Austin-Seymour M, Munzenrider J, Goitein M, et al: Fractionated proton radiation therapy of chordoma and low-grade chondrosarcoma of the base of the skull. J Neurosurg 1989;70:13–17.
7. Miller DW: A review of proton beam radiotherapy. Med Phys 1995;22: 1943–1954.
8. Kondziolka D, Lunsford LD, Flickinger JC: The role of radiosurgery in the management of chordoma and chondrosarcoma of the cranial base. Neurosurgery 1991;29:38–46.
9. Muthukumar N, Kondziolka D, Lunsford LD, et al: Stereotactic radiosurgery for chordoma and chondrosarcoma: further experiences. Int J Radiat Oncol Biol Phys 1998;41:387–392.
10. Chua DT, Sham JS, Hung KN, et al: Stereotactic radiosurgery as a salvage treatment for locally persistent and recurrent nasopharyngeal carcinoma. Head Neck 1999;21:620–626.
11. Tate DJ, Adler JR Jr, Chang SD, et al: Stereotactic radiosurgical boost following radiotherapy in primary nasopharyngeal carcinoma: impact on local control. Int J Radiat Oncol Biol Phys 1999;45:915–921.

Chapter 14

Stereotactic Radiosurgery for Refractory Trigeminal Neuralgia

Kris A. Smith, C. Leland Rogers

Introduction

Trigeminal neuralgia (TN), or tic douloureux, is a chronic, progressive, facial pain syndrome, which most often begins in the sixth or seventh decades of life but may also occur in younger patients. It affects about 4.3 per 100,000 people annually.[1] The severity of the pain can be debilitating or even cause suicide. Trigeminal neuralgia can involve one or more divisions of the trigeminal nerve and is characterized by five classic features as described by White and Sweet: paroxysmal, provokable, unilateral, confined to the trigeminal nerve domains, and unassociated with gross trigeminal motor or sensory loss.[2]

The etiology of TN has been ascribed to a blood vessel compressing the trigeminal root at its junction with the pons, thus altering axonal transmission.[3] The absence of demonstrable compression on imaging studies does not rule out this pathophysiological anatomic relationship because the nerve irritation could be caused by vessels too small to be resolved by magnetic resonance imaging (MRI). Other known causes of TN include multiple sclerosis and, rarely, mass lesions such as tumors or aneurysms. High-resolution, thin-slice MRI should therefore be obtained from patients with TN to rule out a mass lesion, or to identify patients with multiple sclerosis before nonpharmacological therapy is considered. Clearly evident vascular compression may sway the surgeon to recommend microvascular decompression (MVD).

From Pollock BE (ed). *Contemporary Stereotactic Radiosurgery: Technique and Evaluation.* Armonk, NY, Futura Publishing Company, Inc. © 2002.

Treatment of Trigeminal Neuralgia

Several potentially successful therapeutic maneuvers are available for patients with TN. Pharmacological therapy is considered the appropriate initial modality. Carbamazepine (Tegretol) and gabapentin (Neurontin) are the most effective medicines. An initial response to these medicines when narcotics have failed helps to assure the diagnosis. Phenytoin (Dilantin), amitriptyline (Elavil), and Baclofen have also been helpful in some patients. With medical treatment, many patients experience only partial relief, develop recurrent pain after an initial favorable response, or suffer intolerable side effects such as lethargy, imbalance, ataxia, or even bone marrow suppression. An invasive neurosurgical procedure, open or percutaneous, is often the next line of treatment and alleviates pain in most individuals. The most common procedures are (1) MVD performed through a small retrosigmoid craniotomy; (2) percutaneous glycerol rhizotomy; (3) percutaneous radiofrequency thermal rhizotomy; and (4) percutaneous balloon compression.

Each treatment has distinct advantages and disadvantages and a proven track record in alleviating pain. Only MVD addresses the cause of the pain and is therefore potentially curative. The other procedures are palliative and rely on selectively damaging the nerve to decrease its sensitivity to external stimuli and thereby diminish or eliminate the pain. Microvascular depression provides excellent pain relief without damaging the nerve itself. Facial numbness is thereby avoided. Microvascular depression, however, is an open surgical procedure involving critical structures and is therefore associated with the highest risk of all the options. Still, the risk of serious complications such as stroke or death is less than 1%. The recurrence rate associated with MVD is also less than that associated with the palliative procedures.

Since the percutaneous procedures damage the nerve on purpose, they cause some degree of facial numbness. Needle insertion through the face into the foramen ovale of the skull base is used for all these procedures and is associated with a slight risk of infection, bleeding, or other complications. The most feared complications of these procedures are related to the degree of anesthesia produced as a result of the nerve damage. Loss of the corneal blink reflex risks the development of keratitis. Rarely, painful numbness or anesthesia dolorosa occurs and is a miserable condition with no effective treatment. Thermal rhizotomy is associated with a pain-free response rate (90%) that rivals MVD. However, this procedure produces the most numbness and has the highest risk (1–2%) of keratitis and anesthesia dolorosa. Depending on the volume of glycerol injected, glycerol rhizotomy produces less numbness than these other procedures and is associated with a low risk of complications. However, its recurrence rate is high, and repeated treatments are often required. Balloon compression has not gained widespread popularity, possibly due to a reportedly high rate of mastication muscle dysfunction, but it is the treatment of choice in some centers.

Recently, Gamma Knife radiosurgery has emerged as a viable therapeutic option for TN. It may accomplish similar rates of pain relief with lower rates of morbidity than invasive techniques. Indeed, one of stereotactic radiosurgery's earliest applications was for TN when Lars Leksell treated several patients with this disorder[4] using a prototype device in the early 1950s. The current Gamma Knife system uses the same convergent beam technology originated by Dr. Leksell.

Significant improvements, however, permit easy and precise targeting and delivery of a small 4-mm isocenter to the trigeminal nerve root entry zone. Advances in MRI technology that permit high-resolution, thin-slice imaging with three-dimensional reconstruction and stereotactic registration and localization make this procedure possible. Such pinpoint precision depends greatly upon quality control of MRI, including precise shimming to assure a lack of magnetic distortion. Some centers have recommended coregistration with computed tomographic (CT) scanning to assure a lack of distortion. We have performed CTs on some patients for this purpose and found it unnecessary when MRI is performed carefully.

The Leksell stereotactic frame is critically important for the procedure. The frame serves as the basis of the stereotactic coordinate system for targeting the nerve. Skull radii measurements are also based on the frame to ensure accurate calculations of the radiation absorption and therefore accurate dosing for each patient. Furthermore, the frame eliminates movement of the patient's head during treatment.

The Gamma Knife Procedure

We place the stereotactic frame while the patient is briefly anesthetized intravenously by an anesthesiologist, usually with a combination of midazolam (Versed) and propofol (Diprovan). Local anesthetic, a 50% mixture of 0.5% lidocaine, 0.5% bupivacaine, and 1:400,000 epinephrine, is infiltrated into the subcutaneous tissue at the pin insertion sites. No hair is cut or shaved, and no head preparation is required other than morning shampoo and Betadine gel at the pin entry points. With this protocol, the patient experiences no pain or discomfort, and frame application typically requires only several minutes. We have had no frame- or anesthesia-related complications in more than 800 (total indications, including 127 for TN) patients treated at our center.

The patient undergoes MRI immediately after the frame is placed and may be further sedated if claustrophobic. The MRI protocol is a nonenhanced, spoiled grass, gradient echo axial format with contiguous 1-mm thick slices for three-dimensional reconstruction. Quality control measurements are taken on the MRI console directly to assure correct measure-

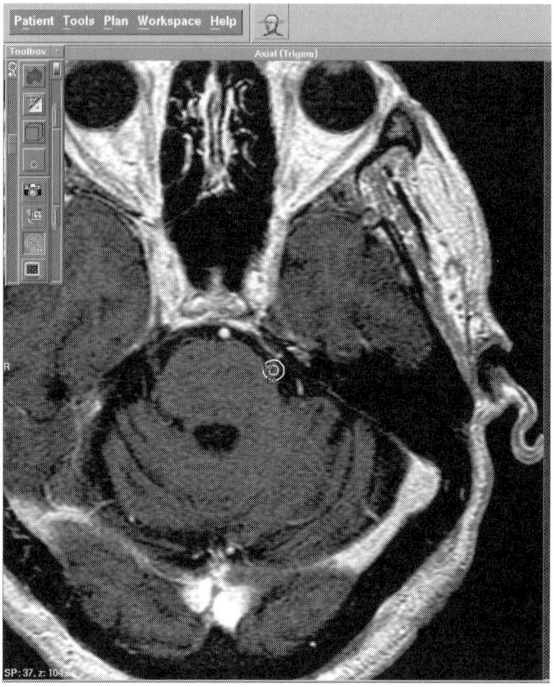

Figure 1. Gamma plan for a typical patient with trigeminal neuralgia. The trigeminal nerve is clearly visualized in the axial, sagittal, and coronal planes. The 4–mm isocenter is placed so that the 50% isodose line grazes the brainstem, and the 90% isodose line is centered on the nerve in all three planes.

ments of the known intrafiducial distances on the attached localizing fiducial box. The box is attached to the frame temporarily during the MRI. These measurements assure that the periphery of the image is undistorted.

The images are transferred over the network to the Gamma Knife workstation, which utilizes the GammaPlan™ software. The images are then registered stereotactically and checked. The software enables a highly magnified image to be viewed in all three planes simultaneously. The trigeminal nerve root entry zone is easily identifiable for targeting. The dose matrix is centered over the target so that the computer can calculate the dose. A single 4-mm isocenter is placed so that the 50% isodose line touches the pons, and the 90% line is central on the nerve in all three planes (Fig. 1). Lens plugs are placed so that any beams that would pass directly through the lenses of the eyes can be blocked separately to minimize the risk of cataract formation. The dose is then chosen, and the computer calculates the time required for the prescribed dose to be delivered. Typical treatment times range from 40 to 60 minutes depending on the dose, size of the patient's head, and age of the cobalt sources in the Gamma Knife unit.

Barrow Neurological Institute Experience

We reviewed our initial experience with Gamma Knife radiosurgery for patients with TN, with regard to efficacy, complications, factors that could influence the likelihood or extent of pain relief, and the incidence or severity of complications. These preliminary results have been published elsewhere.[5] The series is reviewed below, including a new objective rating scale that improves the assessment of the comparative efficacy of this treatment.

Methods

The Gamma Knife facility at the Barrow Neurological Institute (BNI) became operational on March 17, 1997. As of October 2000, 822 patients had been treated, 127 for TN. Four patients with a mass lesion in the trigeminal pathway associated with their facial pain were excluded from this analysis. The first 54 patients (33 females, 21 males) with idiopathic TN (i.e., no obvious anatomical abnormality) treated through March 31, 1999 were the subject of the preliminary report (Table 1).[5] The median duration of follow-up was 12 months (range, 3–28 months). The median age at the time of Gamma Knife treatment was 67 years (range, 43–89 years). Forty-three (80%) patients had typical trigeminal pain, and 11 (20%) had atypical pain defined as any deviation from the features described by White and Sweet.[2] The most common atypical feature was persistent baseline pain in addition to the paroxysmal exacerbations. Ten patients (19%) had multiple sclerosis.

All patients were unresponsive or refractory to optimal or maximal pharmacological therapy or were experiencing unacceptable side effects. Twenty-five (46%) patients had undergone one or more prior invasive treatments (Tables 1 and 2), whereas 29 (54%) received Gamma Knife radiosurgery as their first treatment after pharmacological management failed.

Table 1
Number of Prior Invasive Procedures in 25 Patients with Trigeminal Neuralgia

No. of Prior Procedures	*No. of Patients (%)*
1	8 (32)
2	8 (32)
3	5 (20)
4	3 (12)
≥ 5	1 (4)

Table 2
Types of Prior Invasive Surgery in 25 Patients with Trigeminal Neuralgia

Type of Prior Procedure	*No. of Procedures*
Microvascular decompression	9
Thermal rhizotomy	20
Glycerol rhizotomy	19
Balloon compression	3
Lytic peripheral nerve procedures	5

Patients were treated in a uniform fashion according to two sequential protocols. The first 41 received 35 Gy at the 50% isodose via a single 4-mm collimator targeting the ipsilateral trigeminal nerve adjacent to its root entry zone (i.e., the proximal extent of the affected trigeminal nerve at its juncture with the pons). Given the lack of adverse events observed with 35 Gy, the prescription dose was systematically increased to 40 Gy beginning December 1, 1998. The isodose (50%), collimator size (single 4 mm), and target location remained constant.

Outcome was evaluated by a standardized questionnaire filled out by each patient, independent of input from physicians or other care providers. The questionnaires were mailed to each patient at 6-month intervals and also given to patients at follow-up visits. The response rate was 100%. All patients, except one who died of unrelated causes, are still alive and under continued follow-up care. Pain was gauged by each patient according to the BNI Pain Intensity Score developed for this study (Table 3). Patients assigned themselves a Pain Intensity Score before Gamma Knife treatment, at each follow-up assessment after Gamma Knife, and before and after any previous invasive surgical therapy. Before treatment, all patients reported a BNI Pain Intensity Score of V (severe). A BNI Facial Numbness Score (Table 4) was also developed.

Table 3
Barrow Neurological Institute Pain Intensity Score and Distribution of Post-Treatment Scores

BNI Score	*Criteria*	*No. of Patients (%)*
I	No trigeminal pain, no medication	19 (35)
II	Occasional pain, not requiring medication	3 (6)
III	Some pain, adequately controlled with medication	26 (48)
IV	Some pain, not adequately controlled with medication	4 (7)
V	Severe pain/no pain relief	2 (4)

BNI, Barrow Neurological Institute.

Table 4
Barrow Neurological Institute Facial Numbness Scale and Distribution of Post-Treatment Scores*

BNI Score	*Criteria*	*No. of Patients (%)*
I	No facial numbness	0
II	Mild facial numbness, not bothersome	5 (14)
III	Facial numbness, somewhat bothersome	0
IV	Facial numbness, very bothersome	0

BNI, Barrow Neurological Institute.
*Based on 37 patients with no facial numbness before treatment.

Clinical follow-up was scheduled at 6-month intervals. Imaging evaluations were not routinely undertaken because no patient with a mass lesion in association with TN was included in the study group. Statistical analysis was completed using the MEDLOG Clinical Data Management System (Information Analysis Corp., Incline Village, NV). The Fisher's exact test was used to determine differences between proportions, and the nonparametric Wilcoxon test was used to determine the statistical significance of differing distributions among variables.

Several variables that might be expected to influence outcomes were subjected to univariate analysis: age, gender, pain features (typical vs. atypical), prior invasive procedures, number of prior invasive procedures, response to prior invasive procedures, multiple sclerosis, number of trigeminal divisions involved, presence of numbness before Gamma Knife treatment, and new or worse numbness after Gamma Knife. Each was analyzed for a possible correlation with initial response, recurrence, and complications.

Results

Initial Pain Response

Of the 54 patients, 52 (96%) reported that their level of pain improved after Gamma Knife treatment (Table 3). Nineteen (35%) were rendered pain-free and were able to stop all TN medications. Three patients (6%) required no medications and experienced only occasional tolerable pain. Twenty-six patients (48%) remained on medications but considered their pain adequately controlled. Four patients (7%) reported that their pain had improved after Gamma Knife treatment, but they did not regard it as adequately controlled. Pain failed to improve in two (4%) patients.

If pain relief is based on patients' no longer needing medication, 22 (41%) patients had a dramatic response (BNI Pain Score I or II). Another

16 (30%) patients decreased their medication intake by at least 50% of their pretreatment dose.

Patients who reported complete resolution of their pain, but who remained on TN medication, were assigned a BNI Pain Score of III, even if they were tapering medication intake. Of the 26 patients with a BNI Pain Score of III, 19 reported that their pain had fully resolved after Gamma Knife treatment. They continued on pharmacological therapy due to their apprehension about recurrent pain without medication.

Pain Response Timing

Patients were questioned about the timing of the initial onset of pain relief and of maximal relief. The timing of initial relief ranged from immediate (24 hours) to 192 days, with a median of 15 days. The timing of maximal relief ranged from immediate to 253 days, with a median of 63 days. Seventeen patients (31%) reported that their pain improved immediately after radiosurgery. Of these 17 patients, nine (53%) had BNI Pain Scores of I and stopped their TN medication immediately. One (6%) patient had a BNI Pain Score of II, six had BNI Pain Scores of III, and one had a BNI Pain Score of IV.

Pain Recurrence

Recurrence was defined as any worsening of pain from the maximal level of relief. Any patient who resumed pharmacological therapy after having stopped TN medications was considered a recurrence, even if pain was later controlled again. By these criteria 11 patients experienced a recurrence. Two patients who did not respond to Gamma Knife treatment were excluded, creating a gross recurrence rate of 21%. The actuarial rate of pain recurrence at 2.5 years for the entire patient group was 36%.

Patients with a good initial response were less likely to develop recurrent pain than patients who responded less favorably. Among the 19 patients with a BNI Pain Score of I, only one developed recurrent TN. Of the three patients with a BNI Pain Score of II, none developed recurrent pain. Of the 26 patients with a BNI Pain Score of III, six experienced a recurrence as did each of the four patients with an initial BNI Pain Score of IV. Of the 22 patients (5%) who stopped TN medications after Gamma Knife treatment, only one (5%) has had recurrent trigeminal pain compared to 10 of 30 patients (33%) who were unable to stop pharmacological therapy. This difference was significant at $p=0.030$.

Complications

The only complication observed with any of the 54 patients was delayed, partial facial sensory loss (Table 4). Before Gamma Knife treatment, 17 (31%) of the 54 patients had facial numbness from a previous invasive procedure, seven (41%) of whom rated their numbness as BNI Facial Numbness Scores of III or IV. None of these 17 patients reported a worsened facial numbness score after radiosurgery. Of the 37 patients who had no facial numbness at the time of Gamma Knife treatment, five (14%) developed new numbness. Each rated their new numbness as a BNI Facial Numbness Score of II ("mild facial numbness, not bothersome"). No patient without preexisting numbness has reported a BNI Numbness Score of III or IV as a result of Gamma Knife treatment.

Univariate Analysis

No statistically significant relationships were identified using overall response (BNI Pain Score I–IV), pain recurrence, or complications as endpoints. This result likely reflects the size of the patient population (n=54), the small number of patients with no response (n=2), and the relatively few patients with either recurrent pain (n=11) or complications (n=5).

When a univariate analysis was undertaken with dramatic response (BNI Pain Score I or II) as the endpoint, three variables worthy of mention emerged. There is a suggestion that the number of trigeminal divisions involved may be predictive outcome (p=0.065). Patients with pain in a single trigeminal division had a 53% dramatic response rate compared to 41% in patients with two divisions involved and 13% of those with all three divisions involved.

Two variables reached statistical significance. Patients with typical pain features had a 49% dramatic response rate compared to 9% of those with atypical features (p=0.040). The univariate finding with the greatest degree of statistical significance was the development of new facial numbness. Patients with new numbness after Gamma Knife treatment experienced a 100% rate of dramatic pain relief compared with 35% of patients with no new numbness (p=0.019).

Discussion

Several surgical treatments can be used to treat TN refractory to medical therapy with excellent success rates. These treatments, however, lead to different complications and rates of pain recurrence (Table 5). Although each of the standard invasive alternatives has documented efficacy, the anatomical location of the surgical "target" along the trigeminal pathway has varied.

Surgical Treatment

As many as 50,000 craniotomies for MVD have been undertaken[3] to address a vessel compressing the trigeminal nerve, the putative offending

Table 5
Treatment Results from Pooled Large Series

Outcome	*Radiofrequency Rhizotomy (n = 6205) (%)*	*Glycerol Rhizotomy (n = 1217) (%)*	*Balloon Compression (n = 759) (%)*	*Microvascular Decompression (n = 1417) (%)*	*Gamma Knife* (n = 54) (%)*
Initial pain relief	98	91	93	98	96
Pain recurrence	23	54	21	15	21
Facial numbness	98	60	72	2	9
Anesthesia dolorosa	1.5	1.8	0.1	0	0
Corneal anesthesia	7	3.7	1.5	0.05	0
Perioperative morbidity	1.2	1	1.7	10	0
Mortality	0	0	0	0.6	0

Adapted and modified with permission from Taha and Tew.[23]
*Present series.

anatomical anomaly. The "target" is a vessel that will be surgically separated from the trigeminal nerve near its junction with the pons (i.e., the trigeminal root entry zone). The concept of neurovascular compression was first described in 1934 by Dandy,[6] but has been advanced most ardently by Jannetta.[7] The actual intraoperative incidence of finding a significant offending vessel ranges from the 96% reported by Jannetta[8] to 11% described by Adams et al.[9] As reviewed thoroughly by Hamlyn,[3] most series report vascular compression in about 80 to 95% of cases (median, 88%), lending credence to a neurovascular etiology and to the nerve root entry zone as an appropriate target.

Other surgical options, now predominantly percutaneous, involve some degree of damage to the trigeminal nerve. Thermal lesioning, glycerol injections, and balloon compression are each accomplished by introducing a needle percutaneously into the buccal soft tissues, through the foramen ovale, and into Meckel's cave. There, the Gasserian ganglion is lesioned thermally, chemically, or mechanically.[10] Although percutaneous treatments do not directly address an explicit etiology for TN, their target, the Gasserian ganglion, is located about 2 cm anterior to the trigeminal root entry zone.

Radiosurgical Treatment

In 1949 Lars Leksell applied his first-generation radiosurgical device to the treatment of TN and initially targeted the Gasserian ganglion. He anecdotally reported long-term pain relief in several patients.[4,11,12] As data from more centers and larger patient groups have become available, radiosurgery is being accepted into the standard armamentarium. Young et al[13,14] from the Northwest Neurosciences Institute and Kondziolka et al, reporting the experience of the University of Pittsburgh[15,16] and of a multicenter study,[17] have documented the safety and relative efficacy of Gamma Knife treatment. In these reports, as in the present series, the radiosurgical target was the trigeminal root entry zone, mirroring the microsurgical experience.

The optimal target, the appropriate dose, and the mechanism of treatment effects are issues that need further elucidation. Inconsistent results from radiosurgical series targeting the Gasserian ganglion led to the conclusion that the ganglion may be an inappropriate target.[18,19] Moreover, Barbaro et al[20] reported that dose to the root entry zone correlated with pain response. Patients were treated with a 4-mm collimator and 70-Gy maximum dose to the trigeminal nerve adjacent to the pons. These investigators recognized some variation in individual doses to the root entry zone itself and found that patients who received a higher dose to the point of calculation were more likely to have an excellent pain response after treatment.

Hochman[21] published a case report suggesting the need for a dose ceiling. He identified a patient with paroxysmal involuntary jaw clenching 6 months after the second of two Gamma Knife procedures within a 6-month period. The combined radiosurgery maximum dose was 160 Gy, each prescribed as 40 Gy at the 50% isodose with a 4-mm isocenter at the root entry zone.[21] The patient had failed radiofrequency lesioning before the first Gamma Knife treatment. After the second Gamma Knife treatment, the patient's pain completely ceased but new delayed facial hypesthesia developed. The total dose reported by Hochman exceeds the doses typically used for second Gamma Knife procedures. Young has used 35- to 40-Gy maximum doses for second procedures[22] compared to 80 Gy in the Hochman report. Anecdotally, we have treated a single patient to a total maximum dose of 150 Gy (35 Gy at 50% isodose with a 4-mm isocenter for initial treatment and 40 Gy at the 50% isodose for recurrence) with no such sequela and no other overt adverse events. The issue of dose will require careful refinement over time.

Taha and Tew published the long-term outcome of their extensive experience with radiofrequency rhizotomy and surveyed the literature, combining results from larger series on posterior fossa exploration (MVD and/or partial surgical trigeminal rhizotomy) and percutaneous techniques (Table 5).[23] We lack the extended follow-up compiled by Taha and Tew but have defined pain relief and recurrence conservatively. Patients in the larger radiosurgery series (Table 6) were treated in similar fashion: 70 to 90 Gy (maximum dose) were delivered through a single 4-mm shot directed toward the trigeminal nerve near its junction with the pons. Pain

Table 6
Comparative Gamma Knife Series

	No. of Patients	*Maximum Dose (Gy)*	*Median Follow-Up*	*% Pain-Free*	*% Good Relief BNI I–III*†*	*Onset of Pain Relief*	*% Relapse*	*% Complications*
Young et al[13]	110	70–80	19.8 mos‡	76	88	14 days‡	34	2.7
Kondziolka et al[15]	106	70–90	18 mos	60	77	4 wks	10	10
Kondziolka et al[17]	50	60–90	18 mos	58	94	1 mo	6	10
Rogers et al§	54	70–80	12 mos	35*	89	15 days	21	9

*Includes approximations of percentages of patients with BNI Score I–III relief from other series.

†BNI Pain Intensity Score (see Table 2).

‡Mean.

§BNI, present study.

relief (by estimation) was good (BNI Pain Score I–III) in 88 to 94% of the patients: 35 to 76% of patients became pain-free. The lowest figure is from our series and likely reflects the stringent requirement that patients scored as pain-free (BNI Pain Score of I) no longer take medications for TN. If this criterion is eliminated, 70% of our patients were rendered pain-free after Gamma Knife treatment (19 patients with a BNI Pain Score of I and 19 patients with a score of III who reported no pain but who remained on TN medication).

Complications of Treatment

The complications of invasive treatments for TN include facial numbness, corneal anesthesia, the formidable and essentially untreatable anesthesia dolorosa, and the uncommon but certainly not negligible general perioperative risks for morbidity and mortality. In contrast, the risks of complications from radiosurgical series have been consistently low and limited to delayed, partial facial sensory loss. Moreover, these alterations in facial sensation have been mild (Table 2). Neurological complications other than facial hypesthesia have been noticeably lacking. Anesthesia dolorosa has not been reported as a consequence of Gamma Knife treatment. However, a few patients with dysesthetic facial sensations after Gamma Knife treatment were discussed at the meeting of the American Association of Stereotactic and Functional Neurosurgery Society in Snowbird, Utah in 1999. With the exception of the single case of jaw clenching reported by Hochman,[21] no other neurological sequelae have been reported, as have no systemic sequelae.

In our series, five patients developed new facial numbness after radiosurgery. However, none of the 17 patients with numbness from prior invasive procedures reported worsening numbness after Gamma Knife treatment. In fact, the only complication—new numbness—as positively correlated with an excellent response and thus may be considered desirable. None of the five patients with new numbness found it bothersome. Each stopped all TN medications and experienced excellent pain relief. This association between facial numbness and improved outcome corroborates the experience with percutaneous techniques but begs the question of whether higher doses might improve initial response rates and the duration of response without causing an unpleasant degree of hypesthesia.

Predicting Outcomes

Pain features may also predict initial response rates. Patients with atypical pain were less likely to have a dramatic response (BNI Pain Score I or II) to Gamma Knife therapy and to stop TN medications than those with typical trigeminal pain (9% vs. 49%, respectively; $p=0.040$). This relationship was suggested by Young et al[13] but was not found to be significant. Our data also suggest that the number of trigeminal divisions involved may influence response (p=0.065). This finding is perhaps intuitive, but needs further follow-up and confirmation. Conceivably, these and other factors could eventually be grouped to identify patients who would most benefit from radiosurgery or those who might profit from individualized treatment (e.g., higher doses or targeting a greater length of the nerve).

These concepts are presently being tested clinically. We have increased the dose to the trigeminal root entry zone to 45 Gy at the 50% isodose without altering the location of the target. Although increasing the prescription dose effectively broadens the length of nerve that is treated, we have not specifically attempted to target longer lengths of the nerve. This latter approach is being evaluated in a trial at the Mayo Clinic.

Conclusion

With many available therapeutic options, it is sometimes difficult to choose a treatment for an individual patient. Although Gamma Knife radiosurgery is a safe and effective treatment for refractory TN, it is not necessarily the best initial treatment for all patients. For younger patients, MVD may still be the best initial treatment because the possibility of recurrent pain requiring multiple treatments over the remaining life expectancy would be undesirable. This consideration would be especially important if each additional treatment increased the degree of facial numbness or the risk of anesthesia dolorosa. Microvascular depression is also associated with a higher initial rate of being pain-free and a lower recurrence of pain than Gamma Knife treatment. Furthermore, patients are more likely to be medication-free after MVD. This issue may be important for younger patients at greater risk for developing long-term cumulative side effects such as cerebellar atrophy from medications, especially when decades may elapse before the side effects manifest.

However, Gamma Knife radiosurgery is also an effective treatment, especially for older patients, those with a medical condition that would increase their risk of morbidity or mortality from a surgical procedure, or those unwilling to undertake the higher risks associated with an open surgical procedure. It is the least invasive nonpharmacological treatment for TN and has the most favorable side-effect profile for both recurrent or persistent pain after prior invasive therapy or as the initial treatment. It carries a small risk (10%) of delayed facial sensory loss, typically mild, and of minimal consequence to patients. It has no other apparent sequelae when administered in the manner described. Ironically, the only side effect that we have observed (mild, new facial hypesthesia) may be desirable because it correlates with an excellent pain response. Ultimately, the treating neurosurgeon must present all viable options to patients and make an individualized recommendation so that patients understand the relative risks and benefits of each treatment option and are comfortable with their choice.

Further investigations are needed to answer questions about dosing and targeting and to identify patients likely to benefit from this treatment or its modifications. Additional long-term follow-up data will be important to compare Gamma Knife treatment with the more established treatment modalities in terms of pain recurrence and long-term efficacy. The BNI scoring systems presented here for pain intensity and facial numbness have proved simple and reliable, facilitating data collection, rendering analysis more objective, and improving our ability to discuss results with colleagues and patients.

References

1. Bowsher D: Trigeminal neuralgia: an anatomically oriented review. Clin Anat 1997;10:409–415.
2. White JC, Sweet WH: Pain and the Neurosurgeon: A Forty-Year Experience. Springfield, IL, Charles C. Thomas, 1969, pp 123–178.
3. Hamlyn PJ: Neurovascular relationships in the posterior cranial fossa, with special reference to trigeminal neuralgia. 1. Review of the literature and development of a new method of vascular injection-filling in cadaveric controls. Clin Anat 1997;10:371–379.
4. Leksell L: The stereotaxic method and radiosurgery of the brain. Acta Chir Scand 1951;102:316–319.
5. Rogers CL, Shetter AG, Fiedler JA, et al. Gamma knife radiosurgery for trigeminal neuralgia: the initial experience of the Barrow Neurological Institute. Int J Radiat Oncology Biol Phys 2000;47:1013–1019.
6. Dandy WE: Concerning the cause of trigeminal neuralgia. Am J Surg 1934;24:447–455.
7. Jannetta PJ: Cranial rhyzopathies. In Youmans JR (ed): Neurologic Surgery. 3rd Edition. Philadelphia, WB Saunders, 1990, pp 4169–5182.
8. Jannetta PJ: Treatment of trigeminal neuralgia by micro-operative decompression. In Youmans JR (ed): Neurologic Surgery. 3rd Edition. Philadelphia, WB Saunders, 1990, pp 3928–3942.
9. Adams CB, Kaye AH, Teddy PJ: The treatment of trigeminal neuralgia by posterior fossa microsurgery. J Neurol Neurosurg Psychiatry 1982;45: 1020–1026.
10. Shetter A: Denervating neurosurgical procedures for trigeminal neuralgia. In Carter LP, Spetzler RF (eds): Neurovascular Surgery. New York, McGraw-Hill, 1995, pp 1101–1106.
11. Leksell L: A stereotactic apparatus for intracerebral surgery. Acta Chir Scand 1949;99:229–233.
12. Leksell L: Sterotaxic radiosurgery in trigeminal neuralgia. Acta Chir Scand 1971;137:311–314.
13. Young RF, Vermulen S, Posewitz A: Gamma knife radiosurgery for the treatment of trigeminal neuralgia. Stereotact Funct Neurosurg 1998;70(suppl): 192–199.
14. Young RF, Vermeulen SS, Grimm P, et al: Gamma Knife radiosurgery for treatment of trigeminal neuralgia: idiopathic and tumor related. Neurology 1997;48:608–614.

15. Kondziolka D, Perez B, Flickinger JC, et al: Gamma knife radiosurgery for trigeminal neuralgia: results and expectations. Arch Neurol 1998;55: 1524–1529.
16. Kondziolka D, Lunsford LD, Flickinger JC: Gamma knife radiosurgery as the first surgery for trigeminal neuralgia. Stereotact Funct Neurosurg 1998; 70(suppl):187–191.
17. Kondziolka D, Lunsford LD, Flickinger JC, et al: Stereotactic radiosurgery for trigeminal neuralgia: a multiinstitutional study using the gamma unit. J Neurosurg 1996;84:940–945.
18. Lindquist C, Kihlstrom L, Hellstrand E: Functional neurosurgery: a future for the gamma knife? Stereotact Funct Neurosurg 1991;57:72–81.
19. Rand RW, Jacques DB, Melbye RW, et al: Leksell Gamma Knife treatment of tic douloureux. Stereotact Funct Neurosurg 1993;61(suppl):93–102.
20. Barbaro N, Sneed P, Ward M, et al: Radiosurgical treatment of trigeminal neuralgia: pain relief correlates with root entry zone dose (abstract). Neurosurgery 1999;45:737.
21. Hochman SM: Jaw clenching following gamma knife treatment for trigeminal neuralgia (letter). Neurology 1998;50:1193–1194.
22. Young RF: Jaw clenching following gamma knife treatment for trigeminal neuralgia (letter). Neurology 1998;50:1194.
23. Taha JM, Tew JM Jr: Comparison of surgical treatments for trigeminal neuralgia: reevaluation of radiofrequency rhizotomy. Neurosurgery 1996;38: 865–871.

Comment

Chapter 14

Kim J. Burchiel

In this chapter, Smith and Rogers have reviewed the literature on Gamma Knife radiosurgery for the treatment of trigeminal neuralgia and contributed new data from their clinic at the Barrow Neurological Institute.

I must say at the outset that I am fairly dubious of the unique merits of Gamma Knife radiosurgery for this condition. This chapter highlights some of the issues that make this treatment still somewhat controversial, at least in my mind.

The authors emphasize that procedures other than MVD are "palliative and rely on selectively damaging the nerve to decrease its sensitivity to external stimuli and thereby diminish or alleviate the pain." They assert that these percutaneous procedures "damage the nerve on purpose" and have the mixed benefit of alleviating the pain and occasionally, when used in excess, produce deafferentation pain, i.e., anesthesia dolorosa, or rarely corneal keratitis. The point that has mystified me most about the discussions of Gamma Knife radiosurgery for trigeminal neuralgia is that somehow it is treated as other than a neurolytic procedure, which it clearly is. The degree of deafferentation from Gamma Knife radiosurgery is minimal to moderate as is the pain response. In my opinion, Gamma Knife radiosurgery follows the same rule that any neurolytic procedure does. That is, the more numbness that is produced by the neurolytic procedure, the longer the period of pain relief and the higher the level of complications from deafferentation. In my own experience, corneal keratitis is almost unheard of with a percutaneous procedure, but can certainly be seen after complete trigeminal rhizotomy. Thus, the benefits of a neurolytic procedure are quantitative. It comes as no surprise to the experienced neurosurgeon that damaging a substantial part of the trigeminal nerve results in relatively little sensory loss. This is borne out by experience with both percutaneous radiofrequency rhizotomy and open posterior fossa rhizotomy. It is also well known that minimal injury to the nerve can result in prolonged pain relief, exemplified by the Taarnhoj procedure where the nerve was simply stroked or compressed, rather than cut. Clearly, minimal injury to the nerve is capable of alleviating the pain for periods of years.

The data from BNI suffer from a lack of interpretable presentation and short follow-up. The authors cite a "median duration of follow-up" of 12 months (range, 3–28 months). Without presenting a life table analysis

(Kaplan Meier curve), this data is simply misleading. In an aggressive and expanding program, short follow-up periods often dominate the population.

The outcome from Gamma Knife radiosurgery at the BNI is also quite modest. Only 41% of patients had a dramatic enough response to no longer require medication. Forty-eight percent of their population remained on medication but "consider their pain adequately controlled."

As with other series, there was latency period in the response to Gamma Knife radiosurgery, with a median of 15 days. Again, the reader is left "in the dark" about the actual temporal distribution of pain responses.

Despite a short follow-up, 11 patients experienced recurrence with a cumulative recurrence of 21%. The actuarial rate of pain recurrence at 2.5 years for the entire patient group was 36%. As with other treatments for trigeminal neuralgia, patients with typical pain features had a better response than those with atypical features.

In terms of complications, five patients in this series developed new facial numbness after radiosurgery. This complication "was positively correlated with an excellent response and thus may be considered desirable." The neurolytic effect is clearly beneficial in this series, as it has been in any other ablative procedure used for the treatment of trigeminal neuralgia, as noted above.

The authors conclude by stating that "further investigations are needed to answer questions about dosing and targeting to identify patients likely to benefit from this treatment or its modifications." I could not agree more. What continues to baffle me about the use of Gamma Knife radiosurgery is that a clearly ablative procedure, with all the attendant risks and benefits, can be considered "one of several viable neurosurgical options" for trigeminal neuralgia. The noninvasiveness of the procedure is somewhat misleading and, at the same time, seductive. The cost of the procedure will certainly never compare favorably to an outpatient radiofrequency lesion or glycerol injection. No author claims that Gamma Knife radiosurgery is curative; however, many patients undergo this procedure for primary surgical treatment of their trigeminal neuralgia and will never have a potentially "curative" operation (MVD) performed as a result. There is no doubt that further studies are required, but the efficacy of this procedure should be compared with that of other ablative operations, and possibly even MVD, with regard to both long-term outcome and cost.

Chapter 15

Stereotactic Radiosurgery for Epilepsy and Movement Disorders

Douglas Kondziolka, Dhruv Singhal, Ajay Niranjan, L. Dade Lunsford

Introduction

The origin of stereotactic radiosurgery parallels the developmental history of functional neurosurgery. Leksell initially conceived the idea of closed-skull, single-session irradiation of a precisely defined intracranial target in 1951.[1] He applied this concept immediately to functional neurosurgery. At that time, functional destruction of normal brain required thermal energy, or chemical injection such as phenol. Leksell crossfired photon or proton radiation beams to achieve a similar goal. The initial radiosurgical concept was to create *small,* precisely defined focal destruction of a functional target, which was defined by image guidance. Contrast encephalography provided relative identification of such targets. Leksell first coupled an orthovoltage x-ray tube to his early generation stereotactic frame.[2] Later, he worked with physicist Borje Larsson to crossfire proton beams generated by a cyclotron or photon beam produced by a modified linear accelerator.[3]

The first Gamma Knife collimator helmets created a discoid volume of focal irradiation that could "section" white matter tracts or brain tissue in a manner similar to a leucotome or other instrument. Not until 1975 were circular collimators used to create more spherical radiation volumes better suited to the management of brain tumors or vascular malformations. The genesis and initial goals of radiosurgery were concentrated on the development of a new tool for functional neurosurgery. This chapter

From Pollock BE (ed). *Contemporary Stereotactic Radiosurgery: Technique and Evaluation.* Armonk, NY, Futura Publishing Company, Inc. © 2002.

will review the use of radiosurgery for the established indication of movement disorder surgery, and for a new indication, epilepsy management. Both indications aim to affect discrete regions of neuronal hyperactivity.

Dose Selection for Parenchymal Radiosurgery

The radiosurgical ablative dose for brain tissue had been estimated using animal models.[3–5] Initial patients who had radiosurgery for tissue ablation received maximum doses of 100 to 250 Gy. At small volumes, doses in excess of 150 Gy provided consistent tissue necrosis in animal models.[4,5] Correspondingly, patients treated in initial studies received doses at or above that level and Steiner et al recommended doses of 160 to 180 Gy for creation of thalamic lesions in cancer patients.[6] Although information was available on dose effects, little was known regarding the time required for necrosis to occur. Clinical data showed that pain relief occurred usually within 3 weeks after radiosurgery. In rat experiments with 200 Gy using a single 4-mm isocenter, we found a consistent dose-volume relationship that substantiated observations from the human study.[7] Doses of 200 Gy using a 4-mm collimator were delivered to the rat frontal brain and the brain was subsequently studied at 1, 7, 14, 21, 60, and 90 days after irradiation. At 1 and 7 days, the brain continued to appear normal. By 14 days, the parenchyma appeared slightly edematous within the target volume. However, by 21 days, a complete circumscribed volume of necrosis was identified within the radiation volume. This remained consistent thereafter (Fig. 1). Thus, the clinical observation of pain relief at 21 days noted by Steiner et al was correlated with laboratory findings at the 200-Gy dose.

The ablative radiosurgery lesion appears as a punched-out, circumscribed volume of complete parenchymal necrosis with cavitation. Within a 1- to 3-mm rim that characterizes the steep fall-off in radiation dose, normalization of the tissue appearance is found. In this zone, blood vessels appear thickened and hyalinized, and often protein extravasation can be identified. The brain is edematous in this region, either from an increase in extracellular fluid, or from the intracellular swelling of gliosis. Acute or chronic inflammatory cells are present. Magnetic resonance imaging (MRI) demonstrates all of these features after radiosurgical thalamotomy–a sharply defined, contrast-enhanced rim that defines the low-signal lesion (on short TR images) surrounded by a zone of high-signal (on long TR images) brain tissue.[8] Friehs and colleagues collected imaging data from four centers that created functional radiosurgery lesions (n=56).[9] They found that maximum doses in excess of 160 Gy were more likely to produce lesions larger than expected and recommended a single 4-mm isocenter and doses below 160 Gy.

Although a higher dose creates necrosis more rapidly, such a dose is not *necessary* for necrosis. Because patients who undergo functional radio-

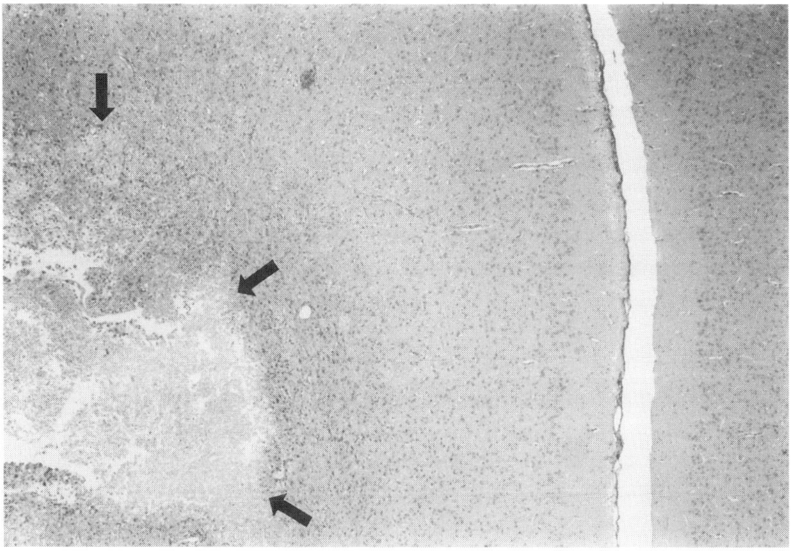

Figure 1. Coronal section of the frontal region of the rat brain 150 days after 150–Gy radiosurgery using a single 4–mm isocenter (H & E, 10x). A 4-mm diameter area of focal necrosis is identified (arrows) with a sharp border between the target and the surrounding normal brain.

surgery (for movement disorders, psychiatric disorders, or noncancer pain) have a chronic illness, it may be that lower and potentially safer doses are warranted. In both large and small animal models, doses at or above 100 Gy cause necrosis, but it takes longer for the necrosis to develop.[7,10,11] To identify the effect of increasing volume, we used an 8-mm collimator in a baboon model. We found that half of the animals developed an 8-mm diameter necrotic lesion at doses as low as 50 Gy.[11,12] Dose, volume, and time are the three key factors that determine the nature of the functional ablative lesion. Once created, this lesion remains stable over years.[4,13]

The limitation of radiosurgery technology as a "lesion generator" stems from the inability to reliably control the effects of dose and volume. When a larger brain target may be desirable, the sharp fall-off in dose outside the target becomes less steep with increasing volume. The risk of adverse radiation effects outside the target volume becomes problematic.[14] At small volumes (ie., single 4-mm collimator), the radiosurgery-created lesion appears reliable.

Imaging in Functional Surgery

Since physiological information is excluded from the targeting component of a functional radiosurgery procedure, high-quality stereotactic neuroimaging must be performed. The imaging must be accurate since small volumes are irradiated. In addition, the imaging must be of sufficient resolution to identify the target structure but also show important regional tissues. Magnetic resonance imaging is the preferred imaging tool for functional radiosurgery.[15–17]

Accurate stereotactic MRI-based localization should be confirmed at each institution.[16] Although some centers fuse MRI data with computed tomography (CT) data, many groups believe this unnecessary once the accuracy and precision of MRI is confirmed at the users center. Computed tomography poorly shows most functional targets such as the trigeminal nerve, basal ganglia, or thalamus, and should not be used as the sole method of planning unless the patient has a contraindication to MRI. Contrast-enhanced, volume acquisition MRI sequences divided into 1-mm slice thicknesses provide graphic definition of nerve and brain structures. The addition of fast inversion recovery MRI sequences helps to separate gray and white matter structures and has been an important improvement in thalamotomy and pallidotomy targeting for radiofrequency electrode-based surgery or radiosurgery. Despite these imaging improvements, the targeting of physiologically abnormal brain regions such as groups of kinesthetic thalamic tremor cells using imaging alone remains indirect. Dose planning during radiosurgery for patients with epilepsy is based on anatomical information derived from MRI.

Radiosurgical Thalamotomy

Ventrolateral thalamotomy for the management of tremor related to Parkinson's disease remains a proven and time-honored procedure within functional neurosurgery. Traditionally, thalamotomy has involved imaging definition of the thalamic target, placement of an electrode into the thalamus, physiologic recording and stimulation at the target site, and creation of a lesion. Radiosurgical thalamotomy by definition avoids placement of the electrode and evaluation of the physiologic response. In radiosurgery, imaging definition alone is used to determine lesion placement. Through the use of contrast ventriculography, CT, and more recently stereotactic MRI, thalamotomy using the Gamma Knife has been performed at centers around the world.[15,17–23] Many surgeons currently believe that although *adequate* results might be obtained by radiosurgery, *better* results are likely after radiofrequency electrode ablation. Insufficient data exists to resolve this discussion. The challenges inherent in choosing the best possible ablative target using imaging are significant. Radiosurgical thalamotomy, if performed, should be performed by surgeons experienced in radiofrequency thalamotomy.

Due to the absence of electrophysiological information, the inability to stop or vary the lesion volume during surgery, and the latency until the clinical response, most surgeons use radiosurgery primarily for patients with associated medical risks (i.e., coagulopathy). In such cases stereotactic electrode placement may be too risky. Ohye first advocated radiosurgical thalamotomy contralateral to a prior radiofrequency lesion, or to enlarge a previously mapped lesion.[18] Others have investigated the utility of radiosurgical thalamotomy for Parkinson's tremor or essential tremor in order to eliminate the hemorrhagic risks occasionally seen after conventional thalamotomy. Duma et al reported a 5-year experience with 38 Gamma Knife thalamotomies.[15] Complete tremor abolition was noted in 24%, excellent relief in 26%, good improvement in 29%, and little to no benefit in 21%. The median time to improvement was 2 months. They used a dose range of 110 to 165 Gy with better results at higher doses. Such higher doses may exert effects on a larger surrounding tissue volume of kinesthetic tremor cells (outside the sharply defined necrotic volume). The larger volume translates into tremor reduction and overcomes any limitations in target selection. Young et al reported that 88% of 27 patients who had radio surgical thalamotomy for tremor (120–160 Gy) became tremor-free or "nearly" tremor-free.[17] Hirato et al also found tremor suppression after Gamma Knife thalamotomy in a small patient series.[18] Friehs et al reported an experience of radiosurgical thalamotomy (n=3) and caudatotomy (n=10) with clinical improvement in most patients and no morbidity.[24]

Between April 1996 and August 2000, 36 Gamma Knife thalamotomy procedures were performed in 35 patients at the University of Pittsburgh. Eighteen patients had essential tremor, five had multiple sclerosis-related tremor, and 15 had Parkinsonian disease.[20] The median age of patients was 75 years (range, 38–92) and the median duration of tremor was 10 years (range, 1–25). Target localization of the ventralis intermedius nucleus of the thalamus was determined by the coordinates based on the position of the nucleus relative to the anterior commissure-posterior commissure (AC-PC) line. This target was localized on 1-mm thick, gadolinium-enhanced MRI slices. Further target adjustments relative to the internal capsule as projected on axial and coronal fast inversion recovery images were made. The final target coordinates for radiosurgery were validated using GammaPlan® software.

The usual target position was one-fourth of the AC-PC distance anterior to the PC. In the left-right dimension, we selected a point at half the width of the third ventricle plus 11 mm from the AC-PC line. The radiosurgery isocenter (4-mm collimator) was placed 2-mm superior to the AC-PC line, so that the inferior portion of the radiosurgery lesion would extend inferiorly to the AC-PC line. The 30% isodose line was placed medial to the edge of the internal capsule. Radiosurgery thalamotomy was performed using the Leksell Gamma Knife Model U (Elekta Instruments, Atlanta, GA). A median dose of 140 Gy (range, 130–150 Gy) was delivered.

The onset of response was noted between 1 week and 6 months (median, 6 weeks) after radiosurgery. Two patients died of unrelated illness

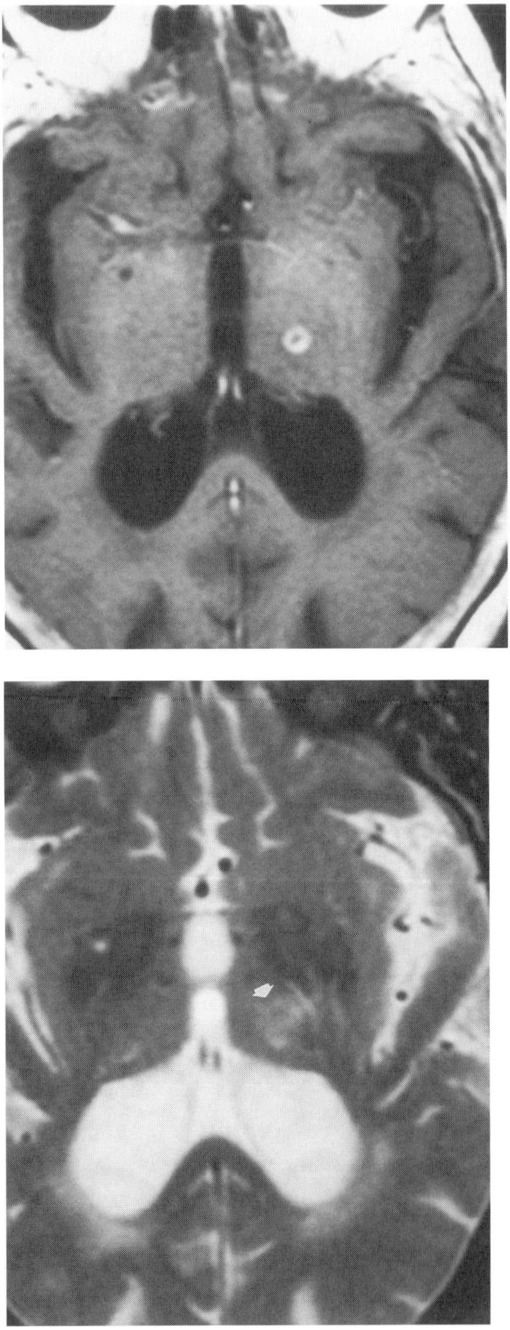

Figure 2. Axial (**Top**) short TR and long TR (**Bottom**) MRI 4 months after Gamma Knife radiosurgery with 140 Gy (one 4-mm isocenter) for a ventrolateral thalamotomy in a 92-year-old woman with essential tremor. She had significant improvement in tremor and resumed handwriting. Note how the signal change on the long TR image (arrow) is larger than the necrotic volume and may impact positively on tremor cells.

after radiosurgery. Eighteen of 27 evaluable patients (67%) reported excellent tremor control (complete arrest or more than 90% relief) (Fig. 2). Seven of 27 (26%) had good control of tremor (50–90% improvement). One patient had no improvement at 6 months. One patient who had significant tremor relief at 3 months and had improvement in daily activities (eating, dressing) began to notice recurrent tremor that returned to the initial state after 9 months. Three patients noted transient weakness of the contralateral upper limb (6–8 months after radiosurgery), which improved with temporary corticosteroid medication.

Radiosurgical Pallidotomy

The increased use of electrode-based stereotactic pallidotomy for patients with advanced Parkinson's disease has received great attention since 1992. Some investigators have performed Gamma Knife pallidotomy using image-guidance alone as an alternative to electrode techniques. Rand et al reported their preliminary results after radiosurgical pallidotomy and noted relief of contralateral rigidity in 4 of 8 patients.[25] No patient in their series sustained a complication. Friedman et al reported on four patients after Gamma Knife pallidotomy (180 Gy) with improvement in only one patient.[26] They noted heterogeneity in lesion volumes on MRI, a finding also documented by others. In contrast to the thalamus, where small radiosurgery lesions appeared consistent, pallidotomy lesions may be more variable due to effects on perforating arteries that supply that region of the basal ganglia. It has been suggested that iron deposition (a potential radiation sensitizer) in the pallidum of elderly patients might lead to variability in the lesion volume. The lesion volumes and contrast-enhancement patterns seem less consistent.[17] At our center only one radiosurgical pallidotomy has been performed. That patient had a basal ganglia venous malformation that precluded placement of an electrode. In our experience, the low morbidity of conventional pallidotomy, deep brain stimulation, or thalamotomy has not provided an argument for a less invasive surgical procedure that excludes information provided by electrophysiological mapping.

Radiosurgery for Epilepsy

Epilepsy affects 1% of the population. Eighty percent of epileptic patients will respond to medical treatment, and the remaining 20%, who have medically intractable epilepsy, should be considered for surgical evaluation. Thirty-three to fifty percent of medically intractable epilepsies can be successfully treated with surgery.[27] Classification of the different forms of epilepsy is important for surgical consideration. In accordance with the International Classification of Epilepsies and Epileptic

Syndromes, epilepsy is categorized as focal, generalized, of undetermined origin, or due to other syndromes.[28] The difference between focal and generalized epilepsy is of particular importance in the consideration of surgery. Focal epilepsies, also called partial epilepsies, originate from a lesion or localized region which is usually restricted to one hemisphere of the brain. Generalized epilepsies are bilateral and cannot be localized to any particular focus or foci.

The goal of surgical intervention is removal of the epileptogenic zone. Surgery for focal epilepsy usually involves resection of a focus. Radiosurgery would involve irradiation of that focus. Surgery for generalized epilepsy may include disconnection procedures such as corpus callostomies and multiple subpial transections. According to the International League Against Epilepsy global survey report from 1997, 91% of surgical procedures are performed for epilepsy of focal origin.

Techniques for Localization of the Epileptic Focus

Optimal success in focal epilepsy surgery is achieved by removing the least amount of cerebral tissue while completely removing the epileptogenic zone.[29] Localization techniques are crucial in determining the location and extent of the epileptogenic zone. Different localization techniques are used to converge on the lesional zone, primary epileptogenic zone, functional deficit zone, and the irritative zone. Although the lesional zone and epileptogenic zones tend to be closely related, it is possible that these zones are exclusive of one another. The tissue around visible pathology, and not the pathology itself, is often the zone of epileptogenesis. Localization techniques help to clarify these zones. These distinctions may be particularly important in radiosurgery, since irradiation of larger tissue volumes can be associated with increased risk.

Magnetic resonance is the superior imaging technique for patients with focal epilepsies.[30] MRI is useful for visual imaging of structural abnormalities other brain disorders such as mesial temporal sclerosis (MTS). Thin-section coronal images of mesial temporal structures can distinguish between different degrees of atrophy which correlate with actual pathology. High-resolution MRI has become important in localizing the epileptic zones in cases of hippocampal atrophy and dysplastic lesions of the cortex which were previously diagnosed as cryptogenic epilepsy. MRI can also be used as a predictor of outcome. In cases of temporal lobectomies, for example, if the MRI and ictal electroencephalogram (EEG) agree on the location of the epileptogenic zone, there is a 95% cure rate versus a 50% cure rate if the two diagnostic tests are inconsistent. These techniques will be important inclusion criteria for epilepsy radiosurgery protocols.

Other imaging techniques that are sometimes utilized in localization of epileptic foci include CT, positron emission tomography (PET), magnetic resonance spectroscopy (MRS), and single-photon emission computed tomography (SPECT). MRS is a technique that is being considered for use in the localization of focal epilepsies. MRS-measured phosphocreatine and adenosine triphosphate levels have been shown experimentally to shift during seizures in animals. In MTS, increased pH and inorganic phosphate have been noted at the epileptic focus interictally, and the level of these metabolites can also be detected by MRS.

Electroencephalograms (noninvasive or invasive) are useful in diagnosing temporal lobe epilepsies and interhemispheric epilepsies. Subdural strips and grids are used for extratemporal neocortical epilepsies. Foramen ovale electrodes are used for localization and lateralization of mesial temporal lobe epilepsy. Noninvasive and invasive localization techniques together are crucial during presurgical diagnostic evaluation of patients with medically intractable epilepsy. However, there is no current consensus as to what techniques and results should be definitive criteria for a recommendation of epilepsy surgery.

Mesial Temporal Lobe Surgery

Approximately 60% of epilepsy surgeries are anterior temporal lobe resections. The anterior temporal lobectomy includes resection of the amygdala, portions of the hippocampus, entorhinal cortex, and part of the temporal pole. This procedure is considered when seizure onset unilaterally involves the temporal neocortex, especially lateral, and limbic structures. Often there is also structural pathology in the affected temporal lobe. Selective amygdalohippocampectomy is a minimally invasive alternative to the anterior temporal lobectomy. Amygdalohippocampectomy involves resection of the amygdala, hippocampus, and parahippocampal gyrus. The indication for this procedure is a focal onset in the mesial temporal lobe unilaterally. The function of the contralateral side should be intact. Clinical symptoms should coincide with the focal side. Mesial temporal lobe epilepsy is caused by hippocampal sclerosis and is the most responsive condition to epilepsy surgery and the most unresponsive to medical treatment. The procedure for MTS is a selective amygdalohippocampectomy. Stereotactic radiosurgery is currently being explored as a new technique to affect this brain tissue without resection.

The second most common surgical procedure for epilepsy is the extratemporal resection. This procedure makes up 13% of all epilepsy surgeries. Surgery for extratemporal-related epilepsy is not performed often unless a lesion has been recognized. In considering extratemporal resections, the focal onset should be localized to a definitive area and the lesion should be identified. In the future, radiosurgery may be suitable for such patients if the focus can be localized accurately and is of small volume.

Seizure Outcome

The Second International Palm Desert Conference (1992) compiled results of epilepsy surgeries from 1986 to 1990. The data showed that those undergoing temporal-lobe resections (n=3579) became free of seizures 68% of the time, had a 90% seizure reduction in 23%, and less than 90% improvement in 9% of the patients. The results for the selective amygdalohippocampectomy (n=413) were essentially identical. According to the Zurich Epilepsy Series (1994), 65% of patients undergoing selective amygdalohippocampectomies (n=304) were seizure-free versus 49% of those patients undergoing anterior temporal lobectomies (n=66). Data compiled since the late 1980s have shown that the amygdalohippocampectomy and temporal lobe resection offer similar postsurgical results in seizure outcome. Many investigators argue for amygdalohippocampectomy because it can be less invasive.

The best prognosis for epilepsy surgery has always been given for those with MTS. In patients undergoing surgery for MTS, 62% were seizure-free at 2 years and 50% at 5 years. However, current follow-up data notes that when follow-up is extended for greater than 30 months, seizure relapses are primarily seen among the MTS surgical patients. After 10 years, 37% of patients who had undergone mesial temporal lobe surgery relapsed versus only 15% of those who underwent extratemporal resections.[31] The high incidence of relapse in MTS is associated with two phenomena. First, those patients with relapse have shown a high incidence of the epileptigenic focus at the remaining portions of the lateral temporal neocortex. Second, sclerosis of the hippocampus can be a bilateral process without symmetry in 90% of patients. It may be that irradiation of this tissue, rather than resection, will be associated with a different short- and long-term outcome.

Parrent and Blume performed stereotactic radiofrequency ablation amygdalohippocampectomy sparing the parahippocampal gyrus.[32] Patients selected to undergo stereotactic amygdalohippocampectomy were divided into two groups. One group (n=5) received 4 to 11 lesions while the second group (n=15) received 12 to 54 lesions. Sixty percent of those from the second group showed "favorable seizure outcome" versus 20% from the less invasive group. Ninety-three percent of patients from the more invasive stereotactic procedure experienced reduced seizure frequency.

Resection and Morbidity

Comparisons between medically and surgically treated epilepsy patients indicated better seizure control in the surgery group, but the occurrence of neurological complications was 23% in the surgical group versus 3% in the medical group. Of those patients with neurological deficits, half of these deficits affected function.[31] Unintended neurological complications in localized resective surgery occurs infrequently (<5%). Of these complications, the majority are transient and resolve within weeks or months.

Following temporal lobe resection, hemiparesis is a complication reported to be transitory in 4% of cases and permanent in 2%. Clinically undetectable visual field defects have been noted in 50% of patients, while 8% had symptomatic deficits. Approximately 5% of patients have been noted to have postoperative cranial neuropathy. Transient aphasia is common after dominant temporal lobectomy, but this condition persists infrequently.[31] Neurobehavioral complications of anterior temporal lobe resections include anomia, dysphasia, memory deficits, and depression. After temporal lobectomies, 1 to 4% of patients suffer significant memory deficits. Postoperative depression is noted in approximately 4 to 9% undergoing epilepsy surgery. Epilepsy patients undergoing surgery are at a 25 times greater risk of committing suicide than the general population. Psychosis is reported in 10 to 25% of patients preoperatively and 10 to 50% of patients postoperatively. Anteromesial temporal lobectomy can result in a complications of verbal memory. On the other hand, hippocampal resection actually improves the memory of many patients who had suffered from memory deficits preoperatively. Similar positive behavioral effects were noted in our rat hippocampal radiosurgery model.

The Role of Radiosurgery for Epilepsy

There is current interest in the use of radiosurgery for patients with focal epilepsy. The observation that brain irradiation (via radiation therapy or radiosurgery) could lead to cessation of seizures has spurred several groups to work in this field. In 1985, Barcia-Salorio et al reported on six patients with epilepsy who had low-dose radiosurgery.[33] The epileptic focus was localized by means of conventional scalp EEG, subarachnoid electrodes, and depth electrodes. Radiosurgery (a 10-mm collimator to deliver an estimated dose of 10 Gy) was performed using a cobalt unit coupled to a stereotactic localizer. They hypothesized that this low radiation dose provided a specific effect on epileptic neurons, without inducing tissue necrosis. In 1994, these investigators provided a long-term analysis in a series of 11 patients using a dose range of 10 to 20 Gy.[34] Five patients had complete cessation of seizures, and an additional five were improved. Seizures began to decrease gradually 3 to 12 months following radiosurgery. They noted that the main difficulty in this approach was correct localization of the epileptogenic focus. Following this work, Lindquist and colleagues at the Karolinska Institute began to perform epilepsy radiosurgery using advanced localization techniques that included magnetoencephalography to define interictal activity.[35,36] In some patients, the epileptic dipole activity identified on magnetoencephalography before radiosurgery later resolved along with seizure cessation.

Radiosurgery for MTS was first performed in 1993. Four patients with MTS underwent radiosurgery targeting the head and anterior part of the hippocampal body, the amygdalofugal part of the amygdala, and the entorhinal area.[37] All four patients experienced a significant reduction of seizures after 3 to 18 months and eventual seizure cessation 32 to 36 months follow-up. From 1996 to 1998, a larger study, which included 21 patients with mesial temporal lobe epilepsy, analyzed the effects of radiosurgery.[38] All patients with greater than 10 months follow-up were seizure-free.

Current issues that remain important for epilepsy radiosurgery include dose selection (necrotizing vs. non-necrotizing), localization methods for nonlesional epilepsy, the target volume necessary for irradiation, and the expected short- and long-term outcomes. It is not known what kind of tissue effect is required to stop the generation or propagation of seizures. Some groups have used low doses (i.e., 10–20 Gy) where few if any histologic changes would be expected. Others have used doses as high as 100 Gy that cause target necrosis and regional brain edema.[39]

To study the effects of radiosurgery on experimental epilepsy, we used a rat kainic acid model of chronic hippocampal epilepsy. In two separate studies, rats were randomized to control or radiosurgery arms (20, 30, 40, 60, or 100 Gy) and then evaluated with serial EEG, behavioral studies, functional MRI, and histology (Fig. 3).[40,41] To date, we have found

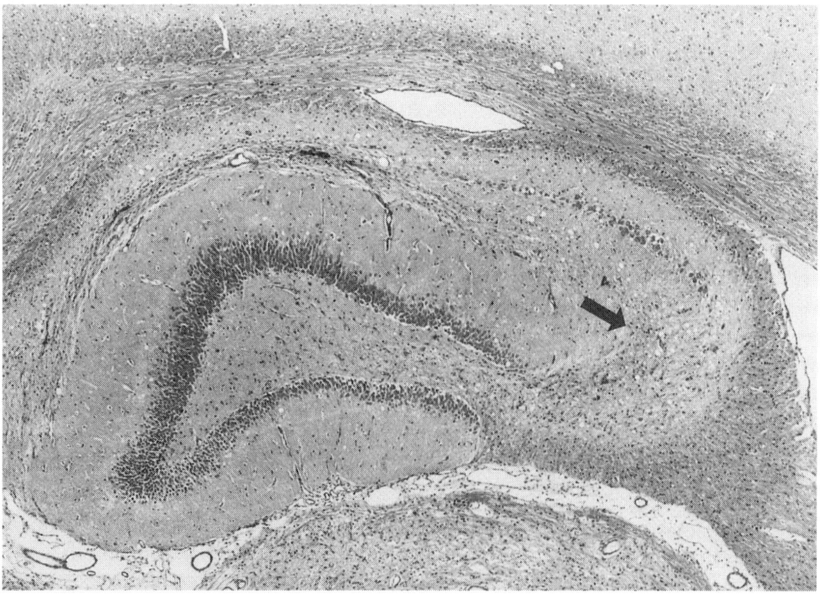

Figure 3. The rat hippocampal region following kainic acid injection and Gamma Knife radiosurgery (60 Gy). Loss of CA-3 neurons can be seen due to kainic acid injection (arrow), but no adverse radiation effects are noted.

that increasing radiosurgery doses has caused greater reductions in the number of seizures without inducing tissue injury. If focal hippocampal (or any other brain tissue) irradiation can eliminate seizures without the need for complete tissue destruction, then radiosurgery may become an important therapy for patients with intractable epilepsy.

Our current goal is to use radiation at subnecrotic doses to impact positively on epilepsy, yet minimize therapeutic risk. A new human study includes investigators from the University of California, San Francisco, University of Virginia, Northwestern University, Yale University, and the University of Pittsburgh. All patients will be resection candidates with MTS, but will undergo Gamma Knife radiosurgery. They will be randomized to receive maximum radiosurgical doses of 40 or 48 Gy targeted by MRI to the amygdalohippocampal region. The safety and efficacy of this approach will be tested by investigators at Epilepsy Centers within these universities.

Radiosurgery for Epilepsy from Hypothalamic Hamartomas

There is published experience in the use of radiosurgery for the focal treatment of hypothalamic hamartomas, known to be associated with gelastic seizures and precocious puberty.[42] Hamartoma resection has been reported, but can be associated with significant risk when complete resection is attempted.[43] In the last few years, several groups have performed Gamma Knife radiosurgery on hypothalamic hamartomas in an attempt to treat patients with gelastic seizures with secondary generalization. Several case reports have been published with encouraging results.[44,45] At the University of Pittsburgh, we have performed radiosurgery in two patients with medically intractable epilepsy and small-volume hamartomas. In both patients, a radiation dose was delivered that respected the optic apparatus adjacent to the hamartoma. Margin doses of 18 and 16 Gy were administered (Fig. 4). Both patients have had improvements in their seizures, at 18 and 6 months of follow-up.

Functional Imaging and Radiosurgery

Improvements in functional imaging eventually will have an impact on radiosurgery. Functional MRI to localize cortical function prior to radiosurgery has been evaluated in pilot studies. Localization of hand motor function, leg motor function, and speech areas surrounding arteriovenous malformations and brain tumors before radiosurgery has assisted dose planning.[46] This information can be used to restrict the radiosurgery dose away from functional areas. Advancements in functional imaging may improve the localization of epileptic foci, and perhaps even regions of

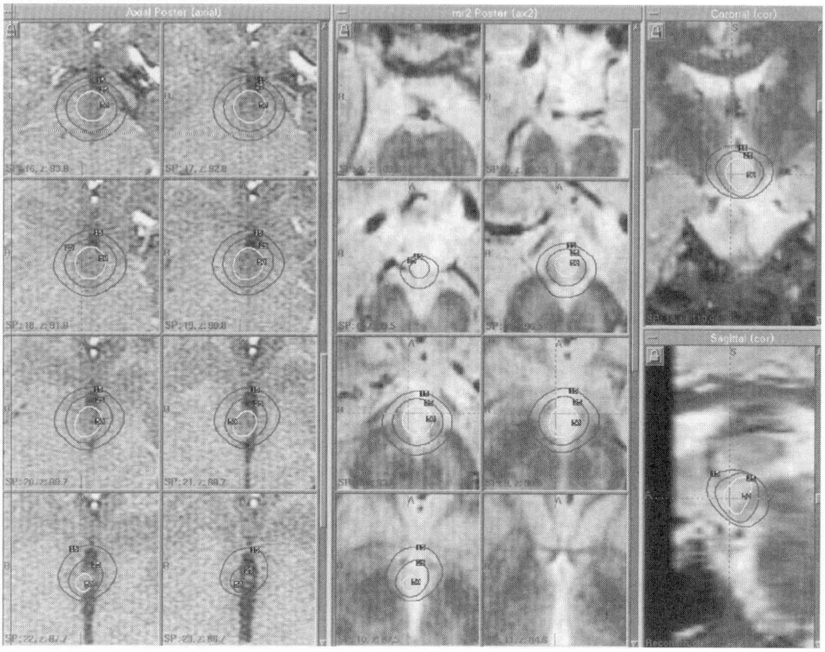

Figure 4. Radiosurgical dose plan showing short TR (relaxation time) and long TR axial images of a patient with a hypothalamic hamartoma and gelastic seizures. Coronal and sagittal views are shown on the right. This hamartoma was irradiated to a margin dose of 16 Gy and a maximum dose of 32 Gy using one 8-mm and two 4-mm isocenters.

excitation in the basal ganglia. Perhaps in the future, imaging studies will be able to identify volumes of thalamic tremor cells. Such physiologic information would impact on the use of radiosurgery for functional disorders by providing a noninvasive physiologic link between image definition and radiosurgical ablation.

References

1. Leksell L: The stereotaxic method and radiosurgery of the brain. Acta Chir Scand 1951;102:316–319.
2. Leksell L: Stereotaxic radiosurgery in trigeminal neuralgia. Acta Chir Scand 1971;137:311–314.
3. Larsson B, Leksell L, Rexed B, et al: The high-energy proton beam as a neurosurgical tool. Nature 1958;182:1222–1223.
4. Andersson B, Larsson B, Leksell L, et al: Histopathology of late local radiolesions in the goat brain. Acta Radiol 1970;9:385–394.
5. Rexed B, Mair W, Sourander P, et al: Effect of high energy protons on the brain of the rabbit. Acta Radiol 1960;53:289–299.

6. Steiner L, Forster D, Leksell L, et al: Gammathalamotomy in intractable pain. Acta Neurochir 1980;52:173–184.
7. Kondziolka D, Lunsford LD, Claassen D, et al: Radiobiology of radiosurgery. Part I. The normal rat brain model. Neurosurgery 1992;31:271–279.
8. Leksell L, Herner T, Leksell D, et al: Visualization of stereotactic radiolesions by nuclear magnetic resonance. J Neurol Neurosurg Psych 1985;48:19–20.
9. Friehs G, Noren G, Ohye C, et al: Lesion size following gamma knife treatment for functional disorders. Stereotact Funct Neurosurg 1996;66(suppl 1):320–328.
10. Kondziolka D, Linskey ME, Lunsford LD: Animal models in radiosurgery. In Alexander E, Loeffler JS, Lunsford LD (eds): Stereotactic Radiosurgery. New York, McGraw-Hill, 1993, pp 51–64.
11. Kondziolka D, Lunsford LD, Altschuler EM, et al: Biological effects of stereotactic radiosurgery in the normal primate brainstem. In Lunsford LD (ed): Stereotactic Radiosurgery Update. New York, Elsevier, 1992, pp 291–294.
12. Lunsford LD, Altschuler EM, Flickinger JC, et al: In vivo biological effects of stereotactic radiosurgery: a primate model. Neurosurgery 1990;27:373–382.
13. Kihlstrom L, Hindmarsh T, Lax I, et al: Radiosurgical lesions in the normal human brain 17 years after gamma knife capsulotomy. Neurosurgery 1997; 41:396–402.
14. Kihlstrom L, Guo WY, Lindquist C, Mindus P: Radiobiology of radiosurgery for refractory anxiety disorders. Neurosurgery 1995;36:294–302.
15. Duma C, Jacques D, Kopyov O, et al: Gamma knife radiosurgery for thalamotomy in Parkinsonian tremor: a five-year experience. J Neurosurg 1998; 88:1044–1049.
16. Kondziolka D, Dempsey PK, Lunsford LD, et al: A comparison between magnetic resonance imaging and computed tomography for stereotactic coordinate determination. Neurosurgery 1992;30:402–407.
17. Young RF, Shumway-Cook A, Vermeulen S, et al: Gamma knife radiosurgery as a lesioning technique in movement disorder surgery. J Neurosurg 1998;89: 183–193.
18. Hirato M, Ohye C, Shibazaki T, et al: Gamma knife thalamotomy for the treatment of functional disorders. Stereotact Funct Neurosurg 1995;64(suppl 1):164–171.
19. Lindquist C, Steiner L, Hindmarsh T: Gamma knife thalamotomy for tremor: report of two cases. In Steiner L (ed): Radiosurgery: Baseline and Trends. New York, Raven Press, 1992, pp 237–243.
20. Niranjan A, Kondziolka D, Baser S, et al: Functional outcomes after gamma knife thalamotomy for essential tremor and multiple sclerosis-related tremor. Neurology 2000;55:443–446.
21. Niranjan A, Jawahar A, Kondziolka D, Lunsford LD: A comparison of surgical approaches for the management of tremor: radiofrequency thalamotomy, gamma knife thalamotomy, and thalamic stimulation. Stereotact Funct Neurosurg 1999;72:178–184.
22. Otsuki T, Jokura H, Takahashi K, et al: Stereotactic gamma-thalamotomy with a computerized brain atlas: technical case report. Neurosurgery 1994;35: 764–768.
23. Pan L, Dai J, Wang BJ, et al: Stereotactic gamma thalamotomy for the treatment of Parkinsonism. Stereotact Funct Neurosurg 1996;66(suppl 1): 329–332.
24. Friehs G, Ojakangas CL, Pachatz P, et al: Thalamotomy and caudatomy with the gamma knife as a treatment for Parkinsonism with a comment on lesion sizes. Stereotact Funct Neurosurg 1995;64(suppl 1):209–221.
25. Rand RW, Jacques DB, Melbye RW, et al: Gamma knife thalamotomy and pal-

lidotomy in patients with movement disorders: preliminary results. Stereotact Funct Neurosurg 1993;61(suppl):65–92.
26. Friedman J, Epstein M, Sanes J, et al: Gamma knife pallidotomy in advanced Parkinson's disease. Ann Neurol 1996;39:535–538.
27. Awad IA, Nayel MH: Epilepsy surgery: introduction and overview. Clinical Neurosurg 1992;38:493–513.
28. Engel J Jr: Surgical Treatment of the Epilepsies. New York, Raven Books Press, 1987.
29. Engel J Jr: Surgery for seizures. N Engl J Med 1996;334:647–652.
30. Laxer K, Garcia P: Imaging criteria to identify the epileptic focus. Neurosurg Clin N Am 1993;4:199–209.
31. Spencer SS: Long-term outcome after epilepsy surgery. Epilepsia 1996;37: 807–813.
32. Parrent AG, Blume WT: Stereotactic amygdalohippocampotomy for the treatment of medial temporal lobe epilepsy. Epilepsia 1999;40:1408–1416.
33. Barcia-Salorio JL, Roldan P, Hernandez G, et al: Radiosurgical treatment of epilepsy. Appl Neurophysiol 1985;48:400–403.
34. Barcia-Salorio JL, Barcia JA, Hernandez G, et al: Radiosurgery of epilepsy: long-term results. Acta Neurochir 1994;62(suppl):111–113.
35. Hellstrand DE, Abraham-Fuchs K, Jernberg B, et al: MEG localization of interictal epileptic focal activity and concomitant stereotactic radiosurgery: a non-invasive approach for patient with focal epilepsy. Physiol Meas 1993;14: 131–136.
36. Lindquist C, Kihlstrom L, Hellstrand DE: Functional neurosurgery: a future for the gamma knife? Stereotact Funct Neurosurg 1991;57:72–81.
37. Régis J, Peragut JC, Rey M, et al: First selective amygdalohippocampal radiosurgery for mesial temporal lobe epilepsy. Stereotact Funct Neurosurg 1995;64(suppl 1):193–201.
38. Regis J, Bartolomei F, Rey M, et al: Gamma knife surgery for mesial temporal lobe epilepsy. Epilepsia 1999;40:1551–1556.
39. Whang CJ, Kim CJ: Short-term follow-up of stereotactic gamma knife radiosurgery in epilepsy. Stereotact Funct Neurosurg 1995;64(suppl 1):202–208.
40. Maesawa S, Kondziolka D, Dixon E, et al: Subnecrotic stereotactic radiosurgery controls epilepsy produced by kainic acid injection in rats. J Neurosurg 2000;93:1033–1040.
41. Mori Y, Kondziolka D, Balzer J, et al: Effects of stereotactic radiosurgery on an animal model of hippocampal epilepsy. Neurosurgery 2000;46:157–168.
42. Kuzniecky R, Guthrie B, Mountz J, et al: Intrinsic epileptogenesis of hypothalamic hamartomas in gelastic epilepsy. Ann Neurol 1997;42:60–67.
43. Stewart L, Steinbok P, Daaboul J: Role of surgical resection in the treatment of hypothalamic hamartomas causing precocious puberty. J Neurosurg 1998;88:340–345.
44. Arita K, Kurisu K, Iida K, et al: Subsidence of seizure induced by stereotactic radiation in a patient with hypothalamic hamartoma: case report. J Neurosurg 1998;89:645–648.
45. Unger F, Schrottner O, Haselsberger K, et al: Gamma knife radiosurgery for hypothalamic hamartomas in patients with medically intractable epilepsy and precocious puberty: report of two cases. J Neurosurg 2000;92:726–731.
46. Witt TC, Kondziolka D, Baumann S, et al: Preoperative cortical localization with functional MRI for use in stereotactic radiosurgery. Stereotact Funct Neurosurg 1996;66:24–29.

Comment

Chapter 15

Aviva Abosch, Andres M. Lozano

In this chapter, Kondziolka and colleagues provide an in-depth review of the field of radiosurgery as it applies to the treatment of movement disorders and the epilepsies. Although the use of radiosurgery to treat disorders of the central nervous system is not new, it has been revisited in the last decade by several groups interested in examining radiosurgery vis-à-vis traditional surgical approaches. Kondziolka et al discuss the relative merits of Gamma Knife radiosurgery with respect to thalamotomy, pallidotomy, mesial temporal lobe epilepsy, and hypothalamic hamartomas.

Benefits of Radiosurgery

The benefits of radiosurgery in the treatment of movement disorders include the point that it is less invasive than traditional surgical approaches, thereby eliminating the possibility of infection and hemorrhage, which remain small but finite risks of the open procedures.[1] Gamma Knife is also less time-consuming than microelectrode-guided radiofrequency lesioning, which can contribute to lower procedural costs and better patient tolerance. Additionally, radiosurgery might be the only option in patients with underlying medical problems (such as coagulopathies) in whom an invasive procedure would incur greater risks. Finally, single-dose radiosurgical procedures are less expensive than the current cost of deep brain stimulation (DBS), and have none of the hardware problems associated with DBS, e.g., risk of infection, hardware breakage, or finite battery life.

Problems with Radiosurgery

Target modification by microelectrode recording data or by macroelectrode stimulation is impossible in the setting of radiosurgical approaches to the treatment of movement disorders. Unlike traditional surgical techniques, Gamma Knife ablative surgery requires 2 to 3 months to "mature," such that an insufficient lesion cannot be recognized at the time of treatment. Furthermore, the modification of effect that remains possible with an implanted DBS is not possible once a lesion has been generated–either by radiofrequency or by radiosurgery. This latter point is relevant in considerations of pallidal surgery and surgery of the subthalamic nucleus; both are locations in which the modifications afforded by DBS might provide improved clinical outcome relative to lesion generation.

There is no consensus yet on the optimal radiosurgery lesion dose to use. Some of the data presented suggest that radiosurgery influences neuronal function beyond the area of radionecrosis. Could radiosurgery modulate the activity of neurons beyond the lesion? The optimal target must be offset in order to avoid damage to the internal capsule in the setting of thalamotomy and the optic track in the setting of pallidotomy.[2] Finally, the ultimate lesion size is unpredictable and can lead to unintended consequences.[2] The same may be said for radiofrequency-generated lesions, but there is greater security in lesion generation when the targeting is guided by microelectrode recording and macrostimulation.

Assessing the Benefits and Risks of Radiosurgery for Epilepsy and Movement Disorders

Any comparison between an established therapy and a novel one–or a novel indication for a preexisting therapy–must deal both with relative efficacy as well as with adverse effects. The evaluation of efficacy should be based on standardized outcomes scales, such as the Engel Classification of post-treatment seizure frequency,[3] and the Unified Parkinson's Disease Rating Scale for Parkinson's disease. Unfortunately, many of the published studies of radiosurgery in the treatment of movement disorders base outcomes analyses on clinical assessments as opposed to formal validated ratings. This is particularly important in conditions that fluctuate from day-to-day and hour-to-hour, and in which patient effort and motivation can have a profound influence, as occurs in the movement disorders. This issue of the quality of the outcome evaluation in radiosurgical trials is particularly important as the investigators are reporting benefits that sometimes are similar or indeed superior to those attainable with careful anatomical and physiological targeting.

The evaluation of efficacy must also take into account the biases inherent in the studies that are compared. Both patient and investigator biases in treatments under investigation must be taken into consideration. Patients want to improve and desire to please their doctors, and of course the doctors want patients to derive benefit from their treatments. Additionally, there can be a substantial placebo effects resulting from treatment that should be factored into the analysis of outcome. These issues can be resolved in large part by study design, with double-blinded, randomized studies as the gold standard. Unfortunately, in addition to radiosurgery, most surgical studies that deal with the treatment of movement disorders or epilepsy have not been conducted in a double-blinded fashion; either the patients, or the investigators, or both are aware of the nature of the therapy. Part of the difficulty has been the prospect of subjecting patients to sham surgeries. DBS surgery offers the possibility, at least in theory, of double-blinded evaluation of the patient with the stimulator off or on.[4,5] Gamma Knife treatment would lend nicely to double-blinded studies, given the noninvasive nature of the technique, as well as the delayed and gradual onset of the clinical results. Nonetheless, a search of the literature reveals no such blinded studies of the efficacy of Gamma Knife therapy for the treatment of movement disorders or epilepsy.

Conclusions

The use of stereotactic radiosurgery in the treatment of epilepsy and movement disorders is growing in popularity. Although less invasive than traditional surgical approaches, the adoption of radiosurgery in these settings will depend on its ability to match the surgical results of resection, lesioning and DBS, with respect to long-term efficacy in controlling the symptoms of these disorders, as well as to the demonstration of equivalent or lesser morbidity.

References

1. Schuurman PR, Bosch DA, Bossuyt PM, et al: A comparison of continuous thalamic stimulation and thalamotomy for suppression of severe tremor. N Engl J Med 2000;342:461–468.
2. Young RF, Jacques S, Mark R, et al: Gamma knife thalamotomy for treatment of tremor: long-term results. J Neurosurg 2000;93:128–135.
3. Engel J Jr: Outcome with respect to epileptic seizures. In Engel J Jr (ed): Surgical Treatment of the Epilepsies. New York, Raven Press, 1987, pp 553–571.
4. Kumar R, Lozano AM, Kim YJ, et al: Double-blind evaluation of subthalamic nucleus deep brain stimulation in advanced Parkinson's disease. Neurology 1998;51:850–855.
5. Pahwa R, Lyons KL, Wilkinson SB, et al: Bilateral thalamic stimulation for the treatment of essential tremor. Neurology 1999;53:1447–1450.

Index

Acoustic neuromas. *See* Vestibular schwannomas, stereotactic radiosurgery of
American Association of Physicists in Medicine, QA programs for Gamma Knife and LINAC-based systems, 32
American Association of Stereotactic and Functional Neurosurgery Society, 321
Arteriovenous malformations (AVMs), stereotactic radiosurgery of
  AVM obliteration, 60–61
  AVM risk management, 61–63
  AVM Treatment Board, 76
  cumulative incidence of postradiosurgical complications, 101–102
  delayed radiation-induced complications, 97, 100–101
  delineating the region of interest (ROI), 85
  dose planning modalities, 84
  dose selection for, 60–63, 86–90
  example of dose distribution within AVM nidus volume, 54–55, 56
  factors associated with successful AVM radiosurgery, 91
  factors correlating with AVM obliteration, 60
  hemorrhage after AVM radiosurgery, 96–97, 98, 99
  histopathology for AVMs after radiosurgery, 77–83
  history of AVM radiosurgery, 76–77
  incidence and natural history of AVMs, 75
  obliteration process of radiosurgically treated AVMs, 80, 83
  rates of angiographically confirmed obliteration, 90–91
  recommended treatment regimen for AVMs, 106–107
  seizure and headache control with, 93, 96
  smooth muscle actin (SMA) positivity in AVMs, 77–83
  stereotactic head frame placement for, 83
  stereotactic localization and dose planning, 83–86
  treatment failure and retreatment, 91–93, 94, 95, 96
  treatment modalities for, 75–76
  treatment results of, 90–101
AVM Treatment Board, 76

Brain metastases, stereotactic radiosurgery of
  advances of stereotactic radiosurgery (SRS) and, 262–263
  advantages of radiosurgery compared with surgical resection, 250–251
  indications for aggressive intervention, 246–247
  Karnofsky Performance Score (KPS), 245
  maximum dose to prescribed dose (MD/PD), 249–250

Mini-Mental State Examination (MMSE), 258
patient evaluation and management, 247–249
Radiation Therapy Oncology Group (RTOG) trials, 245, 249, 250, 253
radiosurgery versus surgical resection, 256–257
recursive partitioning analysis (RPA) evaluating patient survival, 245
results of brain metastases radiosurgery, 249–256
usefulness of whole brain radiation therapy (WBRT), 258
whole brain radiation therapy (WBRT), 246, 247, 249, 253, 256–258, 262

Cavernous malformations (CMs), stereotactic radiosurgery of
complications in, 148–149
conceptual difficulties with CMs radiosurgery, 145–146
confirming pathology, 145
controversy of radiosurgery for treatment of CMs, 153–154
Harvard University, results of published series, 145
optimal radiographic studies to evaluate follow-up, 146
patients appropriate for radiosurgery, 140
radiobiology of CMs and optimal radiosurgery dose, 146
radiosurgery target delineation, 145–146
rate hemorrhage response, 146–148
rationale for radiosurgery, 140
results of published series, 140–145
role of surgery for CMs, 149
Stanford Series, results of published series, 140–144, 146, 147, 148–149
as subset of angiographically occult vascular malformations (AOVMs), 139
University of Pittsburgh, results of published series, 144–145, 147
Chordomas
external beam radiation therapy (EBRT) in treatment of, 284–289
stereotactic radiosurgery of, 283–289, 305–306
Computed tomography (CT)
in AVM radiosurgery dose planning, 84, 85
imaging for localization of epileptic focus, 334
in radiosurgical dose planning for pituitary adenomas, 216
in radiosurgical treatment planning of DAVFs, 116
role in stereotactic radiosurgery, 1
Cranial stereotactic radiosurgery (CSRS), physical aspects of
with circular collimators, 26–27
description of process, 17–18
dose delivery uncertainties, 29–31
dose planning, 20–23
equipment acceptance testing, 31
facilities planning for, 32
fiducial localization, limitation in dose delivery, 30
image/isodose delivery limitations, 30
imaging, limitations in dose delivery, 29–30
isodose calculation, limitation in, 30
with Leksell Gamma Knife, 24–25

with a linear accelerator (LINAC), 25–29, 35
with mini-multileaf collimation (MMLC) system, 27–28, 35
multi-isocenter dose distributions, 21–23
with OUR Rotating unit, 25
with a poured shape collimation system, 27
quality assurance (QA) in, 31–32
radiation delivery modalities and techniques, 23–29
with robotic LINAC system, 26, 28–29
single isocenter dose distributions, 20–21, 22
with standard LINAC, 25–26
stereotactic frame and localization systems, 18–19
treatment, influence of dose delivery, 31
using cobalt-60, 24
using protons, 29
variation in maximum dose matrices, 22–23

Digital subtraction angiography (DSA), for stereotactic head frame placement, 83, 84, 85
Dose selection and prediction of stereotactic outcomes
absorbed dose, defined, 53
in AVM obliteration, 60–61
and AVM risk management, 61–63
description of treatment dose, 57–58
differential and cumulative DVHs, 54
dose of best risk/benefit ratio for each patient, 53
dose selection for arteriovenous malformation (AVM) radiosurgery, 60–63, 70–71
dose-volume histograms (DVHs), 54–55
factors correlating with AVM obliteration, 60
gray (Gy), international standard unit of, 53–54
making a good dose plan, 59, 70
for malignant tumors, 66–67
radiation absorbed dose (rad), 53
risk of complications treating benign tumors, 64–66
target volume distribution, 55–57, 70
Dosimetric considerations. *See* Radiobiological and dosimetric considerations in stereotactic radiosurgery
Dural arteriovenous fistulae (DAVFs), stereotactic radiosurgery of
basic fibroblastic growth factor (bFGF) in surgical specimens, 110
cavernous sinus DAVFs, results of treatment, 118–120
characteristics of DAVFs, 115
comments on DAVF radiosurgical treatments, 127–138
complications in, 121–122
DAVF treatment at Mayo Clinic Radiosurgery program, 114–138
with embolization, 116–117
follow-up with, 118
illustrative cases, 122–129
natural history of DAVFs, 111–112, 137
pathogenesis of DAVFs, 109–111
patients with DAVFs, 114–115
presentation of, 112
radiosurgical treatment planning, 116
transverse-sigmoid DAVFs, results of treatment, 120–121
treatment options, 112–113
treatment rationale, 113–114

Eastern Cooperative Oncology Group performance status (ECOG), 292, 297
Epilepsy and movement disorders, stereotactic radiosurgery of
  assessing benefits and risks of radiosurgery in, 344–345
  benefits and problems with radiosurgery, 343–344
  depression and suicide risk after epilepsy surgery, 337
  dose selection for parenchymal radiosurgery, 328–329
  epilepsy from hypothalamic hamartomas, radiosurgery for, 339
  functional imaging and radiosurgery, 339–340
  imaging in functional surgery, 329–330
  International Classification of Epilepsies and Epileptic Syndromes, 333–334
  mesial temporal lobe surgery, 335
  mesial temporal sclerosis (MTS), 334, 335
  radiosurgery for epilepsy, 333–339
  radiosurgical pallidotomy, 333
  radiosurgical thalamotomy, 330–333
  resection and morbidity, 336–337
  role of radiosurgery in epilepsy, 337–339
  Second International Palm Desert Conference, 336
  seizure outcome, 336
  techniques for localization of the epileptic focus, 334–335
  Zurich Epilepsy Series, 336
External beam radiation therapy (EBRT)
  in treatment of chordomas, 284–289
  in treatment of glomus tumors, 291–292
  in treatment of meningiomas, 158–159, 167–168

Gamma Knife (GK)
  current models in clinical use, 83
  delayed radiation-induced complications, 100
  QA programs for, 32
  in treatment of meningiomas, 159
  See also Leksell, Lars
  See also specific diagnosis and stereotactic radiosurgery
Glial tumors, stereotactic radiosurgery of
  Brain Tumor Cooperative Group (BTCG) trial, 265, 274, 280
  Brain Tumor Study Group (BTSG), 265
  categories of evidence-based medicine, 275
  fractionated SRS (FSRS), 271
  Radiation Therapy Oncology Group (RTOG) "shrinking field" method, 269
  radiosurgery for high-grade glioma, 269–270
  radiosurgery for low-grade glioma, 267–269
  radiosurgery for newly diagnosed malignant glioma, 272–274
  radiosurgery for pilocytic and optic nerve tumors, 266–267
  radiosurgery for recurrent malignant glioma, 270–274
  radiotherapy and brachytherapy for malignant glioma, 274–276, 280

RTOG RPA classification of malignant gliomas, 276
World Health Organization (WHO) Grade I pilocytic astrocytomas, 266
World Health Organization (WHO) Grade II astrocytoma, 269
World Health Organization (WHO) Grade III and IV astrocytomas, 269
Glomus tumors
external beam radiation therapy (EBRT) in treatment of, 291–292
stereotactic radiosurgery of, 289–295, 304–305

International Leksell Gamma Knife Society, 213

Karolinska Hospital, 55, 56–57, 60, 65, 66, 76

Larson, Borje, 14
Leksell, Lars, 1, 14, 24
closed-skull single-session irradiation, 327
development of Gamma Knife, 76, 181
first radiosurgical system, 34
treatment of meningiomas, 159
Leksell Gamma Knife, 6
delivery modality in cranial stereotactic radiosurgery, 24–25
"marble" dose plans, 20
Linear accelerator (LINAC)-based systems, 8
delayed radiation-induced complications, 100
"marble" dose plans, 20
treatment of meningiomas, 159
Magnetic resonance imaging (MRI)
in AVM radiosurgery dose planning, 84, 85
in functional surgery for epilepsy and movement disorders, 330
for localization of epileptic focus, 334
in radiosurgical dose planning for pituitary adenomas, 216, 218, 219
in radiosurgical treatment planning of DAVFs, 116, 117
role in stereotactic radiosurgery, 1
for stereotactic head frame placement, 83
Magnetic resonance spectroscopy (MRS), imaging for localization of epileptic focus, 335
Malignant skull base tumors, stereotactic radiosurgery of, 296–299, 306–307
Mayo Clinic
cases of dural arteriovenous fistulae treated with radiosurgery, 114–138
management program of meningiomas, 164–166
radiosurgery on patients with brain metastases, 251–256
radiosurgery statistics at, 4, 6–9, 14, 15
rates of angiographically confirmed AVM nidus obliteration, 90
Meningioma, stereotactic radiosurgery of
advantages of microsurgery, 175–178
complications with Gamma Knife and LINAC-based radiosurgeries, 161, 163–164

and external beam radiation therapy (EBRT), 158–159, 167–168
Mayo Clinic and management of meningiomas, 164–166
meningioma management, 157–159
patient and dose selection for meningioma radiosurgery, 167–168
pitfalls of radiosurgery, 174–175
radiation optic neuropathy (RON), 166–167
radiation tolerance of the optic apparatus, 166–167
radiosurgery of meningiomas, 159
results of LINAC-based radiosurgery, 159–161
risk of complications, 64, 65
role of radiation treatment in management of meningiomas, 172–174
tumor control with Gamma Knife and LINAC-based radiosurgeries, 159–163
Mesial temporal sclerosis (MTS), 334, 335

Olivicrona, Herbert, 14
OUR Rotating Gamma System, 25

Pituitary adenomas, stereotactic radiosurgery of
acromegaly, treatment of, 217, 219–222, 223, 241, 242
adenoma size and extension, 215–216
complications of Gamma Knife treatment of pituitary adenomas, 233–235, 243
corticotropic adenomas, treatment of, 222–229
Cushing's Disease, treatment of, 222–224, 225, 241, 242
Gamma Knife treatment of pituitary adenomas, 214–238
indications for Gamma Knife treatment, 214–215
multiple-fraction stereotactic linear accelerator radiotherapy, 236–237
Nelson's syndrome, treatment of, 224, 226–228
nonsecreting adenomas, treatment of, 230–232
prolactinomas, treatment of, 228–229, 241, 242
radiosurgical dose planning with Gamma Knife treatment, 216–217
single-fraction stereotactic linear accelerator radiosurgery, 236
stereotactic linear accelerator radiosurgery and radiotherapy, 235–237
thyroid-stimulating adenomas, treatment of, 229
Positron emission tomography (PET), imaging for localization of epileptic focus, 334

Quality assurance (QA) in cranial stereotactic radiosurgery, 31–32

Radiation injury, forms of, 64
Radiation Therapy Oncology Group (RTOG)
Dose-Escalation Study, 42–43, 51
"shrinking field" method radiotherapy of high-grade gliomas, 269
studies/trials of, 245, 249, 250, 253
Radiobiological and dosimetric considerations in stereotactic surgery

curves for cure and complications, 37, 38
dosimetric questions, 42
future developments of, 44
hypofractionation techniques, 49–50
limitations of linear-quadratic formula, 39–41, 46–48
linear-quadratic formula, 38–41
Radiation Therapy Oncology Group (RTOG) Radiosurgery Dose-Escalation Study, 42–43, 51
rationale for fractionation, 41, 48–50
"Radiosurgery: A Neurosurgical Approach to Intracranial Lesions," meeting of, 62
Refractory trigeminal neuralgia (TN), stereotactic radiosurgery of
Barrow Neurological Institute (BNI) experience, 313–323, 325–326
BNI Pain Intensity Score, 314
complications of BNI Gamma Knife treatment, 316–317
complications of invasive treatments for TN, 321
dosing plan with Gamma Knife procedure, 312
etiology of TN, 309
initial pain response to Gamma Knife treatment, 315–316
methods in the BNI Gamma Knife facility, 313–315
microvascular decompression (MVD), 309, 310, 314, 317–318, 319, 322, 325
pain recurrence in BNI study, 316
pain response timing using BNI Pain Score, 316
predicting outcomes, 321–322
radiosurgical treatment of trigeminal neuralgia, 318–321
surgical treatment of trigeminal neuralgia, 317–318
treatment of trigeminal neuralgia, 310–311
univariate analysis in BNI Pain Score, 317
using the Gamma Knife procedure, 311–312

Second International Palm Desert Conference, 336
Single-photon emission computed tomography (SPECT), imaging for localization of epileptic focus, 335
Stereotactic radiosurgery (SRS), 182, 183
defined, 1
diligent long-term follow-up, 6
evaluating traditional dose prescription schemes, 6
evolution of radiosurgery practice, 2–3
impact of radiosurgery on neurosurgery, 6–9
impact of the Internet and patient care, 2–3, 16
indications for radiosurgery, 3–5
radiosurgery knowledge, evolution of, 5–6
Studies/trials
Brain Tumor Cooperative Group (BTCG) trial, 265, 274, 280
Brain Tumor Study Group (BTSG) trial, 265
Radiation Therapy Oncology Group (RTOG) Radiosurgery Dose-Escalation Study, 42–43
Radiation Therapy Oncology Group (RTOG) trials, 245, 249, 250, 253

Tic douloureux. *See* Refractory trigeminal neuralgia, stereotactic radiosurgery of
Trigeminal neuralgia (TN). *See* Refractory trigeminal neuralgia, stereotactic radiosurgery of

United States Nuclear Regulatory Commission (NRC), requirements for monthly and annual checks, 31–32

Vestibular schwannomas (VS), stereotactic radiosurgery of
  cancer genesis, concerns with, 195–196
  concerns regarding radiosurgery, 195–199
  debate regarding role of radiosurgery in management of VS, 182
  difficulty of microsurgery after failed radiosurgery, 196–199
  dosimetry considerations, 186–188
  ethical considerations for VS radiosurgery, 201
  imaging and anatomical considerations, 185–186
  Marseille experience, 182–183, 188–192
  microsurgery versus radiosurgery, 192–195
  middle cranial fossa approach, outcomes of, 206–207
  radiobiology of VS radiosurgery, 184–185
  rationale of VS radiosurgery, 183–184
  risk of complications, 64–65
  stereotactic irradiation, outcomes of, 208–210
  technical considerations, 185–188
  translabyrinthine approach, outcomes of, 207–208
  using radiosurgery to preserve hearing, 199–200